THE VITAMIN CURE for Arthritis

ROBERT G. SMITH, PHD
W. TODD PENBERTHY, PHD

Basic Health
PUBLICATIONS, INC.

Basic Health Publications, Inc.

www.basichealthpub.com

Library of Congress Cataloging-in-Publication Data

Smith, Robert G.

The vitamin cure for arthritis / Robert G. Smith, Ph.D., W. Todd Penberthy, Ph.D.
pages cm
Includes bibliographical references and index.
ISBN 978-1-59120-312-4 (Pbk.)
ISBN 978-1-68162-824-0 (Hardcover)

1. Arthritis—Alternative treatment—Popular works. 2. Arthritis—Diet therapy—Popular works. 3. Vitamin therapy—Popular works. I. Penberthy, W. Todd. II. Title.
RC933.S56 2015
616.7'22—dc23
2014043795

Editor: Karen Anspach
Typesetting/Book design: Gary A. Rosenberg
Cover design: Mike Stromberg

CONTENTS

CHAPTER 1

Responsibility for Learning about Health: Your Role

In his book, *Doctor Yourself,* nutritionist Andrew W. Saul, Ph.D. describes the recovery of several of his clients from debilitating osteoarthritis.[1] One, a woman, almost eighty years old, was a housekeeper who worked with her hands. When she came to Dr. Saul, she had several health problems, but her main priority was to do something about her osteoarthritis. She was desperate, and was willing to try anything to regain her health. She was overweight and bent over from arthritis, unable to close her hands, and her knees were swollen and painful. She was sore all over and had lumps on her arms and legs. All of her symptoms were typical of age-related osteoarthritis, so Dr. Saul knew what to do. He advised her to eat only juiced vegetables for several weeks and then continue to eat only raw foods such as vegetables and sprouts. He knew that, typically, few people keep up this type of diet. However, the woman was determined. She tried the diet of juiced vegetables but wished for other foods such as soup and cooked vegetables. Dr. Saul explained that this would be OK, as long as the focus of each meal was vegetable juices. She could have other vegetarian foods such as cooked beans and brown rice, because the main point was to eat better overall. Over the next several months, she continued to contact Dr. Saul intermittently to ask if this or that food would be OK to combine with the raw vegetable diet. And the good news was she was continuing with the regimen. Then, after a year without any word from her, Dr. Saul was shopping in a health food store one day and was surprised to find a tall, rather graceful woman he didn't recognize. But he recalled her voice when she asked, "Do you remember me?" Her arthritis and the lumps on her arms and legs were completely gone. Without any other treatment, she was cured. We hope this can be your story too!

This book is about how to prevent and reverse arthritis through excellent nutrition. There are several types of arthritis, but they all involve degeneration of the joints and tissues surrounding them. It is considered to be a "progressive" disease, meaning that once the symptoms are diagnosed, they tend to get worse. The ends of our leg bones rub upon each other while carrying the weight of the body. In normal joints, they do this throughout a lifetime of constant wear and tear without damage, but with arthritis, the joint becomes inflamed and damaged, causing severe pain. The pain in arthritis can be continual, debilitating, and for some types of arthritis, crippling. The inability to walk or move the hands without pain induces severe stress, both physical and mental. Arthritis affects one in five Americans, and more than 100 billion dollars is spent each year in this country for its treatment.[2] With life expectancy extending significantly further every decade, and without a widely accepted cure, the incidence of arthritis is expected to increase. Millions of people worldwide are motivated to do whatever necessary to be free from their pain. Although drug treatments exist for age-related arthritis, they generally don't cure the disease, and usually can only slow the progression and treat the pain. Thus arthritis is widely thought to be incurable. This prognosis may lead arthritis sufferers into depression and a major life crisis. However, most forms of arthritis can be effectively treated and prevented by an excellent diet and vitamin supplements taken in adequate doses.

TYPES OF ARTHRITIS

Over the last century, the standard explanation for the cause of arthritis has been that over time our joints simply wear out; that is, the cartilage that lubricates the ends of the bones gets worn thinner and thinner until one bone is wearing directly on another. It stands to reason that wear and tear is responsible for some of the damage. As arthritis sufferers know from their pain, excess stress on an arthritic joint can make it worse. Yet arthritis can be reversed, as we will describe below. The degraded cartilage in a joint can regrow.[3] The process of degradation and regrowth in a joint is a dynamic process that continues throughout life. Arthritis results when the joint does not recover from damage.

Osteoarthritis (OA) is the most common form of arthritis, occurring in about 20 percent of adults, and is typically age-related and usually seen in older people. Arthritis affects more than half of adults over sixty-five, and 50 percent more women than men.[4] OA can be caused by an earlier injury to the joint, for example, after an injury to the knee and surgery to repair the meniscus in the knee joint.[5] Among its symptoms is a progressive destruction of the joint's cartilage, which reduces the ability of the joint to move and induces acute pain. In severe osteoarthritis, the bones rub directly against each other, causing damage to the bones and excruciating pain. OA can affect almost any joint in the body, and is commonly found in the hands, feet, hips, knees, and the lower back. The risk of developing OA is currently thought to be a combination of genetic factors, together with the specific shape of the individual's joint and surrounding bones, and its history of weight loading and damage.[6] The pain of OA often starts in one joint before it appears in other joints.

Rheumatoid arthritis (RA) occurs in only about 1 percent of adults and is more common in women. It is similar to osteoarthritis in being a disease of the joints, but typically its onset is in younger adults, usually above the age of twenty, yet sometimes in children as young as four. Often the onset appears to be triggered by an injury or illness. RA often affects the hands, wrists, and feet, usually on both sides of the body. It is caused by an aberrant response of the immune system to attack the joints and other tissues. The immune system attack tends to deteriorate the joint lining and the cartilage, leading to a similar type of degeneration of the bones as in osteoarthritis. In lupus (also known as systemic lupus erythematosus, or SLE), a chronic inflammatory disease, many organs of the body are damaged, including the joints, causing a similar degeneration. Both RA and lupus are typically seen symmetrically on both sides of the body, and they share several similar features. However, lupus typically doesn't cause as much damage as RA. Other symptoms typical of lupus are muscle pain and tendon pain associated with a joint.

Gout, another type of arthritis, is caused by crystals of uric acid that are deposited in the joint, causing inflammation and pain. It is about five times more common than RA.[7] Gout is caused by abnormally high blood levels of uric acid, a byproduct of the metabolism of protein-rich foods that contain purines, which are found in all foods but especially meat and fish. The uric acid precipitates as crystals in the joints and on the tendons and nearby tissues, and this triggers an immune response that causes pain and damage. Gout is more likely to start in the night when the body temperature is lower because this tends to trigger precipitation of the uric acid crystals. It can also be caused by a reaction to a drug, for example gemcitabine taken for cancer chemotherapy.[8]

Another type of arthritis is caused by infections, such as Borreliosis (Lyme disease) and its associated co-infections including mycoplasma and ameba.[9] Lyme disease and its co-infections can present symptoms similar to arthritis, lupus, multiple sclerosis, ALS, or Parkinson's disease.[10] Other types of inflammation that may include arthritic conditions are fibromyalgia and psoriasis. There are many different varieties of these basic forms of arthritis that can be distinguished. They can often be identified by a blood test and the symptoms, including the location of the pain. Your medical doctor can determine which of these conditions you may have, based on an office visit and lab report.

The stiffness and pain from arthritis can be excruciating and very debilitating, leading the sufferer to expect that the joints will be further damaged by activity. The pain and stiffness, along with ignorance of the proper type of exercise for arthritis, often leads to inactivity. Such inactivity is an important risk factor for many other diseases such as heart disease and diabetes, especially in older people. For many types of arthritis, moderate exercise that moves the joint without further damaging it can be therapeutic.[11] Runners typically don't get arthritis in their knees.[12] Pain-killing drugs can contribute to recovery by encouraging exercise, but may have damaging side-effects. In many cases, a warm-up regimen that gradually induces blood flow to prepare muscles and joints for activity is helpful. Although continual inflammation can trigger arthritis, inflammation around the site of damage is a natural part of the body's response. It helps to clean the site and to start the rebuilding process. Thus, it is important for the arthritis patient to grasp some basic information about joints, how they work, how the body maintains them, and what can go wrong in this process. And most important of all, we must understand the role of nutrition in maintaining joint health, for we are what we eat!

STANDARD ARTHRITIS TREATMENTS

The standard treatment for most types of arthritis is to prescribe drugs to make the patient more comfortable and reduce inflammation, thereby preventing acute damage. This type of treatment can help prevent pain, but the drugs currently available don't cure age-related arthritis. They generally help control the acute symptoms and prevent fast joint degeneration and thereby slow progression of the disease. Some drugs are analgesics that can ease the pain. Drugs can modulate the natural responses of the body, but they don't stop the basic disease mechanisms. Some treatments for arthritis depend on food supplements that come from plants or herbs. Although food supplements are often considered drugs they are not, because they provide natural substances that the body has evolved with for millions of years. Therefore, natural substances can be more effective than and preferable to artificial (pharmaceutical prescription) drugs.

The current standard treatment for OA is to address the symptoms of inflammation, stiffness, and pain using prescription drugs. It is typically treated first with acetaminophen or nonsteroidal anti-inflammatory drugs (NSAIDs) such as aspirin or ibuprofen. Injections of corticosteroids into the joint can give symptomatic relief by reducing acute inflammation, but this therapy is thought to lessen the potential for healing when taken long term. These drugs have many side effects and can cause ulcers and bleeding in the gut, liver disease, and renal failure.[13] The most commonly used analgesic, acetaminophen, can cause liver damage in doses only a few times higher than recommended.[14] Further, aspirin and NSAIDs can actually worsen joint damage. They inhibit the regrowth of cartilage in joints with OA.[15] Artificial synovial fluid can be injected into the joint, which may help for several months.[16]

Treatments for RA include prescription drugs to fight pain and inflammation, but also include drugs to block some functions of the immune system in the hope that the joint inflammation caused by an aberrant immune system can be prevented. Doctors often advise the importance of immediately reducing the acute symptoms of inflammation before severe joint damage can occur. These treatments do not cure the underlying disease, but in some cases they can slow its progression and relieve the acute symptoms. However, drug treatments invariably generate side effects that in some cases can be as bad as or worse than the original arthritic condition. Treatment for gout usually focuses on administering drugs that lower the uric acid level in the blood, so uric acid crystals don't form in and around the joints. Again, these drugs cannot cure, but they do provide some benefit by lessening acute inflammation and preventing the joint damage that can incur as a result. However, they invariably cause side effects that can prevent their unrestricted use by some patients. Some drugs utilized to treat osteoporosis may be beneficial for slowing the degradation of cartilage.[17] There are new treatments today that use stem cells, which are very effective and have few side effects. We will describe these in Chapter 6 below.

For arthritic symptoms caused by bacterial infections such as Lyme disease or mycoplasma, the standard treatment is a course of antibiotics long enough to clear the bacteria from all the infected joints. Many cases of Lyme go undiagnosed and untreated because the proper lab tests have not been run. These include several types of blood test for antibodies to Lyme, as well as blood and urine PCR (polymerase chain reaction) tests that look for DNA from the Lyme spirochete. These types of infection-caused arthritis can be successfully treated with antibiotics, but only if the infectious organism can be correctly diagnosed.[18] And it will help to take adequate doses of vitamins, including antioxidants such as vitamin C, to improve the functioning of the immune system.

For most types of arthritis, doctors advise that lifestyle changes and simple nonsurgical procedures can make a big difference. Application of heat or cold to a joint can help in some cases. Getting enough sleep, losing extra weight, and carefully avoiding more injury will all reduce stress on the joint and to help it recover. In some cases, nonsurgical injections can help reduce ligament and tendon pain. One treatment that has shown promise for reducing pain in a tendon or ligament is to give an injection near where it attaches to the bone. The injection can contain growth factors and glucose (blood sugar). This attracts blood vessels and allows the area to heal faster. Another way is to inject platelet cells from the patient's own blood (Platelet rich plasma, PRP). These cells contain biochemical growth factors and can speed recovery and reduce pain when injected into a joint. The cartilage on the ends of bones does not contain any nerves, so the pain caused by arthritis comes from the heavily innervated surrounding tissues, including bones and the ends of ligaments and tendons. A related problem is that some types of sciatica (sciatic nerve irritation and inflammation) are caused by arthritis in which bone spurs or inflammation of the tissues surrounding the joint impinge upon a nerve. In many cases of back and hip pain, it can be difficult to discover the source of the problem.[19] Physical therapy can help, including stretching the spine and relevant joints to relieve the pressure and irritation of the sciatic nerve. Several good books are available that describe effective treatments for this type of persistent pain.[20]

For acute damage to cartilage in the joint, such as a ruptured disk in the spine or a torn meniscus in the knee, arthroscopic surgery can remove nonfunctional pieces of cartilage that cause pain, get in the way of the joint, and limit its mobility. Good outcomes have been reported for arthroscopic knee debridement (removal of damaged tissue) after a period of healing.[21] But repair of cartilage in the joint is generally difficult, because cartilage usually heals very slowly after surgery. Prolotherapy, or injections of biochemicals or stem cells to stimulate the healing response, is designed to promote healing and growth of the ligaments and tendons surrounding the joint. Another standard option is joint replacement for knee or hip. In severe cases of damage to the spine, joint fusion can prevent inflammation and pain.

Caveats for Current Medical Treatments

Mainstream medical science today is a powerful resource for studying the arthritic disease process because the tools of biochemistry and genetics can be utilized to discover the disease mechanisms and suggest the cause and a potential treatment.[22] However, modern medical practice is often focused mainly on treating the acute symptoms of arthritic disease instead of working to prevent the disease in the first place. Thus, as described above, medical treatments for arthritis are often prescription drugs or invasive procedures such as surgery that can have serious and sometimes even disastrous side effects. Pain management can help to get you moving again, but it cannot cure. Surgery for knee or hip joint replacement has worked wonders for some patients, but it is a last resort and can induce severe side effects such as infection or heart attack.[23] Individuals' reactions to any drug may differ. Therefore, a typical medical doctor will often use a process of trial and error to discover which drugs may help an arthritis patient, testing to see how well each one relieves the inflammation and pain, and how the patient tolerates the side effects. When one drug doesn't work well, another one is prescribed, and sometimes several at once, and so on, until the patient has been tested with a series of expensive and dangerous drugs that cannot cure in any case.[24] If these don't work, the arthritis patient may be referred to a different specialist, sometimes ending up with a surgeon and joint replacement.

NUTRITIONAL TREATMENT

A nutritionist, in contrast to a conventional medical practitioner, will utilize knowledge of biochemistry and nutrition to determine the nutritional deficiencies that cause a progressive disease like OA or RA, and will attempt to help the patient overcome these deficiencies to prevent further progress of the disease or even reverse it.[25] The nutritional approach is more effective and far safer than using drugs such as NSAIDs.[26] Deficiencies in nutrients are common, but once they are determined they are fairly easy to remedy. A nutritionist will recommend an excellent diet that provides robust levels of all the essential nutrients, along with supplements to ensure adequate levels of all the nutrients critical for addressing the disease. Typically, leafy green vegetables are on the top of the list, along with raw vegetables, sprouts, and cooked vegetables such as squash, beans, and legumes, and whole grains. For those who may not be getting enough of the essential nutrients in their diet, a nutritionist might add supplements of vitamins B_1-B_6 (20–100 milligrams (mg) per day), vitamin C to bowel tolerance (3,000–10,000 mg per day up to the point that you get a laxative effect), vitamin D (5,000–10,000 international units (IU) per day), a natural mix of vitamin E with tocopherols and tocotrienols (400–1,200 IU per day), vitamin K_2 (100 micrograms (mcg)), zinc (50 mg), selenium (100 mcg), copper (2 mg), calcium (300 mg), and magnesium (300 mg). The nutritionist works with the patient's other medical professionals to select the right combination of high-nutrient items to prevent any problems with food sensitivities or drug therapy. The nutritionist recommends an excellent diet for all patients with any signs of disease, even young adults, instead of waiting until they get worse later in life and require treatment for an established illness. Nutritional treatment aimed at helping arthritis-related disease is effective for treating pain, but goes beyond the palliative care offered by traditional medicine to promote cartilage healing and regrowth in the joint. We will discuss this approach in detail in the chapters below.

This basic paradigm of preventing disease and helping recovery instead of treating the acute symptoms with drugs is not new—it has been practiced for thousands of years by aboriginal healers. But with modern scientific methods, biochemistry has identified many of the metabolic pathways necessary for correct functioning of the body's tissues. Over the last century this research has identified several essential nutrients, such as vitamins, omega-3 and omega-6 fatty acids, minerals such as calcium and magnesium, and other trace elements such as iron and selenium, that must be obtained from the diet. Deficiencies in essential nutrients such as vitamins and minerals are strongly implicated as a cause of progressive age-related diseases such as heart disease, cancer, and arthritis. Wholistic and integrative medical practice attempts to prevent progressive diseases such as heart disease and arthritis by addressing the whole person including their nutritional deficiencies.[27] This type of treatment is becoming more widely included in conventional medical practice. Moreover, integrative medicine can combine the best treatments from nutrition with the best treatments of conventional pharmaceutical medicine. They are not exclusive. However, nutritional treatments for age-related disease are safer, and most often less expensive and more effective. In the next chapter, we describe the essential nutrients from the perspective of the nutritional treatment of arthritis.

RESPONSIBILITY FOR LEARNING

We live in a complex world, where many different governmental entities, organizations, and corporations much larger than ourselves vie for our attention and money. The government claims it wants to set up a better health care system, but takes in taxes to pay for standardized care that in many cases is too inflexible. Medical insurance companies claim they want to provide a security net for everyone by averaging their medical expenses over large groups, but they effectively control and limit which treatments doctors are allowed to provide. The multinational food corporations claim they want to improve our health by giving us more food choices, but sell us high-priced processed food that lacks adequate nutrition.[28] The giant drug corporations claim they want to cure disease by inventing new drugs to give us more clinical options, but sell us expensive drugs that can't cure and have dangerous side effects. We are served by a health care industry that gives us continuing "disease care" without cures, but makes huge profits.[29]

Yet, the decisions you make about how you live your life are up to you: what you ask and tell your governmental representatives, what insurance policies you patronize, what you purchase in the supermarket, what you ask for in the doctor's office, and what you look up, read, and learn. These responsibilities are all important. If you are advised by a doctor to take a drug, you may benefit by learning more about the causes for your condition or illness, and about all the effective treatments, including dietary and nutritional supplements. It is up to you to utilize the doctor's advice wisely.[30] You and your doctor will likely both benefit. In a similar way, if you go to the supermarket and don't understand what is in the food that you are purchasing, it is up to you to learn more about the processing and additives it contains, for you are what you eat. This can make a great difference in how your body stays healthy and recovers from disease. If you ask for more healthy foods at your supermarket, and discuss healthy food choices with people you know, your words are likely to stimulate changes. You and your community, including the market, will likely benefit. And if you don't understand what is proposed by the politicians for government programs, it is up to you to learn more about these complex systems. If you vote wisely by your choices, you will continue to be a responsible citizen of a complex world. We will all benefit.

Learning about nutrition is one of life's crucial continuing lessons. Each of us must learn about what foods are best for us from whatever sources of information we can find. This requires us to consider a variety of different types of information: what foods are available, which ones taste good and are the most nutritious, and which ones give the most nutrition for the least cost. These differ for each person, because of our cultural and genetic heritage, our differing daily lives and environment, and our individual biochemical differences. This information is inherently complex, and for an individual there is often no easy way to know what aspect of nutrition and the diet is most important. Studies of nutrition that collect information from thousands of participants cannot determine which dietary nutrients and doses are optimal for an individual. A doctor and a patient can often decide together upon a few good dietary alternatives, but in the end it is up to the patient to try them and determine which are best. Thus, the patient is left with a steep learning curve. We will describe this topic more in later chapters.

For many of the dietary recommendations in this book, there is no "clinical proof" that they are optimal or even work at all. The concept of "proof" doesn't exist in natural science—it is a concept applicable to mathematical logic and the law. Rather, science develops and tests hypotheses in a continuing dynamic process of discovery. We will describe this more in Chapter 2.

Some nutritional research studies attempt to discover the effect of a particular diet among a large population, and can state that the result is "statistically significant." This cannot determine proof for an individual or even for a sizeable group, however, because each person or group is different and is likely to have different nutritional needs. Although we cannot provide "clinical proof" that the concepts in this book are correct, we have attempted to provide plentiful references that we hope will provide the interested reader useful insight.

Who We Are and What We Hope to Accomplish in This Book

We (the authors in this book) are scientists who work with the physiology and biochemistry of cells. I (RGS) work in the field of vision and study how the neural circuits of the retina sense the visual world. I grew up with a profound sense of the power of science to improve lives, and of nutrition to maintain health and prevent disease. As a child, I read *Silent Spring* by Rachel Carson, which explained in detail how chemicals have contaminated the environment. This book was a major influence in the development of the modern environmental movement. As a young adult, I read books by Adelle Davis, who wrote about preventing disease and providing health through nutrition.[31] Her books were full of references to nutrition literature, and this made a big impression on me. I was interested that nutrition science was full of important knowledge about everyday foods that could help everyone be healthy. Later, I read Linus Pauling's *Vitamin C and the Common Cold,* and became more interested in the new science of orthomolecular medicine.[32] And I read *Diet for a Small Planet,* by Frances Moore Lappé, that explained the importance of eating complementary sources of vegetable protein.[33] It also showed how the modern world could produce more nutrition from a vegetarian diet with less expense and use of resources.

These authors were all prescient in one way or another. They taught me about the importance of obtaining healthy food from a healthy environment. I learned that the processed food we eat lacks essential nutrients, but that with careful attention to the food we buy, we can obtain healthy food. Over the last several decades, nutrition science has moved on, but the work of these authors remains as an important inspiration. Recent media stories have downplayed Pauling's nutrition work, saying that it has been discredited. Instead, Pauling's work continues to be widely validated and relied upon today. It stands as an excellent inspiration for modern nutritional science.[34]

Pauling was one of the two most famous scientists of the twentieth century, and certainly was the most famous chemist of his time. His pioneering work on chemical bonds is widely considered an important component of the chemistry of molecules. He established the first conceptual framework for understanding how enzymes function in biochemical pathways.[35] He is widely acknowledged as one of the founders of modern molecular biology.[36] His unequaled knowledge and outgoing intellect inspired generations of scientists to pursue careers in molecular biology.

Over the last decade, I enthusiastically read several books about the power of vitamins and essential nutrients for healing based upon Pauling's work.[37] The modern understanding of the importance of nutrients explained in these books led me to participate actively in orthomolecular nutrition. In *The Vitamin Cure for Eye Disease* I wrote about how proper nutrition can prevent or reverse many age-related eye diseases.[38] I have had knee and hip injuries and mild arthritis, which have healed naturally, and have a strong sense of the power of nutrition for healing and preventing disease.

Over the past three decades, computers and the Internet have accelerated the progress of all science including nutrition. Along with my interest in vision and nutrition, I am an electronics and computer enthusiast, have worked as an electronics engineer, and enjoy designing computer hardware and software. I enjoy playing traditional and contemporary music on the recorder, and also enjoy taking photographs of nature and people. Like many scientists around the world, my research in vision benefits greatly from the research literature that is available on the Internet through PubMed for anyone in the world to read. This is good news for everyone, and a tremendous help for anyone interested in learning. And I enthusiastically applaud the United States Congress for ruling that research funded by the National Institutes of Health (NIH) should be made available for free to the public.

Over the past thirty years, I've cultivated a small vegetable garden in my downtown urban backyard. Every summer I grow spinach, radishes, peas, green beans, carrots, broccoli, collards, kale, tomatoes, and squash. This little garden provides much of my food during the summer. The fresh produce has greatly contributed to my health and my interest in nutrition. I learned how to make green smoothies from my home-grown collards and kale. Gifts of the bountiful harvests have been a great way to make friends with neighbors who've moved onto the block. I've also volunteered at several local neighborhood gardens, advising about how to organize a garden, obtain and generate compost, and cultivate for the best yields.

I (WTP) am a scientist working in the field of nutritional biochemistry and developmental genetics. Among other topics, I have studied the role of the B vitamins in the body's tissues. I have fairly severe osteoarthritis restricted to my left hip, and have a deep sense of compassion for those individuals incapacitated by any form of arthritis. I also have a strong desire to cure my own arthritis. My recent work is focused on the role of niacin in the metabolic pathways of cells for preventing disease. My interest in biochemistry began in high school. My grandmother had just lost her husband to atherosclerosis and realized her mortality was imminent. She soon became interested in health, and got chelation therapy treatments. This completely changed her life. During this time she read the *Life Extension* books of Durk Pearson and Sandy Shaw[39] and showed these books to me. I was particularly struck by the ability of niacin to correct dyslipidemia (abnormal cholesterol and fat levels in blood) while causing an unpleasant side effect (temporary skin rash) that dissuaded many people from taking it. This reminded me of the role of exercise for many sedentary people. It is exactly what they need to feel better, but they sometimes require persuasion because of stiffness or temporary pain.

This impression stuck with me as I went to graduate school to get my PhD in biochemistry. As a postdoctoral fellow I trained for several years working with zebrafish, a model organism that is transparent and useful for performing forward genetic screens as well as small molecule screens. I secured my first position as a professor at the University of Cincinnati in 2004 and collaborated with a Fortune 500 company involved in drug discovery. This was a real eye-opening experience into the realities of the drug discovery process. As an independent researcher I decided to focus primarily on niacin-related research, more specifically the endpoint of niacin within our bodies, nicotinamide adenine dinucleotide (NAD), and also the high affinity G-protein coupled receptor for niacin, GPR109a.[40]

As I learned more about niacin I contacted the legends in the field: Dr. Abram Hoffer for clinical information, and Myron and Elaine Jacobson for basic research information. I became increasingly amazed by how important NAD was for many normal biochemical pathways and diseases. From the worst vitamin deficiency epidemic (pellagra) in the history of the United States to the most recent spate of drug targets of focus (Sirtuins, PARP inhibitors, and CD38 inhibitors), NAD is involved at the central core of many diseases. Further, NAD is involved in more biochemical reactions (more than 450) than any other vitamin-derived cofactor (a nonprotein required for enzyme protein function). It is at the center of human cellular metabolic catabolism (release of energy through degradation) of biomolecules.

From Abram Hoffer's studies I learned about the remarkable effects of increasing the body's NAD concentration. He had been ringing the bell about this for decades. During this time Abram and I became friends. He taught me invaluable information regarding the benefits of niacin in the clinic. In my experience, his generosity and selflessness was unparalleled. He was a walking, talking legend, who was available and ready to help. I performed unique experiments testing the effects of different NAD precursors in zebrafish animal models of human disease. High doses of NAD were fantastic at keeping the fish alive when they were exposed to otherwise lethal stresses.

I became particularly interested in learning more about arthritis because of severe osteoarthritis in my left hip. I read the work of William Kaufman, which involved using high doses of niacinamide to treat arthritis.[41] Kaufman studied patients with moderate pellagra and noted that arthritis was one of the symptoms. He gave these patients niacin and noted that their arthritis symptoms were alleviated. More frequent low doses worked better than single high doses. He theorized that due to individual differences, some people required higher levels than others. Many patients received tremendous relief when they took 250–500 mg of niacinamide every hour or two throughout the day. Kaufman's niacin treatment for arthritis was not widely appreciated, but still remains useful and valid today. We will describe it further in the chapters below. When researchers are heavily involved in the trendy fundable fields of molecular genetics, we often forget what was learned decades ago from the more tangible biomedical research. This history is all too often forgotten as market forces continually beat the drum of new drugs instead of the beat of molecules our bodies have evolved to use.

As I contribute to this book, I begin with a mission. I have a fairly good idea of what triggered my osteoarthritis. All of my life I have been passionately excited by playing soccer. In my teens and twenties I played soccer on a concrete cul-de-sac. I persisted in playing soccer into my late thirties, playing with twenty-somethings. However, each time I played I would experience hip pain and limp for several days before recovering and playing again. I did this for years, but it got intolerable all of a sudden in my forties—I unknowingly destroyed most of my hip labrum.

(The labrum is a thin layer of cartilage lining the inside of the hip joint.) Now I can't run without terrible pain. My right hip is without pain, but I have very painful OA in my left hip. This degeneration can get to a point where doctors recommend hip replacement surgery. I am at that point.

My situation seems like a curse, but is actually a blessing in disguise. It is a curse because I had to stop running and playing soccer with all of my lifelong buddies. Even though I'd like to, I can't run with my young children. It is also a real blessing, because many people will get arthritis in their old age. If I can learn how to cure my hip, then I will be ready for the other problems that I may face in old age. I hope that my example and experience will help other people. Conventional medicine says my only options are pain management in the short term, and an inevitable hip replacement in the long-term. I know full well that corticosteroids are likely to cause further destruction in the hip, and may lead to avascular osteonecrosis. Yet other options exist. Orthomolecular physicians, scientists on the cutting edge, and prolotherapists (who use nonsurgical injection treatments that stimulate healing) utilize techniques that can prevent and reverse OA. I have been pursuing these alternate therapies. I intend to learn everything I can and to describe my best attempt to cure arthritis based on all the evidence through orthomolecular medical approaches. So I contribute to this book with the goal of making some kind of progress in healing my hip.

Learning to Take Responsibility

This book is about learning to take responsibility for our health, our community, and the world we live in. We hope that you will get a sense of how science has proceeded over the past century to learn about the essential nutrients. We hope to make the connection between deficiencies in these nutrients and our long-term health obvious to you. One of the book's themes is that we all need to learn more about the characteristics our bodies share, but we also need to learn how each individual is unique. Each one of us has different genes, and we have different stresses in our daily lives that give us different nutritional needs, but we can all learn to eat wisely.

Throughout this book, you will find plenty of references to substantiate our discussion. We hope you will take advantage of these references by looking them up in a library or online. Most of the reasearch papers are available online in PubMed (www.ncbi.nlm.nih.gov/pubmed).[42] For many of these, a file in pdf format is available free for downloading. In fact, half of all research articles published in 2011 are now available free.[43] There's even an interface for tablets and other small-format mobile devices. You go to PubMed online, search to find an article, and click on the rectangle showing the publisher's name in the upper right corner. This link directs you to the publisher's page, where you can read the full text or download the pdf file. For most of the other articles that are not accessible directly, an abstract (summary) is available free online and a pdf is available through a university library. When you have questions about the details of vitamins or how they can prevent arthritis, we hope you will check out the references at the end of the book. Although the popular media, dominated by the drug industry, continues to downplay the importance of vitamin supplements and eating an excellent diet, the field of orthomolecular medicine is moving rapidly. Many new studies are currently in progress to discover what nutrients are most helpful in preventing disease. In the coming years, many new mechanisms for health through nutrition are bound to be discovered. But we already know the basics. Most forms of arthritis can be prevented—and in many cases reversed—through excellent nutrition. We hope you find this book helpful in explaining how and why!

CHAPTER 2

The Discovery and Importance of Essential Nutrients

This chapter recounts the history of the discoveries of some essential nutrients. As generations of nutrition science investigators have done, everyone can and must search for the foods that provide the nutrients most appropriate for their own needs. The anecdotes we present give a sense of how to search for the best hypotheses in a complex topic such as nutrition. All of the nutrients described are important for maintaining health and preventing arthritis.

Although the details of biochemistry are complex, we find the history of vitamins and nutrients interesting and important for developing insight into nutritional effects on health. We believe that an awareness of the discovery of vitamins will be helpful in guiding your learning experience about nutrition. The researchers looking for the "essential nutrients" over the last century were motivated by horrible epidemics. At first, they didn't realize that these epidemics were caused by nutritional deficiencies. They had to carefully review current knowledge while keeping their minds open to new findings. This led them to perform heroic experiments, on people or animals, in which they tried different dietary variations. The results allowed them to eliminate incorrect theories using the scientific method. This process of trial and error allowed them to find the biochemicals that we now call vitamins and essential nutrients. We believe that this history of the discovery of vitamins is instructive, for it is analogous to the process we must all pursue to learn the best foods for our individual needs. The scientific research on what constitutes a healthy diet and on preventing disease with nutrition continues. And just as science learns more about nutrition, we hope the following sections will help interested individuals develop a new awareness about the importance of essential nutrients for the body.

Some authors have written passionately about the need to eat wholesome food but deny the utility of knowledge about the essential nutrients, saying that the concept of tracking nutrients in food is "reductionism" or "nutritionism."[1] This term is supposed to refer to a "reductionist" concept that started with early nutritional researchers, in which some components of food were thought to be good and some bad.[2] The implication of these "wholistic" concepts is that, because the topic of food and nutrition is so complex, we should not track nutrients, for food is more than the sum of its parts.[3] Moreover, the food industry has apparently utilized this "futile concept" of nutritionism for profit, for we are bombarded every time we shop for food by statements about what a particular food product does or does not contain. In reaction to these ideas, many people are suspicious of the rationale for tracking nutrients. Many popular books and TV shows explain that there is more to food than the nutrients it contains!

But modern research has found that the nutrients we get from foods are indeed the important components. This is exemplified by studies of the Inuit living in the Arctic on a traditional diet, showing that it is possible to be healthy eating mostly meat and fat. If these foods are taken from wild animals, they can provide all the essential nutrients, including vitamins.[4] We mention this interesting and unusual diet to make a point. On first thought, many people in our modern society would believe this diet is unhealthy, noting that it lacks vegetables and fruits and that the high level of fat would be detrimental. Indeed, we do not recommend this diet, because eating the corresponding foods produced by our modern food industry would not provide adequate nutrition. The fat that we get from industrialized meat production is unhealthy because it is mostly saturated. Grass-fed meat provides much higher levels of polyunsaturated fatty acids (PUFAs), vitamin K, and other essential nutrients. The uncooked meat and fat of wild animals provided the Inuit adequate amounts of vitamin A, Bs, C, D, E, K and omega-3 and omega-6 PUFAs that gave them health. This and many other examples show the importance of understanding the roles and proper levels of nutrients for maintaining health.

We applaud the foresight and enthusiasm of popular books that expound the benefits of wholesome food and wholistic ideals and the dangers of the existing drug-based health-care system.[5] We hope the reader can grasp our passion about eating an excellent diet. Nutrition is quite a complex topic, and it affects every one of us deeply. The modern diet contains a significant amount of processed foods. This is indeed the cause of much age-related disease. Although many essential nutrients are now known, it seems possible, even likely, that other essential nutrients remain to be discovered. Most of the essential nutrients cannot easily be studied in isolation because their effects are interdependent and symbiotic. As scientists we firmly believe that knowledge about the essential nutrients will help the reader understand why nutrition is so important for preventing arthritis.

BIOCHEMICAL REQUIREMENTS, FOOD, AND VITAMINS

The body is a collection of different types of cells that work together to function as organs. Each cell is an individual, but sends and receives signals to and from other cells that communicate what jobs need to be performed.[6] Cells in organs cooperate with their neighbors to perform the organ's functions. The organs are maintained by blood flowing throughout the body in blood vessels. The blood carries the nutrients required by the organs and removes waste products. Arteries carry blood from the lungs to the heart and through the body. When they emerge from the heart they bifurcate multiple times and become smaller in diameter. The smallest arteries are called capillaries, which are about seven microns (μm) in diameter, the size of red blood cells. Capillaries in an average human body collectively have a huge surface area, equal to 10,000 square feet, and penetrate deep into the body's organs. The average human body has approximately 60,000 miles of blood vessels. That is more than twice the distance around the earth! This huge surface area allows the nutrients in the blood to readily diffuse, or be transported through the capillary walls to the organ's cells. Interestingly, bones are well supplied with blood by arteries and capillaries like every other organ of the body, because they are living organs that contain cells. However, the cartilage in joints has no blood supply. It must get nutrients and relieve wastes via the special synovial fluid in which it bathes. We will describe these mechanisms in more detail in Chapter 3.

The waste from living cells is passed into the bloodstream and eliminated by the kidneys. By default, the kidneys send all of the blood serum (the liquid component of blood) on the path to excretion, but they retrieve all the essential molecules, including water, salt, sugar, proteins, and vitamins, and pump them back into the blood. Any molecule that is not pumped back into the blood by the kidneys is carried out of the body in the urine. This elimination of wastes and regulation of essential nutrients in the bloodstream may seem miraculous, but it makes our lives possible.

Cell Machinery

Modern biology has determined many of the intricate details of how cells work.[7] Each organ comprises one or more specific types of cell. With only a few exceptions, each cell contains a full copy of our genetic material, called DNA (deoxyribonucleic acid). This genetic material instructs the cell precisely how to synthesize different protein biochemicals such as muscle fibers; collagen for the skin, hair, and cartilage; enzymes to metabolize food to generate energy; and other biochemicals necessary for the cell's function. The genetic material in DNA is copied ("transcribed") into a different molecule called RNA (ribonucleic acid), which specifies the sequence of amino acids in protein molecules. (In biological terminology, RNA "is translated into" or "codes" the protein molecule.) A cell takes in its building blocks—absorbed from the food we eat—from the bloodstream. The cell then synthesizes most of the biochemicals it needs using "metabolic pathways" that consist of a sequence of enzymes and cofactors. So, fundamentally, these enzymes chemically transform food molecules into the biochemicals required for cell function.

Animals and plants are dependent on basic chemical building blocks that originate from the soil or atmosphere of planet Earth; for example, some forms of carbon and nitrogen and minerals such as sodium, potassium, calcium, and magnesium. Plants can generate energy and most of the biomolecules they need from sunlight, carbon dioxide from the air, and water and minerals from the soil. But all animals are dependent on plants or bacteria (or indirectly by eating herbivores) to supply the basic biochemicals required by all life, such as the eight essential amino acids for protein and carbohydrates and oils for energy.[8] The energy and basic chemical building blocks necessary for life, that we get from eating meat, originated in plants. Animal cells, unlike plant cells, cannot synthesize all the molecules they need and must derive these biochemicals from food. The ability to move with fins, legs, or wings requires a lot of energy, readily provided by eating plants and other animals. You might say we're addicted to (dependent on) food! Green plants have their own addictions—they require sunlight!

Besides obvious biomolecules such as proteins and carbohydrates, animals need other nutrients typically found in their food. Some of the biomolecules that our tissues require as cofactors for our metabolic enzyme pathways cannot be made by our bodies, and we must get them from other species. This dependency started early in the development of life on earth, in which a complex set of interactions developed between different species.[9] Essential nutrients were required by some species and supplied by others. The same dependencies between different species exist today.

Plants require and can synthesize many of these essential cofactor molecules. Bacteria and other microbes synthesize the rest. These essential nutrients were always available to our ancient ancestors, so they never evolved the ability to synthesize the essential nutrients. That is why our ancestors became dependent on these nutrients millions of years ago.[10] It may seem incredible that vitamins are required for all life, including bacteria and plants, and that these same vitamins are exactly what animal cells need. But we have much in common with plants, including many of the metabolic pathways that all living cells use to grow and maintain themselves.

Over the past 100 years, science has discovered the identity of more than a dozen of the essential nutrients that we must get from our diet. These include the vitamins, essential minerals such as sodium, potassium, calcium, magnesium, micronutrients such as zinc, copper, iron, cobalt, and selenium, and other biomolecules like the omega-3 and omega-6 fatty acids, and lutein and zeaxanthin—and very possibly several others still unknown. We derive a distinct advantage from not needing to synthesize vitamins and other essential biomolecules because this synthesis requires energy, which can be devoted to support other functions of the cell when these biomolecules are found in the diet.[11] This is why animal cells have evolved without the ability to synthesize the essential biomolecules. However, a deficiency in some of these biomolecules slows or completely stops some of a cell's metabolic pathways, which causes the cell to lose some of its normal functions. Further, although many of the minimum molecular requirements for cellular survival are known, current understanding of molecular complexity in disease physiology is limited. This becomes evident when a disease such as diabetes or cancer strikes without warning.

Some nutrients, such as vitamins A, B_{12}, and D, are required in tiny amounts and can be stored over long periods in the body, so they are not essential to eat every day. Vitamin D is not an enzyme cofactor but is considered to be a hormone required by many tissues throughout the body. It is stored in the fatty tissues of the body for several months, with a half-life of six to eight weeks,[12] so if enough is obtained from exposure to midday sun during the summer months its level can remain sufficient in some cases until the next spring, in spite of the lack of ultraviolet light (UV) in winter sunlight. But other nutrients, such as vitamin C and niacin, are not stored over long periods in the body and are required in larger amounts, so a continual supply of these essential nutrients is necessary every day. The B vitamins are typically only stored in the body for a few days, and after a large dose of vitamin C, levels typically drop by half in four to eight hours.[13] Therefore vitamin C is best taken in smaller doses, for example, 1,000 milligrams (mg) per meal, or alternately 1,000 mg every two to three hours throughout the day. We will provide more details about vitamin doses in Chapter 7.

Nutrition Requirements Vary with Age

The nutritional needs of each individual differ, because our genes differ, our daily lives and stresses differ, and our diet and ability to absorb nutrients differs.[14] Some people may not want to admit this fact because it may appear to disrupt the commonly accepted wisdom about the importance of following the standardized medical decisions and treatments they have been taught. A genetic mutation in a cell's DNA can cause it to partially or completely lose function in one or more of its metabolic pathways so that the pathway becomes less efficient or completely blocked. Thus, an individual's genetic heritage interacts with the ability of cells in the different organs to perform their functions utilizing different types and quantities of nutrients. Further, the diet of an individual may affect the expression or importance of their particular genetic characteristics.[15] Moreover, we know very little about how different mutations to a gene affect the cell's ability to function when essential nutrients are deficient or absent. Our daily requirement for vitamins varies between individuals, and varies within an individual from one day to the next. Those who have a lot of physical stress on their joints, for example warehouse or industrial workers and runners, may need higher levels of nutrients such as vitamins C, D, K, calcium, and magnesium. Psychic stress, anxiety, and many prescription drugs can cause the body to lose magnesium, which must be replaced to prevent disease.[16]

Aging Bodies Need Extra Nutrients

The amount of specific nutrients our bodies need changes with age. The aging process is thought to originate in limitations to maintenance of the body's tissues.[17] Aging is not preprogrammed, but depends on many factors that cause damage to the body.[18] Some organs in the body (for example, the skin and stomach) are renewed over a period of weeks to months. This requires their cells to grow and divide using the specifications in their DNA. But cells gradually build up damage in their DNA and other macromolecules (large biomolecules) such as enzymes.[19] The damage occurs largely through oxidative stress and other mechanisms that change the atomic structure of the molecule and limit the cell's ability to function. These mechanisms are complex and are just beginning to be understood.[20] However, nutrition is a big factor. Young people tend to have voracious appetites that may supply a robust dose of essential nutrients if the diet contains adequate amounts of whole grains, fruits, and vegetables. But as we age, we require higher levels of essential nutrients, for several reasons. Aging bodies require extra nutrients to help repair damage to the tissues accumulated over many decades. Each time the skin is cut or bruised, or when we get a bacterial or viral infection, the immune system is called to the site, which generates more blood flow and inflammation. The body tries to repair the damage, but the healing process is contingent upon an adequate supply of essential nutrients. This is also true of systemwide damage to the organs, for instance, the cardiovascular system, and bones and joints. If essential nutrients are inadequate in the diet, the body may build up damage over decades. The length of the telomeres (protective sequences) at the ends of DNA molecules is an indicator of biological aging. As we age, our telomeres become shorter with each cell division and also with oxidative stress. A diet rich in antioxidant nutrients can prevent this type of biological aging.[21]

Many older people who have been eating an inadequate diet have deficiencies of some vitamins and minerals that progressively get worse over their lives. For example, a deficiency of magnesium is very common. All the organs of the body require magnesium to maintain health. This is especially true for the brain, bones, and joints. The body requires a continuous supply of this essential nutrient. When the diet doesn't contain enough magnesium (300–600 milligrams (mg) per day), the body takes some out of the bones, which then accumulate a deficit.[22] Deficits in other essential nutrients are also common. A deficit of vitamin D can result in decreased bone density. A similar deficit can occur with insufficient calcium in the diet. These deficits can build up over several decades, weakening the bones and causing inflammation and damage to the joints. This is a major contributing factor for arthritis.

Older people also tend to be less active and require fewer calories, and as a result often put on weight. In their struggle to reduce many people simply eat less of the same old processed food that doesn't contain adequate levels of nutrients. Further, as they age many people avoid raw fruits and vegetables because they contain fiber which can be tough to digest. The resulting bland diet can limit their intake of essential nutrients. As we've been often told, fruits and vegetables are extremely important and necessary to provide adequate levels of essential nutrients. For example, berries and fruits such as kiwi contain robust doses of vitamins and minerals.

Moreover, the stomach and gut tend to absorb less of the nutrients in food as people get older. This happens because proper digestion requires adequate levels of nutrients to generate stomach acid and other necessary secretions such as pancreatic enzymes and bile, which are often inadequate in older people. Absorption of vitamin B_{12} into the body requires adequate levels of several special-purpose proteins in the gut and bloodstream. Vitamin B_{12} is made only by bacteria and other microbial organisms. Higher animals get it through the food chain by eating lower organisms that in turn collect it from bacteria. In older people and vegetarians a moderate to severe deficiency of vitamin B_{12} is common, causing symptoms such as migraines, numbness and tingling, sharp pains in the extremities, amnesia, and dementia. If caught early these symptoms can be readily cured by eating foods high in vitamin B_{12} (clams, liver, meat, fish), oral supplements, or nasal spray.[23]

Deficiencies in any of the essential nutrients can be difficult to diagnose. The reason is that any one deficiency can cause many problems throughout the body. Magnesium, for example, is used in virtually all cells of the body for synthesis of DNA, RNA, and protein. A deficiency of magnesium can cause many problems, including high blood pressure, asthma, kidney stones, heart disease, strokes, and arthritis.[24] Because magnesium is missing in many processed foods, deficits of magnesium are very common. The same holds true for other essential nutrients such as vitamin C. We need at least 50 mg of vitamin C a day. Humans can go no longer than sixty days without vitamin C in our our diets before severe scurvy sets in. The symptoms of scurvy include severe pain in joints, swollen gums, and easily bruised skin, among others. Eventually scurvy leads to uncontrolled bleeding and death. When a vitamin C deficit is not acute enough to cause scurvy, it is difficult to detect, but over decades it can be deadly, causing heart disease and stroke.[25] Even worse, simultaneous deficiencies of several essential nutrients are also common, and are even more deadly and insidious. Vitamin C, taken with other essential nutrients can prevent heart disease and stroke.[26] However, deficiencies of these and other essential nutrients are often ignored.

Multivitamins that contain the Recommended Dietary Allowance (RDA) or Dietary Reference Intake (DRI) are helpful. But they are insufficient for most individuals, because an average dose of a set of essential nutrients cannot satisfy the needs of any particular person for all the nutrients their body requires. A nutritionist trained in orthomolecular medicine (the use of natural molecules to cure illness) can help you determine which essential nutrients you should focus on and what doses will help. We will return to this topic in Chapter 7.

THE DISCOVERY OF VITAMINS AND HYPOTHESIS-DRIVEN SCIENCE

In the Greek classical period, Hippocratic physicians had little knowledge of nutrition and believed that the only essential component of food was "aliment." This belief continued until the 1800s, when the essentiality of several minerals was determined. By 1850, sodium, potassium, phosphorus, chloride, calcium, and iron were known to be required in the diet.[27] Gradually over the next century the notion of essentiality of specific organic compounds in food was conceived and formalized.[28] These components were not minerals, but existed in generally small quantities in a variety of foods.

For centuries, scurvy was a horrible consequence of long sea voyages because sailors ate meager rations like biscuits and preserved meats, which contain no vitamin C. Epidemics of scurvy also occurred on land due to a lack of fresh vegetables during the winter. Grains could be stored for long periods but they don't contain much vitamin C. For people of many European countries, vegetables stored in a root cellar or fermented foods like sauerkraut, that contain small amounts of vitamin C, provided some relief. But even with these lifelines, scurvy often arrived with late winter. The introduction of potatoes from South America helped lower scurvy rates throughout Europe because they contain a moderate amount of vitamin C and can be stored over the winter.[29] But epidemics of scurvy killed many, for instance, during the potato famine in Ireland of 1845–1852.[30] The notion that a proper diet could prevent scurvy took many centuries to be widely understood. Gradually it was discovered that a regular dose of raw meat, or raw vegetables and fruits, often including greens or citrus, could cure and prevent the ravages of scurvy.

Lind's Experiment

The identification of a specific diet that prevents scurvy was made by James Lind onboard a ship during an ocean voyage in 1747. In one of the first clinical controlled scientific experiments, Lind gave a dozen sailors with scurvy different treatments to see if any could cure the disease. They were all given the same diet, but were divided into six groups of two to receive different test treatments. Each day, two sailors got two oranges and one lemon, two sailors got a quart of cider, two got twenty-five drops of elixir of vitriol (dilute sulfuric acid) three times a day, two got two spoonfuls of vinegar three times a day, two were given half a pint of sea water, and the last two got a mixture of spices and barley water, at that time commonly thought to prevent scurvy. Within six days the two sailors who had received the citrus were mostly recovered. Those who had received cider weren't recovered but were in better shape than the rest.[31] The experiment clearly showed that citrus fruit can cure scurvy. Unfortunately it took the British Admiralty another half century to adopt fresh citrus juice as part of the standard seagoing diet. In hindsight, our modern perspective may blame the Admiralty for ignoring Lind's work.

However, Lind himself didn't realize the implication of his experiments. Even in his later years, he believed that scurvy came from a problem with digestion and elimination of wastes from the body, which, he imagined, the citrus merely ameliorated.[32] But in fact he was aware that many previous attempts to prevent scurvy on ships had been successful. Over three long ocean voyages, Captain Cook had avoided scurvy on his ships by obtaining a variety of fresh fruits and vegetables from each stop on shore.[33] Vasco da Gama, in 1498, and many other explorers on long ocean voyages had also avoided scurvy by obtaining oranges from on shore.[34] Citing previous folk traditions that had already suggested the use of citrus and raw green vegetables, Lind tried to discover how this collective knowledge could ameliorate digestion to prevent scurvy.

After his classic experiment, Lind spent several more decades, in vain, trying to determine the best treatment, focusing on environmental factors like warmth and lack of humidity, and the variety of foods in the diet. Ocean expeditions that started from England in early spring tended to have cold and damp weather for the first several weeks. These expeditions developed more scurvy than voyages that started during the summer or fall, leading him to the hypothesis that the weather was somehow responsible.[35] However, from the lack of fresh fruit and vegetables available on land during the winter, most of the crew would have started the voyage with a seasonally low level of ascorbate (vitamin C). The idea that there was a substance in citrus, cider, and other fruits and fresh vegetables that could exclusively prevent scurvy did not occur to Lind because of his eighteenth century beliefs about the body and health.[36]

The search for a cure for scurvy continued over the next century. Doubts remained even after the British Admiralty decreed in 1796 a daily ration of fresh citrus that was successful in preventing scurvy. By the 1850s, scurvy was widely considered to be a deficiency disease, and had largely been eliminated, although the cause was still in doubt. Some doubted that citrus juice was the answer because when it was processed and put in barrels for long voyages, the crews on some ships continued to get scurvy and many still died. In retrospect, it is likely that the conditions under which the juice was processed and stored caused depletion of ascorbate.[37] Another theory held that a deficiency of potassium was the cause of scurvy, because fruits and vegetables had generous amounts and people with scurvy did not eat them. But it was pointed out that although dried fruits do not prevent scurvy, they contain the same amount of potassium as when fresh. Another source of confusion was that guinea pigs will develop the symptoms of scurvy on a diet without fresh fruit or vegetables, but on the same diet, rats will not.[38] On arctic explorations, fresh meat was found to prevent scurvy, but preserved or spoiled meat did not. To some, this suggested the hypothesis that scurvy was caused by bacterial poisoning.[39] We now know that fresh meat has just enough ascorbate to prevent scurvy if eaten regularly, but that the ascorbate gets depleted when meat spoils or is cooked at high temperature.

The discovery and wide acceptance of the germ theory of disease in the period 1860–1880 captivated the attention of medical researchers and led them to look for germs instead of a dietary deficiency for illnesses.[40] This exemplifies the directed focus that is typical in medical research even today. Yet, in taking the new germ theory of disease so seriously, researchers were prompted to recheck earlier work on scurvy with more careful studies to find its possible germ cause.[41] From these studies, more modern standards of research gradually emerged. In looking to find germs, researchers did more careful studies, which again showed that a deficiency was indeed responsible for scurvy. However, even by the early 1900s there was still some doubt about the missing substance. Eventually it was found that guinea pigs, monkeys, and apes tend to get scurvy but most other animals do not. This allowed more careful biological tests for the unknown substance that prevented scurvy.

Conclusions Limited by Hypotheses

The moral of this story is severalfold. Lind's experiment, and the ongoing unsuccessful studies over the next 150 years, were obviously not conceived nor performed using modern standards of medical research. Yet Lind's experiment was among the first controlled scientific experiments in nutritional health to compare several different treatments. Its results pointed in the right direction. With our modern sensibilities and informed hindsight, we can recognize the power of this type of health trial. But, importantly, just as Lind could not discern the best treatment for scurvy from his experiments, modern interventional randomized controlled trials (RCTs), when performed without informed observations and hypotheses about disease mechanisms are unable to discover the mechanism for disease or the best treatment.[42]

As Lind understood, the role of nutrition in health is complex. Even with a very strong association between a disease and an environmental condition, it can be very difficult to discern causality.[43] An RCT attempting to determine the outcome of a specific treatment tabulates the difference in outcome between groups of participants. Its interpretation is limited to the specific effect of the given treatment on the specific groups tested. It cannot determine a specific mechanism for disease, nor can its results be readily generalized to determine the best treatment for a different group or an individual.[44] Moreover, it is unethical to perform an interventional RCT that utilizes a placebo (a treatment known to be ineffective) to test the effect of one or more nutrients that are already known to be effective. It is unethical because such an RCT would give substandard treatment (the ineffective placebo) to some of the participants.[45]

The most helpful RCTs are those that start with a hypothesis about a disease mechanism and compare a new treatment with an existing treatment already known to be effective in preventing or reversing disease. For example, an RCT testing arthritis treatments could compare different doses of drugs with different doses of vitamins and minerals. In this case, the nutritional treatment that gives adequate doses would be the one known to be effective. To be even more helpful, an RCT might compare several different (adequate) doses and combinations of essential nutrients. However, this type of study is very rare, apparently because the pharmaceutical corporations that develop drugs have already spent huge sums on their products, and know that nutritional treatments are often very effective, quite possibly more effective than drugs. They have little financial incentive to perform such a trial correctly with adequate doses of nutrients. Indeed, an inadequate dose is a major reason why RCTs testing essential nutrients for efficacy in treating disease often find a negative result. To be effective for an age-related disease, such nutritional studies must be performed over several decades. This type of study is very expensive and is not widely performed, but the need is great.

Evidence-Based Nutrition

Implicit in this discussion of scientific study is the importance of finding the best hypothesis or approximation to the truth. Health studies are most significant and useful when they determine causes for disease and suggest new ways to treat it. Modern RCTs are considered to be the gold standard in "evidence-based medicine" because they are unbiased and objective. Groups are selected at random to be given one interventional treatment or another. The attending physician does not know which treatment was given to a patient. This is supposed to eliminate bias in selection and in treatment. But RCTs have many limitations. A study of a drug or medical treatment in an RCT differs fundamentally from the study of nutrition because, unlike pharmaceutical drugs, essential biochemicals such as vitamins are natural molecules that the body requires.[46] As we have seen, nutritional effects can be very subtle and confounding. Proper tests of nutrients would require huge carefully-planned studies on thousands of people performed over many years, in which nutrients are administered at different doses and in different combinations.[47] But this type of study is difficult to organize and execute, and thus is very expensive. Without good assurance of profit from such studies, they cannot be supported by the pharmaceutical industry. Practically, this means that RCT studies testing the efficacy of nutrient supplements have not been correctly planned and performed. High quality RCT studies of nutrients would require major funding by an impartial organization over decades, which seems unlikely unless funded by the government. Unfortunately, many government-funded studies of nutritional supplements have been influenced by the pharmaceutical industry's bias against the role of nutrition in preventing disease.

A less expensive way to look at the effect of nutrition on large populations is to collect and analyze the data from many other nutritional studies. These so-called meta-analyses, or meta-studies, are often inappropriate and poorly performed. Typically the studies collected into the meta-analysis are selected according to strict yet arbitrary standards that ignore most of the existing evidence.[48] Although the collected studies are typically RCTs, each is invariably performed a little differently on a different population with different nutritional needs and advantages. This complicates the interpretation and may completely confound the overall result, especially when inadequate doses of several nutrients are given. Observational and environmental studies that provide helpful intuition are typically not included, which limits the value and relevance of the meta-analysis.

Instead of "evidence-based medicine,' we need "evidence-based nutrition," which takes into account all types of knowledge about nutrition, including RCTs as well as observational and environmental studies. An observational study determines the association or "correlation" between a treatment and an outcome without actually providing the treatment, for example, those with higher levels of vitamin C or D measured in a blood test also have less risk of age-related diseases such as heart disease, strokes, and arthritis. An environmental study looks at the incidence of a condition or disease under different environmental conditions, for example, the incidence of a deficiency of vitamin D in RA patients associated with the geographical region and strength of sunlight.[49] These studies are much easier and less expensive to perform, and can help develop hypotheses that can then be tested with more rigorous RCTs. Nutritional research should not presume that nutrients work on the body like fast-acting drugs.[50] Many age-related diseases and their nutritional causes require several decades to be revealed. The bottom line is, although some RCTs have not always shown benefits for nutrient supplements, many recent studies, including RCTs and observational and environmental studies, have shown that in the modern world with its processed food, supplements can play an important role in our health.[51]

This interpretation of the discovery of essential nutrients emphasizes the need for hypothesis-driven science in nutrition research.[52] A series of scientific results, such as observational studies about a disease mechanism (scurvy), showing a correlation (eating fresh foods) and RCTs suggesting a specific cause (lack of fruit), can drive the generation of a new hypothesis. In the case of Lind's controlled experiment, the hypothesis evolved that a disease such as scurvy is caused by a deficiency of a substance (citrus juice) in the diet. After many negative results and wrong conclusions, the results from a testing this hypothesis allowed later researchers to imagine a more specific mechanism, which then generated another hypothesis (lack of vitamin C) and an improved prediction about what foods can cure the disease. Many further studies tested these predictions to verify and elaborate the hypotheses about the essential nutrient (ascorbate). Today this progression of ideas continues among many different researchers worldwide, encouraging further discussion of the disease mechanism and requirements for a variety of nutrients. This ongoing process drives the development of further hypotheses and tests. Scientific knowledge (ascorbate is required at higher levels than needed to prevent scurvy) is the result.

Current conceptual limitations, exemplified by Lind's inaccurate belief that scurvy was a problem of digestion, always constrain the process of imagining new disease mechanisms and may slow the creation of new hypotheses.[53] Medicine as a whole, and more specifically the drug-driven medical science so commonly seen in recent decades, is unfortunately constrained by current conceptual limitations in precisely this way. The pursuit of knowledge by testing hypotheses has many blind alleys. We don't get arthritis exclusively from wear-and-tear on a joint or because of a deficiency of a drug. Instead, science has moved on to show that deficiencies of essential nutrients are often responsible for the development of arthritis.[54]

VITAMINS AND THE PRE-INDUSTRIAL DIET

Interestingly, many vitamins were discovered as unintended consequences of the industrial revolution. Food that contains a lot of essential nutrients such as vitamins and minerals can support life, including microbial life, so it quickly spoils and develops mold. Before the industrial revolution, white flour was prized because it could be stored on the shelf for months without spoiling. In hindsight, we understand that white flour cannot sustain life! In Europe during the 1700s white flour was produced by a "gradual reduction" or "high grinding" process of milling, in which the grain was passed through several sets of millstones, with each successive pair set a little closer together.[55] The bran and germ were removed from the coarse ground flour in a winnowing process by blowing air across the grain ground by each set of millstones, much like chaff is removed by the wind when threshed grain is tossed into the air. By the 1840s this method was widely utilized by large mills, some passing the grain particles through a dozen or more sets of millstones. This process could remove most of the bran and germ before the endosperm (the part of the kernel containing mostly carbohydrate) was ground to flour.

But this final product of "almost white" flour was expensive, and most households in Europe and North America could not afford it. Ordinary stone milling with "low grinding" could remove the bran (the hard outside surface of the kernel) but it could not readily remove the germ, which contains most of the oil and protein. The polyunsaturated oils released by milling the whole grain with its germ require refrigeration, because when exposed to the air they oxidize rapidly and go rancid. But refrigeration was not available, and ice boxes were not widely used to store staples such as flour. Thus, the whole wheat flour typically produced before 1840 by a local mill and purchased by most households would spoil in a few weeks, quickly becoming rancid and moldy. To prevent this problem, most farmers stored their grain on the farm and took only small quantities to be milled.[56] In hindsight, it is apparent they did not realize how fortunate they were. Mills were active throughout the year producing "whole grain" brown flour, which unknowingly provided the essential nutrients required for health.

The Industrial Revolution and Food Processing

During the industrial revolution from 1840 to 1880, millers first developed steel milling rollers that could efficiently crush cattle feed and sugarcane. They eventually learned how to make rolls (milling rollers) to remove the bran and germ from grain.[57] Several sets of rollers were typically used, with the distance between the rollers carefully adjusted to remove the coarse bran particles first. For particularly hard wheat, grooved or fluted rollers were more effective because they could break the kernel and crack off the bran and germ before the kernel was finely milled. This process allowed the remaining endosperm, in a further milling step, to be ground into white flour. Various grades of flour could then be produced and marketed that contained different amounts of the "undesirable" germ and bran.

In the United States, the Pillsbury Company was the first to mill grain with steel rollers.[58] By 1880 the milling industry had evolved to produce inexpensive "high-quality" white flour that ordinary working-class people could afford. For the next several decades, many people ate generous portions of white bread made from flour stripped of nutrients. Before the advent of refrigeration, this "modern" white flour was preferred because it didn't spoil and thus tasted better. Processed corn and rice flour were produced in the same way by removing the bran and germ. The milling industry took pride in removing everything from the whole grain that did not contribute to its "good taste."[59] This effort improved sales of the so-called modern white flour and, as our huge multinational food and drug corporations understand so well, also improved the profits.

During the next several decades after this milling revolution, diseases such as beriberi (deficiency of vitamin B_1, or thiamin) and pellagra (deficiency of vitamin B_3, or niacin) appeared widely, and rapidly became epidemics.[60] The symptoms of pellagra are often characterized by the "four Ds": dermatitis, diarrhea, dementia, and death.[61] Many people died horrible deaths during these epidemics. They occurred wherever poor people, who couldn't afford a good diet, ate mostly cheap processed grains.[62] Refined foods such as flour or grits made from wheat, corn (maize), and rice were the main culprits. Epidemics of pellagra occurred in Italy, Romania, and the Old South of the United States. But those who could afford fresh vegetables and meat avoided these epidemics.

Epidemics Traced to Food Processing

An epidemic of beriberi in the 1880s was among the first to be solved. The bacterium responsible for tuberculosis had recently been discovered, so following common sense, beriberi was also hypothesized to be caused by a bacterium. Christian Eijkman, a medical researcher, was sent to the Dutch East Indies (now Java, Indonesia) to discover the source of the epidemic. In a series of controlled scientific experiments, Eijkman showed that when chickens were fed polished rice, they got symptoms of beriberi in several weeks.[63] But when given unpolished rice the symptoms disappeared within a few days. Then it was discovered that the epidemic of beriberi in the prisons of Dutch East Indies could be traced to those prisons that served polished rice. When fed unpolished rice, people with beriberi recovered quickly. Eijkman was able to isolate a component of rice bran that protected against beriberi. Similarly, in 1912, a doctor in Newfoundland hypothesized that beriberi was caused by over-reliance on white flour and a lack of good nutrition including greens.[64] For decades, poor people received handouts of brown unbleached flour, which they sometimes called in a derogatory tone "dole flour." They received sound nutritional advice to eat this flour, but many didn't because it tasted bad and had the stigma of a dole out.[65] Like most people of that era, they preferred "modern" white bleached flour. Brown flour spoiled rapidly because it had more nutrients, but even so, it kept those who relied on it in better health!

ENRICHED WHITE FLOUR AND WHEAT GERM

White flour became popular in the 1880s when the milling industry discovered how to remove the bran and germ inexpensively with steel rollers. But the resulting flour was yellowish due to small amounts of healthy vitamins and carotenoids. To make it even whiter, beginning in the early twentieth century, white flour was bleached, removing all but traces of many essential nutrients. Bleaching also accelerated the aging process that helped to increase the gluten activity. This new inexpensive white flour generated more profits, but the resulting deficiencies caused several horrible epidemics. Nutritionists lobbied for some way to enhance the nutrition found in refined foods, and during World War II the US government started a voluntary campaign to "enrich" white flour with some of the missing B vitamins.[66] In 1941 several large millers started to enrich or "fortify" white flour, but small mills resisted enrichment because it reduced their profits.[67] Because cheaper unfortified white flour could still be purchased, there was a concern that the poor, who were most at risk for deficiency diseases, would continue to get pellagra and other deficiency diseases.[68]

In 1943 the enrichment of bread was made law, and after the war many states made enrichment of all refined cereal grains and bread mandatory.[69] This enrichment promptly terminated the worst epidemics of the B vitamin deficiency diseases, and prevented some cases of arthritis.[70] Public debate about the word "enriched" ensued, for only a few of the necessary nutrients had been added back into white flour. Many other nutritious ingredients could easily be added in small proportions without much affecting its taste and cooking properties.[71] In this way, enriched flour could be made more nutritious. In the following several decades, calcium, iron, and folate were added to the enrichment of white flour. This enrichment with some essential nutrients did help to prevent epidemics of some deficiency diseases, but not all. Deficits of essential nutrients are still common in the modern world.

Most of the B vitamins, vitamin E, and magnesium are removed from the whole grain when the bran and germ are removed during the processing to make white flour. These essential nutrients are readily available in wheat germ. You can purchase wheat germ at your local supermarket to get the relatively inexpensive benefit of its exceptional combination of nutrients. Wheat germ spoils quickly, and according to the label should be kept in the refrigerator. This is because it contains many of the nutrients required for health, including essential polyunsaturated fatty acids. These fatty acids oxidize readily at room temperature, causing the wheat germ to spoil in a few weeks. In contrast, magnesium and other essential minerals don't spoil in storage or cooking. We only need to make sure we get an adequate dose of these minerals in the foods we eat, and that they are well absorbed in the gut.

White rice is processed like white flour, by removal of the bran and germ. Parboiled rice has recovered some of the B vitamins from the bran in a cooking step during processing that occurs before the removal of the bran and is less sticky than plain white rice, but unprocessed brown rice is better for your health. Unfortunately, many people still prefer sticky white rice, white bread, cookies, cake, and pasta made from enriched flour that is missing some essential nutrients, and do not eat generous portions of vegetables and fruits. As a consequence, wherever processed food makes up much of the diet, arthritis and other deficiency diseases are rampant. You should avoid foods made with enriched flour because the magnesium and vitamins it lacks are important in preventing arthritis. To ensure that you get adequate amounts of all the essential nutrients, you can take a multivitamin tablet along with an excellent diet of unprocessed fruits, vegetables, beans, and whole grains.

THE DISCOVERY OF VITAMINS

A similar chain of events allowed other epidemics to be traced to deficiencies of biochemical substances in food. Only after careful controlled scientific studies did it become obvious that the problem was the removal of the bran and germ during the refining process.[72] Over several decades, Eijkman's scientific method of experimentation became widely acclaimed and he was recognized with the 1929 Nobel Prize in Physiology or Medicine.[73] Further investigations by others, including Vedder and Williams, Hopkins, and Funk discovered the exact biochemical that protected against beriberi, which was eventually called thiamine or vitamin B_1.[74] These studies underscore the fact that many investigators contributed to the prevention of the deficiency disease (beriberi) and the discovery of the specific natural molecule that cures it (thiamine).

Originally, pellagra, like other deficiency diseases, was thought to be caused by some type of bacterial infection. By 1910, the industrial refining of maize flour caused a large epidemic of pellagra in the United States.[75] The refined grits sold in the southern states were no longer the traditional "hominy grits" made by processing with an alkaline solution, but were made with the new milling process and sold as hominy grits.[76] However, the new grits were deficient in niacin, which caused the epidemic of pellagra. Maize is thought to have a lower availability of vitamin B_3 (niacin) than wheat or rice, and its niacin is thought to become more available when the maize is processed in an alkaline solution. Further, the amino acid composition of traditional maize is less balanced than other grains. This increases the niacin requirement for those who eat heirloom varieties of maize. Native people unwittingly avoided pellagra by application of lime-water to maize, which allowed it to be ground more easily but also improved the availability of tryptophan, a precursor to niacin.[77] Those who relied on maize without the alkaline treatment developed pellagra. A similar process using alkaline solution is used today in making tortillas, corn chips, and hominy grits.

In 1917, Goldberger showed that a pellagra-like disease in dogs, black tongue syndrome, could be cured by diets containing any of several different foods.[78] Elvejham showed in 1937 that the black tongue syndrome could be cured by niacin or niacinamide,[79] and soon afterward it was found that niacin or niacinamide could cure human pellagra.[80] Niacin was later shown not to be absolutely essential for humans, because it is synthesized slowly from the amino acid tryptophan.[81] Niacin is readily available in small quantities in most whole grains, except maize when it is not alkaline treated.

Careful observation by doctors, along with vigorous public debate[82] and heroic animal experiments over the next several decades, determined that these horrible diseases were caused by deficiencies of essential nutrients, eventually called vitamins.[83] Many of the missing vitamins were identified by medical researchers in the bran and germ of grains. The biomolecule responsible for preventing scurvy was eventually isolated from fresh vegetables and fruits by Szent-Györgyi in 1928. The exact structure of this molecule and its synthetic pathway was determined by Haworth in 1933, and together Szent-Györgyi and Haworth named the substance ascorbate (that is, the anti-scorbutic compound). By then it was also called vitamin C. Their discovery was recognized by the Nobel Prize of 1937.[84] Vitamin C was the first vitamin to be produced synthetically, and it was soon available as a supplement.[85] The artificially-made ascorbate molecule was shown to be exactly the same as the natural one found in foods. It was determined that they both prevent scurvy and other effects of vitamin C deficiency. By the 1930s nutritionists widely recognized that eating foods in proper combinations to supply essential nutrients could greatly improve health and prevent disease.[86]

THE BEGINNINGS OF ORTHOMOLECULAR MEDICINE

After their initial discovery, many nutrition researchers studied the effect of different doses of vitamins because the tests in which they were discovered could not determine which doses were optimal. Szent-Györgyi stated that, from the beginning of his studies on vitamin C, he always felt that scurvy was a "pre-mortal" syndrome—merely taking enough ascorbate to dissipate the symptoms of scurvy would be insufficient for full health. In his view, the needs of the body for ascorbate are much higher than the minimum needed to prevent scurvy.[87] Doctors experimenting with higher doses of vitamin C found they could improve recovery from many types of disease.[88] They found it safe to for most people to take at very high doses. Eventually it was found that the optimal dose varies with the level of disease and stress. This search for correct doses of vitamins was the start of orthomolecular medicine, which has continued to grow and evolve over the past century.[89] The word "orthomolecular" is derived from "ortho-" from the Greek word for "straight," "upright," or "correct," a term used widely in biochemistry and medicine. Pauling coined the term orthomolecular to mean the use of the "right molecules in the right concentration" to prevent and cure disease.[90]

For each essential nutrient, a dose-response curve must be generated to discover what minimal doses prevent acute disease and how higher doses can improve health.[91] Eventually, for very high doses, a plateau is typically reached beyond which further increases give no further advantage. Moreover, every individual has different requirements for nutrients, so their optimal doses will differ.[92] And any potential toxicity at high doses must be fully studied and understood. Although vitamin A and some essential minerals such as iron, copper, and selenium are toxic at high levels, the B vitamins and vitamin C are not toxic at doses even a hundredfold greater than the recommended minimum. With careful observation, and reference to the symptoms of the B vitamin deficiency diseases, doctors often found mild symptoms of these diseases in their patients, who recovered when given the vitamin in higher doses. In the 1930s, Kaufman studied pellagra and found that many patients with pellagra also had the symptoms of arthritis. After white flour was enriched in the early

1940s, the worst cases of pellagra had disappeared, yet his patients continued to have subclinical pellagra and arthritis. Kaufman found that the symptoms of arthritis could be successfully treated with the antipellagra vitamin niacin or niacinamide.[93] We will return to this topic in Chapter 5.

AGE-RELATED DISEASES, GENETICS, AND NUTRITION

In recent decades, we have often heard about the genetic origin of many diseases, for instance, when someone has inherited a gene mutation that causes a tendency for the specific condition or disease. But we all have this problem in one way or another, because we all have genetic differences that affect the ability of the body to be healthy under different conditions in our daily lives.[94] This knowledge is a tremendous relief for some people because it removes any personal culpability for genetically-caused problems, since the genes we have inherited cannot be changed (except by gene therapy).[95] As a consequence, most people only need to deal with the shortcomings of their particular genetic background, which usually gives them just a susceptibility for getting a disease. Unfortunately, some young adults who have arthritis may learn from genetic testing that they have a gene directly associated with the disease. From this they may feel that they are doomed to a life with inflammation in their joints. Tragically, this may be true for some patients with rare genetic diseases that tend to strike the young. For example, a type of osteoarthritis (osteochondritis dissecans) caused by a genetic mutation in aggrecan, one of the molecules of the cartilage in the joint, appears as early as age thirteen in affected individuals.[96] In a study of individuals in a five-generation family, those with the mutated gene had weak and disorganized cartilage, most often leading to osteoarthritis. This is a rare example, but it shows how our bodies are affected by our genetic makeup. All individuals have genetic variations. Some of these variations may cause disease. We will discuss this topic more in Chapter 4.

However, age-related disease is much more widespread. Older patients are also commonly advised that their condition is related to their genetic heritage. Yet, if diseases that originate in genetic differences were inevitable, such age-related diseases would likely strike early in life. In most individuals, genetic variations don't cause disease directly, but only cause a predisposition for disease. Thus, diseases that appear in middle-aged or older people, with or without a known genetic component, are often termed "age-related." This term describes many progressive, supposedly incurable diseases including heart disease, cancer, diabetes, eye disease, and arthritis. We now know that the process of aging contributes to these diseases but does not cause them. There are several factors in aging, but major ones are oxidative stress and nutritional insufficiency.[97] Age-related diseases and the rate of aging are thought to originate in accumulation of damage to macromolecules in cells.[98] The damage accumulates throughout life. But it originates in large part from nutritional deficiencies that tend to get worse with age. These can be prevented by an excellent diet along with adequate doses of essential nutrients.[99]

Triage Theory of Essential Nutrients

To understand why age-related diseases are associated with poor nutrition, biochemists hypothesize that our distant ancestors evolved to thrive in spite of hardships that caused famine and nutrient deficiencies.[100] Most vitamins and minerals are required for more than one function in the body. For example, some vitamins are required for metabolic pathways that produce energy. But they are also required for combating oxidative damage and maintenance such as repair of DNA and tissues that help to prevent age-related disease. However, as animals evolved, keeping tissues alive took precedence over other functions such as maintaining arteries and joints for obvious reasons. In the short term, the body can survive without maintenance, but it must have energy to stay alive. So maintenance functions were given lower priority. Natural selection caused our biochemical pathways to prioritize the cell's nutritional needs and its utilization of essential nutrients. This is called the "triage" theory, and it explains why an excess of nutrients helps prevent age-related disease and arthritis.[101]

The triage theory of essential nutrients is named after the system used to sort patients after a disaster or in the emergency room. The term comes from the French verb "*trier,*" meaning to sort, and was first widely used during World War I.[102] Patients are sorted according to the urgency of their needs, so the ones who urgently need the most care can get it quickly. This system is designed to maximize the number of survivors. Similarly, the triage theory of essential nutrients hypothesizes that, early in history, animals evolved to utilize scarce vitamins and minerals preferentially for critical body functions such as energy metabolism or blood clotting. These same vitamins were also required by other noncritical enzymes responsible for maintenance functions. But the enzymes involved in these critical functions evolved through natural selection to have a greater binding affinity for the essential enzyme cofactors known as vitamins. The binding affinities of the maintenance enzymes evolved to be lower, allowing the vitamin cofactors in times of food scarcity to be utilized preferentially to support the metabolic pathways for energy and other essential functions.[103] This setting of priorities can occur with a genetic mutation that limits the affinity of an enzyme for biochemicals it binds to, such as its reactants (molecules that are transformed by the enzyme) and cofactors (molecules required to help the enzyme).[104] There is good evidence to back up this hypothesis. Premature aging can be caused by damage to DNA in the cell's mitochondria, the cellular energy producers, and the cell's nucleus.[105] This can be caused by modest deficiencies of essential nutrients. Some of the processes of aging, such as protein misfolding or loss of fluidity in cellular membranes, can cause critical enzymes in metabolic pathways to slow down their functioning, with lower affinities for the biochemicals they bind.[106]

For example, the first signs of a vitamin K deficiency are incomplete synthesis of calcium binding proteins outside of the liver, such as in joints and bones. This happens in a mild deficiency of vitamin K even when its function to make proteins in the liver involved in blood clotting (coagulation) is preserved. Accordingly, vitamin K_1 is preferentially distributed to the liver. Evidently this is because the coagulation function performed by vitamin K is more critical for preserving life.[107] But higher intake of vitamin K and other vitamins can allow the enzymes responsible for maintenance functions in joints and bones to prevent this type of damage.[108]

Poor nutrition has a well-known but insidious damaging effect on bone and joint health, which directly implicates it as a cause of arthritis. The progressive nature of inflammation that causes arthritis is related to the damage from long-term deficiencies of essential nutrients such as vitamins C, D, E, K, and the B vitamins, as well as calcium and magnesium and other minerals. Most of these essential nutrients are relatively safe in much higher doses than in ordinary daily multivitamin tablets. For example, we need higher doses of B vitamins, because they are water soluble and are readily excreted, yet our tissues require them in high doses to keep their cellular maintenance and disease prevention mechanisms functioning optimally. Vitamins C and E are antioxidants and can be taken safely by most individuals at very high doses (C: 10,000 or even 50,000 milligrams (mg) per day when necessary; E: 400–3,200 international units (IU) per day) to reduce inflammation and prevent damage. You may benefit by discussing high doses of these vitamins with your medical doctor.

Oxidative Damage

Many things can go wrong with the cellular machinery that synthesizes the biomolecules needed to run the engine that is a cell. Damage to a specific locus (position) in the DNA molecules, called a "mutation," can cause mistakes in the cell's biochemical products that change the functions performed by the cell and its progeny. Some mutations can be beneficial, allowing an organism to function better in its environment. In this case, the organism may survive and procreate more successfully, allowing the population with this characteristic to grow. This process is called "natural selection," and is responsible for the emergence of multicellular organisms, plants, animals, and humans during billions of years of evolution. Most mutations of DNA are detrimental to a cell, however, and they can affect any aspect of its function.[109] For example, a mutation can cause the cell to be unable to generate energy from food, or cause it to grow uncontrollably and cause cancer, or a myriad of other malfunctions. Mutations can be caused by errors in the cell's genetic machinery, or several other mechanisms, including ionizing radiation from cosmic rays from outer space, medical X-rays, or UV light, and toxic or oxidizing chemicals.

Oxidation, the process whereby electrons are removed from molecules by "free radicals," can damage any molecule inside or outside a cell, including the all-important biomolecule, DNA. Free radicals are molecules that have a higher affinity for electrons than most other biomolecules. They simply grab an electron from almost any biomolecule they meet in their random path through a cell's cytoplasm or in their travel through the bloodstream. The result is that the biomolecule is converted into a free radical, which can then proceed to damage another nearby molecule, and so on. The process can generate a long sequence of damaging reactions to the cell's biomolecules, wreaking havoc with the cell's ability to perform its many functions. Ironically, the worst types of free radical include various forms of oxygen, including superoxide, O_2: the hydroxyl radical, OH; ozone, O_3; and hydrogen peroxide, H_2O_2. These molecules all contain an unbound oxygen atom that has a particularly high affinity for electrons to form a chemical bond. Yes, you read this correctly: even though oxygen is necessary to provide energy for life, it can be toxic! Oxygen and many other toxic chemicals can induce oxidative damage to our tissues. So although some normal metabolic pathways and functions of the cell need oxidation reactions, cell survival requires that unrestrained oxidation by free radicals be minimized.

Oxidative stress is thought to be a major cause for many age-related diseases because it is directly associated with inflammation and cellular damage.[110] Oxidative stress lowers the level of available antioxidants in the body. For example, smokers have lower levels of vitamins C and E in their blood.[111] A bacterial or viral infection causes oxidative stress, as does a bruise, a cut to the skin, or high sugar in the bloodstream as in diabetes. Infections that continue for prolonged periods, such as those that may occur with root canal work on teeth, cause toxicity, inflammation, and oxidative stress throughout the body.[112] Damage due to oxidative stress is especially insidious because it is progressive, that is, when it continues over many years the damage accumulates and gets worse. It is thought to be responsible for many serious progressive diseases such as heart disease, cancer, diabetes, eye disease, and arthritis.

ANTIOXIDANTS

To prevent oxidative damage, our cells rely on antioxidant molecules that are able to donate an electron to a free radical, thereby neutralizing it. When an antioxidant molecule donates an electron in this way, it becomes oxidized. The resulting oxidized antioxidant molecule is not as dangerous as the original free radical because even with a missing electron the antioxidant doesn't have a high affinity for grabbing electrons and wreaking havoc. Cells can recycle oxidized antioxidant molecules by "reducing" them back to their original form, or they can generate new antioxidant molecules. Some common antioxidants important for the body include glutathione, lipoic acid, uric acid, melatonin, vitamin C (ascorbate), vitamin E, carotenes found in colored vegetables, and many others, including enzymes such as peroxidases that catalyze a chemical reaction to neutralize the free radicals. Under some conditions antioxidants can cause oxidation, including a "reducing" reaction with iron or other atoms that can then become free radicals.[113] Thus too much iron in the body can cause oxidative damage. But under most conditions, antioxidants do not cause oxidation and are essential for maintenance of tissues throughout the body. Further, some oxidized biomolecules are important for normal function in cells because they act as cellular messengers that relay an important signal to the cell.[114] For example, while free radicals are known to cause mutations that contribute to cancer, they are also thought to be an important signal late in the disease telling cancer cells to die.[115] Oxidative stress caused by damage such as that due to injury or prolonged strenuous exercise and the resulting generation of free radicals is thought to be an important signal to stressed cells to step up their maintenance functions to repair the damage. Free radicals are also utilized by immune cells to destroy pathogens.[116] Yet antioxidants are also known to empower the immune system, which is a major reason why consumption of fruits and vegetables helps to prevent illness.

Glutathione and Lipoic Acid

A cell can generate several important antioxidants. Glutathione (GSH) and lipoic acid are generated by cells through their normal metabolic pathways. Glutathione is thought to be one of the most important antioxidants inside mammalian cells, where it is involved in managing reactive oxygen species (ROS). For example, mice that lack a functional enzyme for producing GSH will die of liver failure within one month. However, these mice are able to survive when they are fed N-acetyl-cysteine in water.[117] Glutathione can be synthesized by a cell's enzymes from the three amino acids cysteine, glutamate, and glycine,[118] and after it is depleted by donating an electron, a cell can readily regenerate it. Glutathione is so deeply involved in this process of preventing oxidative stress that laboratories report the level of depleted glutathione in a tissue as a measure of its oxidative stress.[119] Glutathione is also used by cells as a signal of their level of oxidation to control essential cellular functions.[120] Many age-related diseases such as heart disease and diabetes are associated with low levels of glutathione, and genetic problems with the synthesis of glutathione are thought to be involved in some cases.[121] Lipoic acid is also an antioxidant found inside cells that has a variety of beneficial functions.

Glutathione is symbiotic with other antioxidants such as alpha-lipoic acid and vitamins C and E. These antioxidants can help to increase the level of glutathione, and glutathione can help to increase the level of these and other antioxidants. Neither glutathione nor lipoic acid are essential nutrients because they can normally be synthesized and recycled by the body. But their levels can be depleted by inflammatory progressive diseases like heart disease and arthritis. The level of depleted glutathione is increased in arthritis, likely because of the increased oxidative stress.[122] Consequentially, in rheumatoid arthritis the level of glutathione peroxidase (GSH-Px), the enzyme that utilizes glutathione to remove oxidative stress inside cells, is substantially increased as a compensatory mechanism.[123] Taking ordinary supplements of glutathione won't help, because glutathione isn't well absorbed by the gut. But supplements of N-acetyl-cysteine (NAC), a precursor for glutathione in its synthetic pathway, are well-absorbed and can raise the level of glutathione in the body. Oxidative stress indicated by low GSH levels is associated with a lack of B vitamins including biotin in lame animals.[124] This highlights the importance of the vitamin pathways in preventing oxidative stress.

Vitamin C

Ascorbate (ascorbic acid or Vitamin C) is a powerful antioxidant and an essential nutrient that guinea pigs, monkeys, apes, and humans must get from their diet. It is essential for our health because without it we would develop scurvy in a few months. Vitamin C functions as a cofactor required by a variety of enzymes, and also as an antioxidant that directly interacts with other molecules and antioxidants such as the classic lipid antioxidant vitamin E. Most other animals can make their own ascorbate, so ascorbate isn't a vitamin for them. It is simply one of the molecules that their bodies make when needed. Scientists have hypothesized that early ancestors of apes could make ascorbate, because lemurs (primitive primates found in Madagascar) can make ascorbate. Humans evolved from later apelike primates that lived in tropical jungles and ate lots of fresh fruits containing vitamin C.[125] A large ape such as a gorilla will typically eat twenty pounds or more of greens per day, and this diet contains 4,000 mg or more of vitamin C, as well as the other essential nutrients.[126] The diet of some monkeys contains approximately 50 mg of vitamin C per pound of body weight per day, equivalent to 7,500 mg for a 150 pound human, an amount 20 to 100 times more than the minimum daily requirement.[127] Because our distant ancestors got enough vitamin C from their diet, they were able to survive without the ability to make it. We inherited this inability to make vitamin C from our apelike ancestors. It has been estimated that early humans could obtain up to 3,000 mg per day or more of vitamin C from their diet, which included lots of raw vegetables and fruits.[128] With this dose, it is evident that vitamin C is not a vitamin in the original sense of an essential molecule required at a tiny dose. Vitamin C might be better characterized as an essential macroscopic nutrient, like other major components of food. Like other essential nutrients, it is actively reabsorbed into the bloodstream by the kidneys.[129]

Ascorbate is a relatively small, simple molecule similar to glucose (blood sugar). All vertebrate animals have a metabolic pathway consisting of four enzymes that transform glucose into ascorbate. In most animals, this metabolic pathway functions correctly and provides relatively large amounts of ascorbate, up to 10,000 mg per day for a 150 pound animal.[130] Our DNA contains the genes to make these four enzymes, but the last one in the pathway (L-gulonolactone oxidase, GLO) is nonfunctional because of mutations.[131] Similar mutations have occurred in the same GLO gene in the ancestors of a few other species. As a consequence, humans, monkeys, and apes (and a few other species such as guinea pigs, passerine (perching) birds, some bats, and teleost fishes), cannot make ascorbate as do all other animals.[132] Yet all of these species that lack the ability to make a ascorbate can get it in robust amounts from their diet. This access limited the evolutionary pressure to maintain a functional biochemical pathway to make ascorbate.[133]

The same effect is thought to account for the loss of the ability to make several other vitamins in a variety of species, starting billions of years ago in bacteria through animals living today.[134] The study of genetics shows that as some species of bats and birds evolved, they lost but later regained their ability to make ascorbate, sometimes multiple times.[135] This suggests that the loss of the ability to make ascorbate is not always permanent, but may vary as a species evolves, depending on the diet. Another theory suggests that the inability to make ascorbate along with a diet that supplied it provided an evolutionary advantage. Those individuals lacking the ability to make ascorbate required less glucose and hence less food, which helped them survive when food was scarce. However, as described above, individuals vary, and some guinea pigs and humans can remain healthy with hardly any vitamin C in their diet.[136] This sort of ability may be responsible for the generally good health that allows some people to live to age 100 and beyond.[137] But most of us need at least 100 mg per day of vitamin C, and can be much healthier with much larger amounts (3,000–10,000 mg per day).

Vitamin C Is Recycled in the Body

Because of the importance of vitamin C, most cells contain special transporter proteins, sitting in the cell membrane, that are highly specific for ascorbate.[138] The ascorbate transporter is a type of pump, powered by the gradient (difference in concentration) of sodium, which is at a high level on the outside of cells and low on the inside. The amount of ascorbate transporters is controlled by the level of ascorbate, so that when the ascorbate level goes down, cells throughout the body will make more transporters so they can obtain a sufficient amount of vitamin C. Typically, the level of vitamin C inside cells and tissues is approximately fifty-fold higher than in blood plasma.[139]

In response to the missing enzyme for synthesizing vitamin C, the bodies of primates, including humans, have evolved to adapt to a lower level of ascorbate, and can regenerate it to some extent when it gets depleted. Because vitamin C is synthesized by living organisms (and by vitamin manufacturers) from glucose, it presents a peculiar problem for cells. The oxidized form of vitamin C (dehydroascorbate) is similar in molecular shape to glucose, and is brought into cells by glucose transporters.[140] The main function of most of these transporters is to supply the cell with glucose, but they also transport dehydroascorbate to some extent. Some studies have suggested that because dehydroascorbate is similar in shape to glucose, a high level of blood glucose will compete with dehydroascorbate in binding to the transporter. This will antagonize the uptake of dehydroascorbate and thus lower the ability of red blood cells to recycle it back to vitamin C.[141] However, adult higher primates (including humans) and guinea pigs possess a unique glucose transporter in the membrane of their red blood cells, not found in other adult animals, that allows them to preferentially take up dehydroascorbate into the cell.[142] There, it is regenerated by mitochondria, the energy producers of cells, back to its original active form.[143] The recycled vitamin C prevents oxidation within the cell's cytoplasm, and is also released back to the bloodstream, where it can continue to do its job of donating electrons and preventing oxidative stress.

This duality of function for glucose transporters provides an economy to the cell, but it also allows high levels of dehydroascorbate to compete with glucose for binding to some types of transporter. This mechanism for antagonism between oxidized vitamin C levels and glucose for binding to the transporter may explain why many symptoms of diabetes, in which elevated blood sugar causes damage to tissues, can be ameliorated by vitamin C.[144] It also may explain why elevated blood sugar is so bad for us—for a variety of reasons, it may effectively cause "cellular scurvy." Although oxidized vitamin C is actively recycled in the bodies of humans and apes, both the oxidized and unoxidized forms are also readily excreted in urine. And during times of stress, infection, or diseases such as arthritis, its level can drastically fall. In this case, large supplemental doses of vitamin C can provide a much needed boost to the body's ability to recover.

Rationale for Megadoses

The average human body contains several grams (1,500–3,000 mg) of vitamin C, depending on the amount absorbed from food, and loses only a small amount of it daily when it is not under much oxidative stress.[145] For this reason only a small daily dose of vitamin C is considered necessary by mainstream medicine. Scurvy that develops over a period of weeks to months can be prevented by a small dose, which is captured in the current RDA for vitamin C (50–100 mg per day). However, vitamin C in high doses is effective in helping to prevent and recover from disease because the available pool of vitamin C in the body is limited. When the body is under stress it requires more vitamin C than can be provided by its recycling mechanism or by ordinary foods in the diet. In acute oxidative stress, the dehydroascorbate cannot be recycled fast enough, and the antioxidant function of vitamin C and other antioxidants such as glutathione can be easily overwhelmed.[146] During severe oxidative stress, often caused by illness, supplements of vitamin C can prevent a deficiency.[147] For example, during a bacterial or viral infection or some other type of environmental stress such as breathing smoke or other toxins, the vitamin C level in the bloodstream drops.[148] When patients are recovering from the shock of surgery, trauma, burns, sepsis (severe infection), or critical illness, their vitamin C levels can drop precipitously, causing a crisis for the body. When this happens, the body may need 3,000 mg or more of vitamin C, given through intravenous treatment, to bring the vitamin C level back to normal.[149] This relatively high dose of vitamin C has been verified for safety and efficacy at restoring vitamin C levels. Vitamin C, when taken with other antioxidants such as vitamin E, is a major factor in patient recovery.[150] The equivalent oral dose would be 10,000–30,000 mg or more taken over several hours.[151]

Unfortunately, for many people in our modern society, a high degree of continuous oxidative stress has become the norm. Deficiencies of essential nutrients in the modern diet cause our bodies to be prone to age-related diseases such as heart disease, cancer, diabetes, and arthritis. This is the rationale for large daily doses of vitamin C (3,000–10,000 mg per day in divided doses, and up to 100,000 mg per day when sick). A single large dose (1,000 mg or more) is normally not completely absorbed.[152] But when the body's reserve of vitamin C is depleted, the blood level drops, and it will be actively absorbed from the gut to a greater degree.[153] The total amount absorbed from many small doses (500 mg) taken frequently throughout the day is much greater than the amount absorbed from a single huge dose (10,000 mg). But, because the body's need for vitamin C changes day by day, it's important to know how to determine the optimal dose. We will discuss this topic in Chapter 7.

Vitamin C is one of the most important antioxidants for the body, because it is water soluble and flows throughout the body in the bloodstream, preventing oxidation in blood vessels and inside cells.[154] It is able to regenerate other antioxidants such as vitamin E when they get oxidized (used up) by donating an electron.[155] But the solubility of vitamin C in water means that it is easily lost in the urine. This causes its lifetime in the body, even with the special regeneration and recycling, to be relatively short, with a half-life of four to eight hours.[156] Most animal species, especially those that have little ascorbate in their diet, can make enough in their bodies for their well-being, even though it is water soluble and is readily excreted with a short half-life. They make about 10,000 mg per day (scaled to our body weight), and up to tenfold more when necessary to fight off an infection or recover from stress.[157] This is comparable to the high dose that present-day monkeys and apes get in their natural diet.

An Essential Enzyme Cofactor

Vitamin C is also an essential cofactor in the production of collagen and several (twenty or more) other biomolecules.[158] One essential role of vitamin C is to help generate cross-link bonds between cysteine residues (an amino acid containing sulfur) of long-chain extracellular proteins such as aggrecan.[159] This type of molecular bond allows a cell to generate the long chain proteins with cysteine residues placed at critical points that serve as "tie points" for the molecules. After these protein molecules are synthesized, the thiol (sulfur-containing) side groups of the cysteine residues are cross-linked, forming a strong disulfide bond between adjacent protein fibers. This system allows the long, thin protein fibers to be synthesized inside the cell and readily transported through the cell membrane, then linked together outside the cell into a continuous 3-D matrix. Ascorbate is necessary for this cross-linking of collagen molecules. Each cross-link requires a vitamin C molecule to catalyze a hydroxylation reaction (adding water) onto a proline residue (an amino acid). This reaction strengthens collagen and allows carbohydrate and phosphate groups to be added. Collagen can then aggregate and further cross-link into a 3-D matrix.[160]

Collagen is the most common protein in the body, and is the glue that holds together many organs including the skin, arteries, bones, and joints. A deficiency in vitamin C leads to degradation of collagen throughout the body, and without vitamin C for several weeks, scurvy sets in. With a deficiency of vitamin C, the tendons, ligaments, and cartilage of joints get weak and the arteries and skin break because they are dependent on collagen for their strength. With more severe deficiency, bruising and bleeding occurs and eventually causes death. The maintenance and repair of these tissues with new collagen requires vitamin C at several stages as a cofactor. Without vitamin C, the collagen fibers lack cross-links, which leaves it weak and prone to breakage. The molecules of vitamin C are oxidized by their role in collagen synthesis, so a continuous supply of renewed ("reduced") vitamin C is necessary to keep the body healthy and strong.[161] Vitamin C is also essential for the synthesis of carnitine, which is involved in providing energy for muscles and for a healthy immune system.

Vitamin C is essential for bone and joint health, in preserving the strength of collagen in the cartilage, maintaining tendons and ligaments, adding new calcium into bone, and resorption and removal of calcium when needed by the body.[162] It is also essential to prevent oxidative stress in joints, which can otherwise lead to osteoarthritis.[163] In some cases of scurvy documented in recent medical literature, the initial diagnosis was arthritis, because joint weakness is a consequence of a gradual deficiency of vitamin C.[164] Oxidative stress is a major risk factor for arthritis, and vitamin C is synergistic with other antioxidants such as glutathione in preventing oxidative stress,[165] and thus in preventing arthritis. In many arthritis patients, measures of oxidative stress increase, and the level of antioxidants and measures of collagen metabolism drop. This implies that arthritis causes a huge oxidative stress.[166] It also implies that antioxidants such as vitamin C, taken in adequate doses, can help prevent arthritis.

Vitamin D

Virtually all animal species require vitamin D, with the exception of underground animals. An adequate dose of vitamin D is essential for preventing rickets (bone malformation during childhood). But in addition to this role, vitamin D is also essential for preventing disease throughout the body.[167] Vitamin D was discovered in 1922 in cod liver oil from which the vitamin A had been removed, when it prevented artificially induced rickets in rats.[168] In cod and other non-oily fish, the vitamin D is found in the liver. In oily fish such as salmon, catfish, mackerel, herring, and sardines, it is found throughout the flesh. However, at the time vitamin D was discovered, it was not realized that the biggest source of vitamin D for humans is the skin, where it is produced from a natural derivative of cholesterol by UV rays from direct sunlight. Nocturnal animals must get vitamin D from their food, and some species have a much lower requirement than ours.[169] Animals covered with fur can get vitamin D by licking oil from their fur.

The main function of vitamin D for mammals is the regulation of calcium in the body. It is responsible for maintaining an appropriate level of calcium inside cells and within tissues and the bloodstream.[170] It does this by regulating calcium and phosphorus uptake in the gut, and calcium storage and retrieval in the bones. This is consistent with a recent review of studies of vitamin D supplementation, which found little effect on osteoporosis and bone mineral density.[171] It is also consistent with what is known about vitamin D, which regulates the level of calcium in the bloodstream and tissues by controlling both resorption and regrowth of bone. In people with inadequate calcium intake, vitamin D can function to remove calcium from bones. But in people with adequate calcium intake with a normal calcium level in the tissues, vitamin D does not automatically add calcium into the bones.[172]

Vitamin D is considered to be a steroid hormone because its mode of action in the body is similar to other hormones.[173] It interacts with tissues throughout the body where it binds to specific intracellular receptors that are similar to steroid hormone receptors. The receptor bound with vitamin D interacts with DNA inside the cell's nucleus to control the transcription of certain genes to make proteins that perform various cellular functions.[174] One of these proteins is osteocalcin, which is involved in making new bone.[175] Another of the proteins regulated by vitamin D is the calcium binding protein that is responsible for uptake of calcium in the gut. This mechanism stops absorbing calcium from the gut when the level in tissues is high enough. But when calcium levels fall too far, the vitamin D receptor in bone cells causes them to resorb (degrade) more bone to free up calcium for use by the body. However, many other tissues (more than two dozen) not involved in calcium metabolism have similar intracellular vitamin D receptors. They include immune system B and T cells, and brain, breast, kidney, parathyroid, thymus, and uterus. Some tumor cells have vitamin D receptors, which when bound with the vitamin stop the cells from proliferating.[176] It is thought that although thirty minutes exposure of unpigmented skin to UV sunlight can cause skin cancer by mutations to DNA, the cancer risk is reduced through vitamin D production more than it is increased by UV-generated mutations.

Deficiency of Vitamin D Contributes to Disease

A deficiency of vitamin D during childhood or likely even in adulthood contributes to multiple sclerosis and also to many other age-related progressive diseases such as heart disease, cancer, osteoporosis, and arthritis.[177] Vitamin D produced in the skin by exposure to sunlight will not cause toxicity, because in a process of negative feedback the amount produced by the skin drops when its level in the blood increases.[178] The skin of elderly people creates vitamin D at a reduced rate, and the elderly are more likely to wear sunscreen or stay indoors, so they are at greater risk from the age-related diseases contributed to by a deficit of vitamin D.[179] This sets the stage for osteoporosis and osteoarthritis.

Several clinical trials have studied the effects of vitamin D on the immune system, rheumatoid arthritis (RA), and cardiovascular disease. Vitamin D is known to be a powerful modulator of both the innate and adaptive immune systems. It is thought to be involved in the antimicrobial response as well as wound healing, and is also thought to regulate expression of signal receptors on monocytes (a type of white blood cell) to reduce or prevent autoimmunity. Deficiencies in vitamin D have been linked to RA.[180] In mouse models of RA, vitamin D prevents onset and progression. Symptoms of RA are often linked with cardiovascular disease, which has been linked with a deficiency of vitamin D.

A deficiency of vitamin D can lead to mood disorders such as seasonal affective disorder (SAD). The vitamin D level in many people who live in the United States, who don't supplement with this vitamin, is typically adequate during the summer but drops during the winter months. By the middle of the winter the level is inadequate, which drives mood disorders. This situation is especially serious for older people who don't get outside much and have arthritis pain. The combination of pain, fear of damage to the joints, and mood disorder tend to keep people inside and immobile. Of course, vitamin D along with other essential nutrients and mobility are exactly what can prevent this condition. Vitamin D is a powerful hormone, and we recommend that everyone supplement with it during the winter months. See Chapter 7 for more on this topic.

Vitamin E

While vitamin C is the body's main water soluble chemical antioxidant, vitamin E is the main fat soluble antioxidant. Vitamin E is lipophilic ("fat-loving") and resides in cell membranes, where it donates electrons to oxidized fatty-acid molecules and proteins in the lipid bilayer. This property is important, because vitamin E can neutralize oxidative stress where other water-soluble antioxidants can not: in the membrane and in other nearby molecules.

Vitamin E is not just one molecule but is any of a group of eight closely related compounds (isomers): d-alpha-, beta-, gamma-, and delta-tocopherols, and d-alpha-, beta-, gamma-, and delta-tocotrienols. The form most commonly included in supplement capsules is alpha-tocopherol because it is the most powerful of the eight vitamin E compounds for its role as originally assayed (analyzed).[181] The other vitamin E compounds have lower activity for the original assay, but are thought to have other important roles in the body. Further, the artificially synthesized form, dl-alpha-tocopherol (also called all-rac-alpha-tocopherol), has only about 50 percent of the biological activity as the natural d-alpha-tocopherol. Although both of these forms are powerful antioxidants, only the natural d- form (also called RRR-alpha-tocopherol) is selectively absorbed and utilized by the body.[182] One of the other isomers of vitamin E, d-gamma-tocopherol, is thought to be of specific help in increasing bone formation.

Vitamin E was discovered as a consequence of testing rats for other essential nutrients. Rats were fed a simple diet that included carbohydrate, protein, fat, and salt. This diet allowed them to grow to maturity but they were sterile. Further studies showed that adding greens, additional butterfat, or wheat germ restored fertility.[183] The biological role of vitamin E is still being actively studied. Besides its role in reproduction, it dilates blood vessels, slows platelet aggregation (clotting), and also helps to regulate several important cell signaling pathways.[184] Tocotrienols are similar to tocopherols but are thought to be more powerful antioxidants, and they appear to have a different function in the body.[185] Vitamin E is important for preventing inflammation, and is synergistic with other antioxidants like vitamin C and glutathione. Because vitamin E is located in cell membranes, it is not active in the cytoplasm of cells like other antioxidants. Although the eight vitamin E compounds appear to have different functions, one current hypothesis is that all the different functions of vitamin E originate in its lipophilic antioxidant property.[186] However, they are part of a powerful team of antioxidants in the body.[187]

Vitamin K

Vitamin K was discovered by Doisy and Dam in the 1930s, who

received the Nobel prize in 1943 for determining its essential role in blood clotting.[188] They first discovered vitamin K during experiments that designed to test whether cholesterol was an essential nutrient. Chickens fed on a diet that was depleted of a fatty food component containing cholesterol would die of hemorrhages (uncontrolled bleeding), even when they were supplemented with pure cholesterol. This implied that some other substance was missing. Eventually vitamin K was identified as a nutrient essential for blood clotting. This vitamin is extremely important, for it is critical not to bleed to death when we bump into something. Hemophiliacs, who lack the ability to form blood clots using the vitamin K pathway, will routinely get huge bruises from the slightest fall. Normal people usually don't have problems with clotting disorders associated with a deficiency of vitamin K because the form of vitamin K involved in blood clotting, called vitamin K_1, is efficiently recycled and maintained in the body.

For most of the twentieth century, vitamin K was considered vital only for blood clotting. However, it is now known that several other functions of vitamin K are also important in controlling calcium flow within the body. Further, there are several forms of vitamin K, and they have different localizations and functions in the body. When vitamin K is even slightly deficient, diseases such as cardiovascular disease, osteoporosis, and arthritis are commonplace. In recent decades it has been discovered that vitamin K plays important roles in the control of cartilage and bone development and maintenance, as well as in the brain. Today we now know that there are sixteen proteins dependent on vitamin K: eight coagulation proteins, four bone/cartilage production-regulating proteins, and several others. All of these have essential functions, but they have different sensitivities to a vitamin K deficiency. Thus, it's important to eat an excellent diet that contains a robust amount of vitamin K, and if this is not possible, to take supplements.

Omega-3 and Omega-6 Fatty Acids

Linoleic acid (LA) and alpha-linolenic acid (ALA) are part of the omega-6 and omega-3 fatty acid families, respectively. These two polyunsaturated fatty acids (PUFAs), found in a variety of seeds and nuts, are essential nutrients because the body requires them but cannot synthesize them.[189] They are essential for cell membranes but they also function as precursors for other cell signaling molecules. Omega-6 fatty acids are generally more inflammatory than omega-3. Another molecule, also often labeled ALA, is alpha-lipoic acid. This is an important antioxidant but is unrelated to alpha-linolenic acid. Other omega-3 and omega-6 fatty acids required by the body are not essential because the body can synthesize them from LA and ALA. For example, docosahexaenoic acid (DHA) and eicosapentaenoic acid (EPA) are two long-chain omega-3 fatty acids found in fish oil that are not essential, because they can be made by the body from ALA. But nevertheless they are important for health. To some extent, DHA and EPA can substitute for ALA. Therefore, all of these are considered to be essential omega-3 fatty acids (EFAs) that are important for many cell functions, including membrane fluidity, as cell signaling messengers, and as gene modulators.[190]

The essential fatty acids LA and ALA were discovered from 1928 to 1930 as part of the study that discovered vitamin E, because they are both fat soluble.[191] At that time, researchers were searching for essential nutrients, and they found that a component of fat contained something essential for health. After designing a diet for rats that contained all the known essential nutrients, consisting of carbohydrate, protein, minerals, and yeast, wheat germ, and cod liver oil for vitamins, it was found that rats could not grow or reproduce. But adding liver, lettuce, or lard greatly improved growth and allowed reproduction.[192] Nutrition tests were run on humans and the same components were found necessary. Vitamin E was one of the necessary components. The other unknown components in these foods were found to be linoleic and linolenic fatty acids.[193] They are found in many seeds and nuts, greens, meat, and fish. These omega-6 and omega-3 fatty acids are essential for a variety of cell functions, especially for cell membranes.

All cells are enclosed by a membrane that is composed of a "lipid bilayer." The bilayer contains two layers of fatty acids with the hydrophobic tails pointing inward, and the acid hydrophilic heads facing outward to the extracellular and intracellular spaces. The most common saturated fatty acid in membranes, palmitic acid (found in palm and coconut oil, butter, and animal fat), has a straight hydrophobic tail which tends to form a crystallinelike matrix in the membrane. Thus it is solid at room temperature. Polyunsaturated fatty acids, in contrast, have a bent hydrophopic tail that doesn't fit alongside the straight-tail palmitate and other saturated fatty acids. The result is that the membrane is more fluid, which is very important for many cells in the body. Moreover, the unsaturated carbon bonds in PUFAs are highly susceptible to free-radical oxidation, which damages them. Thus, they require continual replacement. The omega-3 fatty acids are also thought to perform signaling functions, in which they bind to receptors in the genetic machinery in cells. For example, they can inhibit the generation of some prostaglandins. However, EPA and DHA are thought to perform slightly different functions.[194] Also, the ratio between the amount of omega-3 to omega-6 fatty acids is thought to be important.[195] Although omega-6 fatty acids are found in higher amounts in a typical modern diet, a high level of omega-3 fatty acids is thought to be beneficial, and for the most benefit, the ratio of omega-3 to omega-6 levels should be as high as possible.

It's interesting to note that dark-green leafy vegetables such as kale and collard greens as well as summer and winter squash have a high ratio of omega-3 to omega-6 PUFA fatty acids. While their content of PUFAs is low, you can survive quite nicely if you eat only these vegetables because they provide adequate amounts of the essential nutrients. Considering their low calorie content, dark green leafy vegetables are among the most nutritionally dense food sources known!

Calcium, Magnesium, and Phosphate

These minerals are essential for the strength and durability of bones and teeth. They are also essential for all tissues.[196] For example, calcium and magnesium are essential for the signaling functions of the neural circuits of the brain that allow us to sense the world, remember, make decisions, and signal our muscles to move. In muscles, calcium is essential to initiate the muscle contraction, and this process is regulated by magnesium.[197] In heart muscle, calcium and magnesium play an essential role in generating and regulating the heartbeat. Literally every organ has an essential function that involves calcium and magnesium. As described above, calcium levels in the body are regulated by vitamin D, so that when the calcium level is low, more calcium is absorbed from food in the gut, and when it is very low, it is taken from the bones. This process is accomplished by calcitonin, which moves calcium into bones, and parathyroid hormone (PTH) which moves calcium from the bones into the blood. Thus bones act as a reservoir for calcium, which helps the body preserve homeostasis (constant levels for maintaining essential functions).

Magnesium, like calcium, is essential for bone and all other tissues. It is an essential cofactor for more than 325 enzyme pathways in the body that regulate thousands of reactions, including energy metabolism, cell growth and reproduction, regulation of muscle contraction, and neural function in the brain.[198] The magnesium content of normal bone is 1 to 2 percent of its calcium content.[199] At first thought, it might appear that such a minor component of bone would not be important for bone and joint health. But magnesium has a special relationship with calcium, for it helps to keep calcium dissolved in the blood and urine.[200] It also helps to activate vitamin D to maintain calcium levels in the blood.[201] Further, magnesium is a necessary cofactor for the enzymes that metabolize vitamin D.[202] With high doses of vitamin D, more magnesium is required by tissues, so it is drawn out of the muscles. This can cause problems with muscle twitching and cramps.[203] Magnesium helps to activate the hormone calcitonin, which is involved in taking calcium from the tissues and blood into bones for new formation of bone tissue. This lowers the risk of heart attack, kidney stones, and osteoporosis and osteoarthritis.[204] Thus, magnesium is crucial for calcium absorption and metabolism. The bones act as a reservoir of magnesium, much like they do for calcium. However, a magnesium deficit is more likely for most people because it is often lacking in their diet. Further, calcium supplements in the presence of a magnesium deficit can cause deposits of calcium in soft tissues like joints, which can cause arthritis.[205]

Phosphate is essential for all tissues, including bone. It is one of the most abundant minerals in the body; about 1 percent of body weight, mostly in the bones and teeth. Phosphate is taken into cells by special transporters that increase its concentration by a factor of 100.[206] The mineral content of bones consists mostly of calcium phosphate arranged in a larger crystalline form called hydroxyapatite. This material is what gives bones strength. Currently hydroxyapatite is used by surgeons to encourage bone regrowth where it has been excised, and on the surface of prosthetic joints to form a tight biologically-active bond to existing bone. Hydroxyapatite is strong in compression (like concrete) but is brittle and breaks when twisted or pulled apart. Bone also contains collagen fibers which give it some elasticity. Phosphate levels inside and outside cells are closely regulated by a complex set of biochemical interactions with calcitonin and PTH. With a deficit of phosphate, the body cannot grow bones or keep them properly filled with calcium or supplied with blood vessels. The body maintains a relatively constant level of phosphate by regulating the amount that is taken up by the gut, the amount stored into bones, and also the amount that is excreted and taken up by the kidneys.[207]

Calcium, magnesium, and phosphate are stored in the bones, so when the body excretes them in urine without a balancing amount being absorbed by the gut, a deficit results in the bones that can accumulate over many decades. This can cause a deficit of these essential minerals in the tissues, which is a major cause for many age-related diseases such as heart disease, diabetes, and arthritis. When the bones accumulate such a deficit of calcium, magnesium, or phosphate, the result can be osteomalacia (soft bone), osteoporosis (porous bone), and osteoarthritis. Because the level of magnesium is so closely regulated by the body, even when there is a deficit in the tissues and bones, the level in the blood may be within the normal range. To determine whether a deficit of magnesium exists, a dose of magnesium is given while urine is collected over a twenty-four hour period. The amount excreted in the urine is the excess not utilized by the body. If the test shows little magnesium in the urine, this indicates a magnesium deficit.[208]

When the calcium and/or magnesium content of the diet is limited, a major problem for maintenance of calcium and magnesium levels in the body is blockage of uptake by the gut. Tannins in bitter black or green tea can bind to minerals in the gut, preventing their uptake. Oxalate, found in many foods including spinach and chard, and phytic acid (phytate), found in seed hulls and the bran of grains such as wheat and rice, can chelate (bind strongly to) many important nutrients such as niacin, calcium, and magnesium, causing them to be eliminated in the stools.[209] Oxalate in low levels is not a problem, but when the body is dehydrated, a high level of oxalate in the presence of calcium can precipitate in the urine, causing kidney stones. Cooking degrades oxalate, so it is helpful to cook greens such as spinach, kale, and chard to prevent uptake of oxalate and lower the risk of kidney stones.[210] Another way to prevent uptake of oxalate when eating foods with high levels is to eat an excess of calcium-containing foods or supplements, to cause binding and elimination of the oxalate.

Many of us have been given advice to take calcium supplements as we age, to avoid osteomalacia and osteoporosis. However, calcium supplements have recently been shown to be a risk for cardiovascular disease such as heart attacks and strokes. This is especially relevant when there is a deficiency of vitamin K. But it is also known that the efficacy of calcium uptake (from food and calcium supplements) for preventing these bone diseases is improved by adequate magnesium levels. Too much calcium without adequate magnesium can cause many problems including heart attack, osteoporosis, and arthritis.[211] Calcium deficiencies are also common. A high-protein diet can cause calcium excretion in urine, which can cause calcium deficiency. Supplements of magnesium can prevent this type of deficit.[212]

Most people probably know what foods contain calcium: dairy products and green leafy vegetables are good sources. But magnesium is a different story, because many people are unaware that they are deficient. It's easy to be confused, because a deficit in magnesium can cause many symptoms that are also caused by other conditions. Also, a magnesium deficit is often ignored by medical doctors because of the difficulty of diagnosing and testing for it.[213] Two centuries ago, the diet of most people included 500 mg of magnesium per day or more, because refined products were generally not available. The same refining of wheat and rice flour that removes the B vitamins also removes most of the magnesium. A slice of whole wheat bread weighing 25 grams contains 25 mg of magnesium, but a slice of white bread the same size contains only 6 mg, a drop of 75 percent in magnesium content.[214] This is true for all foods made from "enriched flour" such as white bread, "wheat" bread, low-calorie bread, cookies, crackers, cake, and most pasta (whole wheat pasta is OK). Unfortunately the current "enrichment" process that adds some vitamins doesn't add magnesium. Good sources of magnesium include whole grains, green leafy vegetables, tomatoes, beans, legumes, and nuts.

Niacin and Niacinamide

Niacin (nicotinic acid) and niacinamide (nicotinamide) are related biochemicals, and both are termed vitamin B_3 because either one can prevent pellagra. Like all the other B vitamins, they are essential for the metabolic pathways of most cells in the body. Both niacin and niacinamide are converted to an important cofactor called nicotinamide adenine dinucleotide (NAD) that is essential in transferring electrons in the respiratory enzyme pathway inside cells.[215] NAD and its related compound NADP (Nicotinamide adenine dinucleotide phosphate) are universally important for life. They are involved in 450 biochemical reactions, more than any other vitamin-derived cofactor.[216] However, niacin and niacinamide are not interconvertible. Although they can both prevent pellagra, several effects of niacin differ from those of niacinamide.

Niacin was originally called "nicotinic acid". The compound nicotinic acid was first derived from nicotine by oxidation with nitric acid, but nicotine and nicotinic acid are different molecules. However, the name "nicotinic acid" was thought to be too suggestive of nicotine, a different chemical, which is an addictive drug component of tobacco products. Therefore, the name was changed to "niacin" for better public reception.[217] As described above, the amino acid tryptophan can be converted in the body to niacin. Most grains contain some tryptophan, but it is not readily absorbed from maize unless it is treated with alkaline water. This explains why pellagra was such a problem for people who relied on maize without alkaline treatment for a staple food.

In the United States during the period of 1900 to1950, the risk of death from pellagra among women was about twice that of men, and the occurrence of pellagra in women was three to twenty times that in men.[218] This difference may have been due to several factors. Estrogen, the female sex hormone, is known to inhibit the conversion of tryptophan to niacin. In addition, it is thought that during the epidemics of pellagra in the early twentieth century, women ate less nutritious food than men. Typically women would give the most nutritious food such as milk to children first. Also, men earned higher wages so they were able to purchase higher quality food, especially outside of the home.[219]

The Niacin Flush

In large doses, niacin, but not niacinamide, causes a "niacin flush" on the skin that feels warm and can generate a temporary rash that disappears after thirty to sixty minutes.[220] This reaction is not harmful, and some people like the warmth of the flush.[221] The flush is caused by activation of the high affinity G-protein coupled receptors, GPR109a and b, which cause the release of a variety of prostaglandin signaling molecules and results in vasodilation and the flush response.[222] In rare cases other temporary symptoms may occur. Niacin is frequently given to patients with dyslipidemia (low HDL with elevated VLDL, cholesterol, and triglycerides), a risk factor for atherosclerosis.[297] In these patients niacin typically correctly elevates HDL, while decreasing VLDL, cholesterol, and triglycerides. Amazingy, in patients with exceptionally low cholesterol, niacin can also raise their cholesterol.[223] Niacinamide doesn't generate the flush, but it also doesn't give the benefits regarding LDL and HDL cholesterol levels.[224] Occasionally, niacin appears to cause an increase in the level of liver enzymes in a blood test. Many liver enzymes require the cofactor NAD itself for their activity. Because administering niacin increases the level of NAD, this necessarily raises the measured activities of those liver enzymes. But this is not a measure of the liver responding to toxicity. Instead it is merely a measure of enzyme activities available with the excess NAD cofactor to deal with normal body metabolites and toxins. When this happens, it does not necessarily indicate any pathology, for if niacin is stopped for a few days the liver enzymes will usually go back to normal.[225]

Niacin Prevents Arthritis Pain

The connection between niacin and arthritis was made in the early 1940s by Kaufman, who found in his practice of internal medicine that many of his patients had subclinical symptoms of pellagra.[226] At that time, many people ate white bread made from processed white flour that lacked the germ and bran. This caused a variety of ailments in Kaufman's patients that appeared to be mild forms of the vitamin deficiency diseases. Many had a form of dermatitis that he recognized as a subclinical symptom of pellagra without the obvious skin rash. Their light skin was sensitive to the sun, and retained a tan for five months or more after sun exposure. Many of them also had calluses where their skin had rubbed against shoes or furniture, and the callused areas were pigmented dark yellow to brown.[227] Kaufman experimented with taking niacin and niacinamide, and found that he preferred niacinamide because he found the skin flush reaction uncomfortable. He also noticed that, when he took niacin and got a niacin flush, the areas of his skin that flushed were the same as those in which pellagra usually occurs.[228] Kaufman prescribed niacinamide for hundreds of his patients with a variety of preclinical pellagra symptoms. He experimented with doses and found that some patients required higher doses than others. And he found that frequent low doses (divided doses) were more effective than larger doses taken less often, even when they totaled to the same daily amount. When patients took niacinamide in these frequent doses, they regained health within a few weeks, and stayed healthy as long as they continued to take the vitamin. Kaufman also found that with niacinamide therapy, patients were calmer and could work more efficiently, with less mental stress, and an increased sense of well-being.[229] For him this was evidence that many of his patients were in fact deficient in niacin (vitamin B_3).

But Kaufman noticed that, in some of his subclinical pellagra patients that also had osteoarthritis, niacinamide taken at high doses promptly relieved their arthritis symptoms. As a doctor he was rather conservative, but he noticed that for many patients their arthritis persisted when they were treated with lower doses of niacinamide (less than 500 milligrams). So he tried higher doses. Excellent relief of arthritis symptoms was achieved by doses up to 5,000 mg per day, administered as 250 or 500 mg every hour throughout the day. He observed that for the same total daily dose, lower doses administered more frequently were superior to higher doses administered less frequently. He also found that the doses required to relieve the subclinical pellagra in patients who had arthritis were greater than required for those who had no arthritis.[230] High doses of niacin or niacinamide remain among the most reliable and effective treatments for arthritis today.

Kaufman developed an objective metric of arthritis severity by measuring how much it limited the angular range of joint movement. This allowed him to observe even small degrees of improvement or deterioration, and his services became sought after for his very effective program for treating arthritis. However, this discovery happened around the time when cortisone treatments were being promoted, so it was not widely appreciated by the medical community. After 1943, when commercial white flour was enriched with B vitamins, Kaufman noted that the vitamin deficiencies in his patients were less severe. However, his patients continued to have arthritis and limitations in their joint motion, even if they didn't complain of it. The niacinamide treatment usually relieved the pain of osteoarthritis and much of the limitation in joint movement, even in patients with such severe symptoms that recovery seemed unlikely.[231] When these patients stopped taking niacinamide, the arthritis symptoms returned. When niacinamide was given at a lower dose, the symptoms of pellagra or arthritis returned, but at a more gradual rate than if niacinamide was stopped completely.

The same type of malnutrition continues today. People who eat white bread, cake, and pasta made from enriched flour, without enough other nutritious foods in their diet, slowly build up damage from a deficiency of niacin, and other vitamins and minerals and essential nutrients. Because of individual variability, some individuals may have a greater requirement for B vitamins than others, which can lead to long-term deficiencies and damage to their joints.

Remarkably, the niacinamide treatment for arthritis is hardly mentioned by many rheumatologists today. This treatment, which has been proven to work, is often not even considered, mostly out of ignorance. There is little downside and potentially a remarkable life-changing upside to simply trying Kaufman's established treatment.

CHAPTER 3

JOINTS: HOW THEY WORK AND WHAT CAN GO WRONG

This chapter describes the basic structure of bones and joints, how they work, and what goes wrong in arthritis. Because of their structure, joints have intrinsic weaknesses that tend to fail during injury, stress, and poor nutrition. These problems are not unique to arthritis and can be related to many other age-related progressive diseases. Understanding these weaknesses and relationships will clarify that while arthritis is not always associated with aging, it is often related to diet.

Osteoarthritis (OA), one of the most common forms of arthritis, is a disease of the joint, including the cartilage, the underlying bone, the joint capsule and synovial membrane, and the surrounding tissues.[1] This chapter explains what can go wrong with these tissues, and how a lack of nutrients contributes to damage.

BONE HEALTH

We depend on the skeleton to support the body, and generally we only need to think about the skeleton when something goes wrong. The skeleton appears to be a static fixed set of bones. Implicit in this notion is that, after we're fully grown, our bones don't change much. Everyone understands that joints and muscles do the moving. However, the skeleton is a living organ that contains several different types of cell. These cells are continually in action. Bones are continually changing shape and density according to the stresses they encounter in our everyday lives. That includes stresses from exercise, lifting heavy loads (including the body), and from gravity. In outer space, bones change their composition and lose density due to the absence of stress from gravity.[2]

Bone consists of minerals such as calcium phosphate and magnesium that have been deposited by bone cells into an external matrix of proteins as a crystalline submatrix. These minerals are hard and give a rigid structure, but they are formed around a scaffold of flexible protein. The mineral content of healthy bone is about 65 percent, and the other 35 percent is protein, mostly collagen, which gives it elasticity and additional strength.[3] Bone consists of two kinds of tissue. Cortical (or compact) bone is hard and comprises the surface of large bones and the entire volume of small bones in the hand, wrist, and feet. Inside large and flat bones is trabecular (spongy or cancellous) bone, which contains the bone marrow. It contains the same basic components as cortical bone, but is less dense. It can change its content of minerals and other cellular components faster.

Calcuim and Magnesium Remodeling

Bones are a reservoir of calcium and magnesium for the soft tissues of the body, and are responsible for supplying the necessary quantities of these minerals to the tissues when dietary intake is insufficient. Bone is continually being "remodeled" in a process of resorption and formation.[4] When the body's tissues need more calcium or magnesium, special bone cells called "osteoclasts" resorb (break down) some bone tissue, often deep inside the bone where it is porous, and supply the calcium and magnesium to the blood which then carries it to the tissues where it is needed. When excess calcium and magnesium are available in the blood beyond what is needed for the body's tissues, other special bone cells called "osteoblasts" deposit these minerals to form new bone. Incorporation of calcium into bone is regulated by a protein called osteocalcin. Vitamin D stimulates osteoblasts to increase their expression of osteocalcin, which also requires vitamin K to function.[5] Other bone cells called "osteocytes" help in this process. They are the cells that live enclosed within the bone matrix, and they sense the mechanical stresses within the bone and communicate this to the osteoblasts and osteoclasts.[6] They can develop into osteoclasts to assist in removing bone minerals.

The remodeling process happens inside bones, so normally we don't notice any changes. But in older people, bones often lose much of their density of calcium because the regrowth phase is slowed while the resorption phase continues. This can be prevented or slowed by proper nutrition, including an excellent diet, supplements of vitamin C, vitamin D, calcium, and magnesium.[7] Vitamin C in particular is essential for inhibiting osteoclasts from degrading bone and stimulating growth of osteoblasts that create new bone growth. In postmenopausal women, who are at high risk for arthritis, high doses of vitamin C can compensate for the bone loss usually found with cessation of estrogen production.[8]

TYPES, MAKEUP, AND FUNCTON OF JOINTS

The skeleton has several types of joints, classified as fibrous, cartilaginous, and synovial. Fibrous joints connect bones with collagen fibers to keep the bones relatively immobile. Examples of fibrous joints are those that hold the bones of the skull together. Cartilaginous joints connect bones with cartilage that is securely fastened, holding the bones together but allowing some motion. An example is the joint connecting the ribs to the breastbone. Cartilage is a tough but flexible tissue made of collagen, the most common protein in the body. It is responsible for the strength of the skin, arteries, and the firm tissue inside the nose and ears. Synovial joints, found at the hip, knee, ankle, foot, shoulder, elbow, wrist, and hand, don't directly connect bones together, but allow the bones to move or "articulate." Synovial joints are the type of joint afflicted by arthritis.

Articular Cartilage

At a joint, the tips of the bones are covered in a special type of cartilage called "articular cartilage" that is very slippery yet firm (Figure 3.1). It is rubbery and squishy, yet very strong so it can resist a huge weight, and is supplied with a system of lubrication to prevent damage from the weight. Up to 80 percent of the volume of articular cartilage is water, much of it bound in a gel-like matrix. The remainder is made up of collagen and other molecules that give the cartilage its strength and resilience, as well as chondrocytes, the cells that synthesize these molecules. The cartilage is bathed in synovial fluid, which is very slippery (like egg white) and provides lubrication. This fluid also provides nutrition to the living cells in the cartilage and removes their wastes. In the hip, a thin layer of articular cartilage called the labrum lines the bone cavity that receives the head of the femur. It is shaped like a round gasket and helps to keep the femur inside the hip.

Joint Capsule

The bones are loosely connected by the "capsule" that surrounds the joints to hold the synovial fluid. The capsule comprise two layers, the synovial membrane on the inside and the fibrous capsule on the outside (Figure 3.1). Further outside the capsule, ligaments are connected firmly to both bones to keep them within a range of positions, so the bones can articulate without their tips jumping out of position within the capsule.[9] There are several types of synovial joints that allow different types of motion. The shoulder and hip joints are "ball-and-socket" joints that allow motion in any direction, whereas the knee and elbow are hinge joints that only allow motion in one plane.

Moving Bones, Joints, and Balance

To start walking, we lean forward a little to get slightly out of balance by pushing the body with muscles in our legs. Then each leg in turn swings forward, pulling the body forward while the leg moves back. Walking is therefore a process of controlled fall.[10] Unless the legs pull the body forward we would quickly fall face down. Implicit in this process of walking is the ability to balance. When we're not moving, the leg muscles adjust the balance by pushing the body back and forth to prevent falling. If we were still balanced when starting to walk by moving our legs, our legs would pull the lower body forward and the rest of the body would fall backwards. Thus, bipedal walking requires an exquisite sense of motion and balance. In the miracle of bipedal locomotion, two-legged species like us and, for example, birds, can sense acceleration due to movement and also the force of gravity to allow us to remain upright while walking. Our sense of motion comes from vision, and our sense of acceleration comes from the canals of the inner ear. The joints that hold our bones together are necessary to perform this miracle.

Knee Joint

The knee joints are crucial to walking and balance, because they allow the leg bones to be connected yet move while supporting the body's weight. Walking requires the joints to be flexible, and capable of supporting a force of several hundred pounds, yet also be maintainable. It's crucial to be able to recover after injury. The bones that connect at the knee, the femur (thigh bone) and tibia (shin bone), slide across the articular cartilage in the knee joint. The ends of the bones form curved surfaces called condyles. These curved surfaces allow the bones to fit together at the joint and articulate (move) in a bending motion. The condyles are covered by a thin layer of articular cartilage. The cartilage contains living cells called chondrocytes, which synthesize a set of extracellular proteins that give the cartilage its unique properties. The cartilage can bear tremendous weight while allowing the bones to move smoothly. It can do this because it is specially constructed from tough fibers made out of collagen, elastin, aggrecan (chondroitin sulfate proteoglycan 1), and hyaluronic acid (non-sulfated glycosaminoglycan) in a gel-like "ground substance."[11] The collagen is strong but flexible and protects the bone, and the elastin is rubbery and can rebound after being pushed in by the force of a weight. The aggrecan fibers contain many ionic sulfate and carboxyl side-groups that

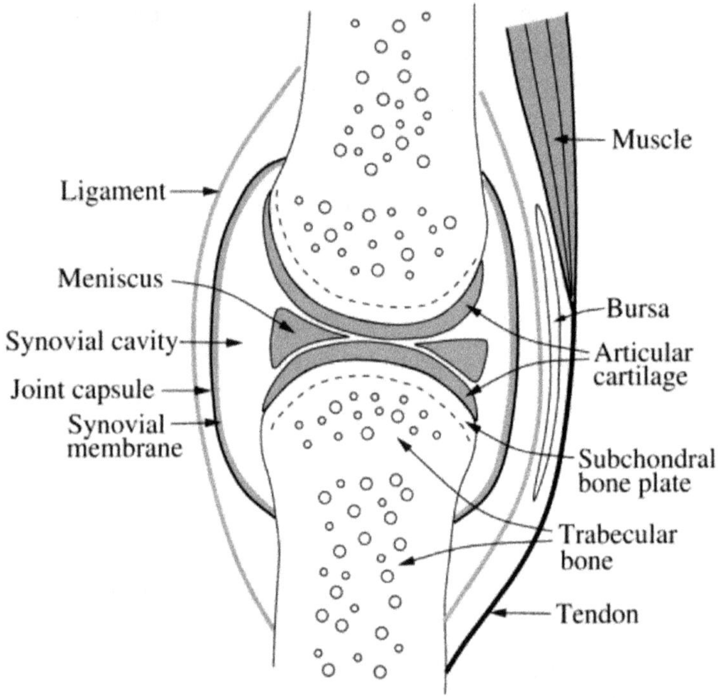

Figure 3.1. Structures of a synovial joint, found in the feet, hands, knees, elbows, shoulders, and hips. The ends of the two bones form curved surfaces called condyles. These are covered with articular cartilage that supports the weight and acts to lubricate the joint during motion. The articular cartilage contains no nerves or blood vessels, but instead is bathed and nourished by synovial fluid contained within the synovial cavity. The meniscus (present only in the knee joint) is also cartilage, but is not directly connected to the articular cartilage. A hard layer of bone underneath the cartilage, called the subcondral bone plate, supports the cartilage and contains many nerves. Beneath the subchondral bone, the bone is porous (trabecular) and contains many blood vessels. A bursa also contains synovial fluid and cushions ligaments, tendons, and muscles. The knee cap (patella) is omitted in this schematic view.

bind water molecules through osmotic attraction. This causes the cartilage to generate a swelling pressure which along with the collagen and elastin fibers can resist a tremendous force.

In addition, the synovial fluid contains several slippery long-chain molecules such as hyaluronic acid and lubricin (proteoglycan 4).[12] These molecules are synthesized by some of the cells in the synovial membrane and also in the surface layer of the articular cartilage. Hyaluronic acid (also called hyaluronan or hyaluronate) is a large molecule that acts as a lubricant in the synovial fluid during walking and a shock absorber during running or jumping. In addition to its lubrication function, it protects against free radicals and suppresses the degradation of cartilage by signaling pathways such as pro-inflammatory cytokines.[13] The overall effect is to lubricate the joint when the bones are moved under load. The articular cartilage in the knee joint doesn't connect the bones together. It protects the ends of the bones while allowing them to slide across each other without damage. The joint is held together by surrounding tissues, including the fibrous joint capsule, its inner synovial lining, and several very tough ligaments. All of these tissues depend on collagen for their strength.

Meniscus

The knee joint also contains two structures made out of cartilage called the menisci (singular: meniscus). They are C-shaped structures that sit between the articular cartilage of the two bones, but curve around the edge of the joint. They are connected to the bone at the ends of the C, and are concave to fit closely around the convex surface of the articular cartilage. The menisci are soft but firm and help to absorb bumps during walking like the shock absorbers in your car. They also help to lubricate the joint and distribute the weight evenly across the cartilage and tips of the bones. The menisci help to increase stability of the joint, and they limit its motion to prevent extreme flexion or extension. Another important role for the menisci is to help provide nutrition for the joint. With recent technological advances in imaging (for example, the MRI scan) medical science has learned a lot about the structure of the joint including the meniscus. The outer third of the menisci that transmit less weight load are fed by arteries, which are very important for supplying nutrition to the synovial fluid and articular cartilage.[14]

A tear or rip of the meniscus is one of the most common types of injury, typically in active young adults but also in older people. Repairing damage to the meniscus is also one of the most common orthopedic surgical procedures. Prompt diagnosis and treatment of any injury to the meniscus is considered very important to prevent later degenerative disease such as osteoarthritis.[15] Even so, related sports injuries such as a torn anterior cruciate ligament in young female soccer players commonly cause osteoarthritis after a decade or more.[16]

MAINTENANCE OF CARTILAGE

The articular cartilage that covers the ends of the thigh bones and shin bones requires nutrition from the body for its maintenance. Most tissues of the body are supplied with nutrition by blood flowing through the arteries and capillaries. For example, bones contain a matrix of blood vessels that provide nutrition and allow the bones to regenerate and reform in response to changes in their load. The blood vessels are supported and protected by the bone tissue. However, the cartilage cannot contain blood vessels because it is squishy and flexible, and they would not be strong enough to withstand the huge pressure on the joint from the body weight it supports. Instead, the cartilage receives its nutrition from the synovial fluid, which is contained within the joint capsule and its inner synovial lining. The synovial fluid must carry the necessary nutrients to the cartilage and must remove its waste molecules. This process is relatively slow compared to the flow of blood, however, so the articular cartilage is only able to grow and maintain itself slowly.

The body must synthesize new molecules for maintenance, but it also must break down existing structures that require reshaping. Overall, these life-sustaining chemical reactions that take place within tissues are called "metabolism." Some of the new molecules are small ones derived by breaking down large molecules in food. Some of these small molecules (for instance, blood sugar or glucose) are used as energy. Others are used as building blocks to make new large molecules to grow or repair the body. The terms "anabolic" and "catabolic" refer to different aspects of this process of metabolism. Anabolism is the process of building up large molecules from small ones, for example, synthesis of proteins such as actin and myosin fibers for our muscles, or collagen fibers needed for making cartilage. Catabolism is the process of breaking down large molecules into smaller ones, for example, breaking apart long-chain carbohydrates in grains into simple sugars. This process continues with sugars getting further broken down into carbon dioxide and water in the aerobic respiration cycle inside cells. Our bodies depend on catabolism of food molecules to gain energy, which can then be utilized to build up other molecules, in the process of anabolism, to make cells and body organs. Plants have a slightly different balance of anabolism and catabolism. Using the sun's energy, plants take carbon dioxide and water and in a process of anabolism synthesize carbohydrates such as cellulose and sugars. At night, in a process of catabolism, plants take some of the molecules they've synthesized and break them down, as animals do, into carbon dioxide and water to generate energy necessary to stay alive.

Resorption and Formation

The bone and cartilage of a joint such as the knee are in a continual process of catabolic degradation and anabolic renewal.[17] This process is a delicate balance, much like the balance we must maintain in order to stand upright and walk. A similar process occurs within bones and within the joint. Normal growth of articular cartilage happens when chondrocytes, the only cells that live in cartilage, release collagen and other proteins that get cross-linked into a robust extracellular matrix. But this process is a balance of degradation and regrowth, in a process similar to the remodeling of bone. Both bone and cartilage are continually being remodeled in response to the body's needs and this requires adequate nutrition.[18] Whenever we perform a new type of exercise in which the joint is stressed in a new way for an extended time, its articular cartilage and the underlying bone tissue get remodeled, according to the stress (force per unit area) and strain (movement under stress) that each part of the joint receives.

Protein biomolecules called cytokines are local signals for degradation and regrowth and are used widely in the body to control many biological processes, such as cell growth, differentiation (making different organs), immunity, and inflammation. Cytokines in the synovial fluid have been widely studied. Some cytokines are pro-inflammatory, that is, they promote inflammation and degradation of cartilage and bone.[19] They attract cells from the immune system to generate local inflammation, which can lead to a vicious inflammatory cycle.[20] These cytokines also increase the production of matrix metalloproteinases (MMPs), enzymes that can degrade all components of extracellular matrix, leading to destruction of cartilage.[21] Other cytokines are anti-inflammatory and promote regrowth of bone and/or cartilage. The balance between pro-inflammatory and anti-inflammatory signaling pathways plays an important role in initiation and recovery from arthritis.[22]

Subchondral Bone Plate

At the base of the cartilage where it attaches to the bone sits a thin layer where the cartilage is calcified to become hard, like bone. Under this bottom layer of cartilage, a dense and very hard layer of bone forms, called the subchondral bone plate, about 1–3 millimeters thick, which is responsible for resisting breakage of the bone tip under extreme pressure.[23] These two dense layers are harder than the articular cartilage above and the porous or "trabecular" bone below. Thus the soft articular cartilage rests upon a hard layer of material it must protect from contacting the bone on the other side of the joint. In a normal joint, the articular cartilage is relatively thick and thus can withstand deformation from a weight. In osteoarthritis, the subchondral bone plate tends to get thinner during the early stages of the disease and then get thicker than normal during the late stages. This is accompanied with thinning and damage to the articular cartilage.[24] Exactly what causes these changes is currently unknown. But they are part of a dynamic remodeling process of the bone and cartilage that comprises a balance between resorption and formation.[25]

One clue to the regrowth of cartilage is its slow progress. Because articular cartilage does not have a direct supply of nutrients from blood, it can only grow with nutrients provided by the synovial fluid. In the middle of the layer of cartilage, the chondrocytes don't get much oxygen.[26] But the bone underneath can grow faster because it is well-supplied by blood vessels. Thus, the hard subchondral bone plate underneath the articular cartilage may appear to take the lead in resorption and regrowth in response to differences in the stress applied to the joint.[27] In response to damage from an excess load on the joint, the articular cartilage may temporarily change the balance from formation to resorption, after which it will attempt to reform new extracellular matrix to strengthen the cartilage layer. But this is only possible when damage is not continual, to give the cartilage enough time to regrow. This may take many months or even several years. And it is also dependent on a sufficient amount and concentration of molecular building blocks and essential nutrients. There are no nerves in cartilage, but the joint capsule, tendons, ligaments, and subchondral bone are well innervated.[28] Thus, once pain occurs in OA, this typically means that the cartilage has already been substantially degraded.[29]

Ligament Injury

The pain of OA differs from pain caused by acute injury, but they may be related. A common injury to athletes is a torn anterior cruciate ligament (ACL). This ligament is very important for stabilizing the knee joint. Injury to the ACL is acutely painful because the ligament contains nerves that sense the damage. This type of injury typically heals slowly. If the ligament is not given adequate protection and time to heal, or not corrected by surgery, the overall knee structure and articular cartilage may become abnormal, often leading to arthritis with chronic pain. Therefore when acute pain is felt in the knee, the cause should be carefully determined. If it originates in damage to the surrounding tendon or ligament tissues, they can heal if they are given protection from further injury along with proper nutrition. The healing process can sometimes be helped by surgery. However, acute pain from a torn ligament or tendon differs from the chronic pain from damage to the cartilage and bone described above that indicates OA has advanced into the underlying bone.

Extracellular Matrix

The extracellular matrix of collagen, aggrecan, and elastin in the articular cartilage sits in a gel that contains proteoglycans and water. The chondrocytes are locked into this gel-like matrix of cross-linked fibers, so to stay alive and functioning, one might imagine they are entirely dependent on passive diffusion of nutrients through the matrix. But this would limit the flow of nutrients from the synovial fluid, slowing the regrowth and remodeling of the cartilage. Although small molecules diffuse quickly through the extracellular matrix, large molecules diffuse slowly. Some are stored in the extracellular matrix.[30] Ironically, the cartilage is dependent upon movement and some weight loading of the joint for a robust supply of nutrients. Even though heavy weight loading of the joint can cause damage to the articular cartilage, some movement and pressure is helpful to provide a flow of nutrients in and waste products out of the cartilage. It is like trying to clean a carpet using a detergent solution and a roller. The detergent solution spread on top will diffuse down into the carpet passively. But repeatedly squeezing the solution in and out by moving the roller back and forth (as in the articular motion of the joint on the cartilage) will push the detergent solution down into the bottom of the carpet and squeeze it out, which will clean it faster. Motion of the joint that pushes the synovial fluid into the cartilage gives its chondrocyte cells more nutrients than simply waiting for them to diffuse passively into the cartilage. Pressure on the joint squeezes out the metabolic waste products from the cartilage, and intermittent removal of weight from the joint allows the cartilage to absorb a new dose of synovial fluid. This is one reason why it helps to warm up before regular daily exercise. Motion of the joint tends to warm up the synovial fluid, which allows it to diffuse into the cartilage more completely, and provide better supply of nutrients and flushing of waste. And, of course, adequate rest is necessary after daily exercise. Sleep allows the body to devote its resources to recovery from inflammation. Keeping weight off the joints during sleep allows the newly supplied nutrients to help regenerate the cartilage.

Remodeling Cartilage and Bone

Because articular cartilage is continually in a balance between resorption and formation, the degradation in cartilage thickness with age is a consequence of both a lower rate of formation as well as a higher rate of resorption. This process of "remodeling" is a consequence of the natural mechanism for healing. With damage, the rate of resorption increases to allow the joint to "resculpt" its cartilage to stress. This allows the joint to adapt to changing stress conditions. Under normal conditions, the type II soft collagen and chondroitin sulfate in the articular cartilage is degraded by an enzyme called aggrecanase, and this is thought to be reversible; that is, new collagen can be readily synthesized to reform the collagen.[31]

To understand how the mechanism works, consider how the load on your legs and joints changes when you are performing different tasks with your legs. When you walk in a field of grass, your legs and joints will have quite a different load than when climbing up and down a winding stone staircase. The gentle walking motion on grass will move the knee joints, with some pressure from the body's weight, lubricating them without much shock. But hard plodding on stone steps will cause shocks to the joints that can damage them. If the steps are high, the joints must articulate to a greater angle. If this angle is near the end of the joint's range of motion, the joint motion may damage the cartilage. When you twist your body quickly to turn while going down winding stairs, the knee joints will twist also. They may be damaged by too much angular and lateral motion. When climbing a mountain, hikers often find that their joints hurt much more going down than going up. The shocks that joints feel are often worse going down because the force of gravity accelerates the shock of the body's weight dropped on them. This is further worsened at the end of the day with tired muscles. Joints are stabilized by muscles, and when they are tired or weak the bones and their cartilage can misalign, causing more wear and tear.

In a normal knee joint, when these motions are repeated day after day, week after week, the joints adapt, reshaping the bones and the cartilage in the joints to better take up the stresses they are given. Cartilage with more stress placed on it will tend to degrade; that is, it will gradually thin because it is resorbed by enzymes released by chondrocytes that remove some of the collagen and elastin and other proteins in the extracellular matrix. The subchondral bone plate underneath the thinning cartilage adapts to this change by removing some of its top surface to allow more space for the cartilage. Then more bone mass is added to the bottom of the subchondral bone plate. Likewise, cartilage in an area of a well-used joint with less stress will degrade less and the subchondral bone plate will sense less stress, so both the cartilage and the bone underneath will gradually thicken. This process of adaptation to the local stresses within the joint keeps the ends of the bones strong and resilient to the pattern of weight loading. The cartilage is continually being formed anew, so that its matrix of collagen and other proteins will slowly regrow. The bone underneath will also resorb and regrow. This remodeling of both cartilage and bone together is a continuous process that happens every day as we move and our joints adapt to the stresses they sense.[32]

In osteochondritis dissecans (OCD), a rare joint disease, the articular cartilage and subchondral bone tend to form cracks. This disease can be caused by a mutation in the gene for the aggrecans molecule.[33] The mutation causes the aggrecans molecule to be misformed, so it cannot correctly serve its function to attract water molecules into the articular cartilage. This weakens the cartilage, allowing cracks to form. The subchondral bone may also die because of loss of blood circulation, called avascular necrosis. The bone responds by resorbing the damaged portion, but the articular cartilage is then left without support so it tends to get further damaged. The bone and cartilage then often will tend to get fragmented and these fragments can move around inside the joint capsule. This can cause further damage and pain.

ESSENTIAL NUTRIENTS TIP THE BALANCE

The resorption and regrowth of cartilage depends on a healthy supply of nutrients to the chondrocytes and removal of their waste products. To grow new cartilage, the chondrocytes need amino acids required for collagen and elastin, vitamins B_1, B_3, and C to allow synthesis of the collagen, and many other micronutrients such as copper and manganese.[34] Bones also need amino acids, vitamin C, and other vitamins, and also a good supply of calcium and magnesium. As mentioned above, in the case of nutrients to support bone growth and remodeling, the body will take calcium and magnesium from bone by resorption to support the more urgent nutritional needs of many other organs such as the heart, liver, skin, muscles, and brain. Magnesium is crucial for more than 300 different enzymatic reactions in the body, so the body appropriates it from the bones when the diet is insufficient to supply enough.[35] Calcium is appropriated in a similar way. If dietary calcium and magnesium or other nutrients such as phosphate are insufficient to reform new bone, the result is osteomalacia or osteoporosis. A diet with a high level of nutrients will allow bone regrowth, so the bone in and around joints can successfully remodel.

The nutrients that support regrowth of cartilage have a similar but worse problem. The chondrocytes that form cartilage require energy and the amino acid building blocks for collagen and the other proteins in the extracellular matrix, along with calcium and magnesium. But since they can't get these nutrients directly from the bloodstream, they are dependent on diffusion and movement of the synovial fluid within the joint capsule to get their nutrients. And they can't do this when the articular cartilage is being continually damaged more and more every day without regrowth.

The balance between damage and regrowth must be tipped in favor of regrowth to allow the damaged cartilage to be resorbed and then regrown more every day. This net positive balance towards regrowth and remodeling is dependent on the essential nutrients that we get from an excellent diet. This dependency occurs in part because long-term deficits of the bone minerals (calcium, magnesium, and phosphate) tip the balance towards bone resorption. But resorption also happens when vitamins B_1-B_{12}, C, and D are not supplied at sufficiently high amounts to provide support for regrowth.[36] In addition, regrowth of cartilage is dependent on the amino acids required for building new molecules of its components. For example, the amount of hyaluronic acid in joints is controlled by the levels of its synthetic and degradative (hydrolytic) enzymes in the synovial fluid. In OA and RA the levels of synthetic enzymes for hyaluronic acid are lower and the levels of degradative enzymes are higher, tipping the balance towards cartilage degradation.[37]

Typically the process of remodeling and regrowth slows in older people with joint damage. But in this case, the remodeling becomes tipped in favor of resorption, which lowers bone density and thins the articular cartilage. But the good news is, eating an excellent diet with proper doses of supplements can help at any age to tip the balance back towards regrowth.

Risk and Benefit of Motion and Pain

Synovial joints are built for action, for the articular cartilage and synovial fluid are very slippery and have hardly any friction. Moreover, the cartilage is finicky, for it depends on motion for its health. If a joint remains inactive for too long, the process of resorption and regrowth will slow down, simply because the supply of nutrients to the chondrocytes in the cartilage, and disposal of their wastes, is dependent upon motion with some weight applied. A joint that is moved without weight will not get the same degree of cleansing and nutrient resupply that keeps the chondrocytes healthy. Yet, on the other hand, it is thought that wear-and-tear on the joint over decades, carrying the body's weight, will damage the cartilage, eroding it and preventing regrowth. The best compromise is to exercise to provide motion under some weight, but not enough motion or weight to damage the cartilage or other surrounding tissues of the meniscus, capsule, and ligaments.

Damage to a tissue will generate free radicals that in many tissues serve as a signal for the body to repair itself. This is especially true of bone. A moderate level of free radicals in bone is thought to direct the bone tissue to regenerate.[38] In tissues such as muscles or bone that are supplied with blood, a complex set of mechanisms set up by the innate immune system cause inflammation around the site of damage and arrange repair of the tissue. The repair cannot function in this way in articular joints such as the knee and hip. Motion of the joint will prevent any inflammation localized to a portion of the articular cartilage, because the synovial fluid is pushed by joint motion across, into, and out of the cartilage. Instead, the entire synovial capsule becomes inflamed, causing synovitis. The joint depends on continual use for its well-being and repair. The damage that occurs in a joint on average every day must be repaired, on average, over a day. Otherwise the joint will slowly fall into disrepair and the cartilage will erode. When blood comes into contact with the articular cartilage, it can cause oxidative stress that can damage the joint. This damage can be prevented by antioxidants.[39]

It is often difficult for the patient to discern where in the joint pain originates. A way to signal the damage to the joint with pain would help, for this would allow the patient to favor the joint to allow it to repair itself. But cartilage doesn't contain any nerves, so the body feels no pain when minor or moderate damage occurs to the articular cartilage. Therefore, it is difficult to determine the best amount of motion or weight for the joint to recover. If pain comes from an injury to the surrounding tendons and ligaments, this is a clue that the joint should be protected from more trauma. However, if the tendons and ligaments have not been injured, pain may originate within the bone. In this case, by the time pain is felt in the joint the damage may have worn through the cartilage into the subchondral bone, where blood vessels and nerves are plentiful. But this may indicate major damage to the cartilage. Often an early clue to damage in the cartilage is an overall inflammation of the joint, including swelling of the synovial fluid within the capsule, and redness around the joint where the blood supply is increased.

STAGES OF OSTEOARTHRITIS

The various stages of OA have been described with a standard assessment of its progression (Figure 3.2).[40] A set of different grades of progression allow doctors to diagnose, compare, and communicate how serious the joint damage has become. Grade

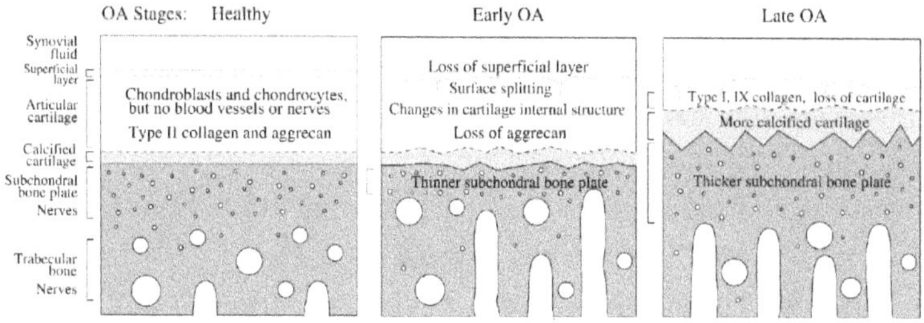

Figure 3.2. The articular cartilage and subchondral bone, showing the changes that occur at different stages of osteoarthritis (OA). Left, healthy joint. The articular cartilage is a rubbery but firm layer of tissue covered in a smooth slippery superficial layer. It consists of chondrocytes ("cartilage cells") and their precursors, chondroblasts, held in an extracellular matrix of collagen and other long-chain molecules such as aggrecan. The chondrocytes synthesize and secrete these molecules which are responsible for the firm yet slippery characteristics of the articular cartilage. The cartilage does not contain any blood vessels or nerves because it deforms when supporting the weight of the body. It is supplied with nutrients by the synovial fluid. The bottom of the articular cartilage is hard and calcified much like bone. The cartilage is supported by a hard layer of bone called the subchondral bone plate. This bone is very dense but contains blood vessels that supply its nutrients. It also contains nerves that can sense weight and damage in the joint. In early-stage OA, damage occurs to the cartilage, which loses its superficial layer and changes its internal structure, losing much of its aggrecan. The subchondral bone plate thins in response to remodeling. In late-stage OA, much of the cartilage is lost or becomes calcified, and the subchondral bone plate thickens dramatically.

0 is normal cartilage, in which the surface is smooth, and the surface, middle and deep layers are constant thickness across the joint. The chondrocytes are elongated towards the surface, without any signs of chondrocyte proliferation that occur with OA. Grade 1 shows the first potential signs of OA. The surface of the matrix is intact, but it may show abrasion and swelling, and microcracks may also appear at the surface. Chondrocyte proliferation may be present, for the cartilage is stressed and is trying to regrow. These changes are evidently a normal response to wear-and-tear by the joint, and don't necessarily represent a progressive degeneration. Grade 2 shows a rough surface, discontinuous

in some areas, and flakes of the surface of the matrix break off, or "spall," due to the lateral forces from the moving joint. Cracks in the surface matrix may extend through the surface layer into the middle layer of the cartilage. At this stage, OA may still be reversible. Grade 3 shows many cracks that extend into the middle and bottom layer of the cartilage. The cracks widen into fissures, which may branch into lateral cracks and subfissures. Chondrocytes die or are disoriented away from the surface.

In late OA, grade 4 shows surface erosion ("delamination"), in which large areas of the surface have been worn away. This can happen when the lateral cracks of grade 3 become enlarged, allowing large flakes of the surface layers to separate. When several cracks or fissures surround ("circumscribe") an area, a large chunk of cartilage can separate, in a process of "excavation." These signs are not purely mechanical but result from damage or death in the chondrocytes. Chondrocyte proliferation is often present as well. Another sign of grade 4 OA is that cysts can form due to continual edema within the cartilage, in a process called "cavitation." This tends to degrade the matrix and allows separation of the surface layer, which can cause delamination or excavation of chunks of cartilage. Grade 5 shows areas where all the soft type II collagen has been removed ("denuded") down to the bottom hard calcified layer. The bone layer nearby and underneath is typically thicker than normal, and is more active, as if it is trying to regrow. This bone tends to contain microfractures which are repaired with fibers of type I collagen. This new fibrous cartilage in some cases can fill in the entire volume of cartilage that had originally been removed, but it is not normal articular cartilage. At this stage, OA is widely thought to be irreversible. Grade 6 shows "deformation," or changes in the contour of the cartilage, accompanied by fractures and regrowth in the subchondral bone plate. These deformations are the result of substantial damage to cartilage and fractures into the bone and fibrous collagen and bone regrowth. In some areas where lateral fracture of the bone causes separation of the overlying cartilage, a large central chunk of cartilage gets shoved into a crack underneath nearby cartilage at the edge of the joint. These may get fused together by regrowth of fibrous collagen, causing further joint deformity.

These six grades of OA show the typical progression of the disease, but don't explain how or why the progression occurs.[41] It is thought that subchondral bone interacts to a large extent with the cartilage above. In the early stages of OA, before much damage or pain occurs in the articular cartilage, the subchondral bone is resorbed (thinned) to a measurable extent. Why this occurs is not known, but antiresorptive drug treatments for preventing osteoporosis, if given early enough, also lower the blood levels of markers of collagen type II degradation.[42] This suggests that if the bone loss can be prevented early in OA, the typical progression of damage to cartilage could also be prevented.

Osteoarthritis and Inflammation

When discussing arthritis, the term " inflammation" may bring to mind rheumatoid arthritis, not OA, because OA has been considered a disease of wear-and-tear on the joints. Yet, OA is now understood to be associated with inflammation. Although the standard signs of joint inflammation (white blood cells in synovial fluid) are usually missing in OA, other more subtle signs are present.[43] Much of this recent progress comes from research in molecular biology, which shows that signaling molecules that play a role in inflammation, such as cytokines and prostaglandins, can upregulate the enzymes in cartilage that degrade the extracellular collagen matrix. Some cytokines are pro-inflammatory, and others are anti-inflammatory. Both types have been studied for their roles in preventing inflammation in arthritis.[44]

These observations have led to a new understanding that OA is usually associated with and potentially caused by systemic inflammation.[45] Although a local inflammatory response may indicate that the immune system is doing its job in removing damaged tissue, systemic inflammation along with chronic pain may indicate a more involved problem. When a joint swells, the synovial membrane becomes painful, especially at night, and by morning the joint may become stiff. This type of synovitis is hypothesized to cause resorption of the cartilage. One theory for the cause of synovitis in OA is that fragments of degraded cartilage contact the synovial membrane and initiate an allergic type of reaction. But there has not been much evidence for such an allergic reaction in OA. The evidence suggests that the cells of the synovial membrane release signaling molecules such as cytokines that cause chondrocytes in the cartilage to resorb more collagen, apparently in an effort to further remodel the joint.[46] The reaction of the synovial membrane in this way is thought to involve macrophages (a type of immune cell) that are present in the synovial membrane. Macrophages are often present in a focal inflammatory response in an attempt to clean up the damaged tissues. Macrophages are part of the "innate immune system" responsible for fighting off infection that is activated by inflammation of the synovial membrane.[47]

Another aspect of inflammation that may cause OA is that advanced glycation end products ("AGEs") can weaken cartilage. This can activate chondrocytes to degrade the cartilage. AGEs are the result of a nonenzymatic reaction of a carbohydrate (e.g. fructose or glucose) and a protein or fat molecule. This compromises the function of the molecule and causes oxidative stress. AGEs are associated with the normal process of aging, but are also caused by diabetes (high blood sugar), and also by cooking sugars and carbohydrates (for instance, French fries) at high temperature. When the extracellular matrix in articular cartilage becomes glycated, it gets stiff and cannot properly absorb the forces of the joint.[48] The production of AGEs can be limited by taking adequate doses of vitamin C, B_6, alpha lipoic acid, and thiamine.

Although being overweight is a big risk factor for knee OA, the additional mechanical stress on the joint from the extra weight is not the only relevant factor.[49] People who are obese also have a twofold increase in risk for OA in their hands. This increase in risk can't be explained by the additional weight, but is explained by inflammatory factors associated with the extra body fat.[50] It is also known that "metabolic syndrome" (obesity with other factors such as high triglycerides, high blood pressure, or high blood sugar) causes the greatest increase in risk for OA. All of these factors indicate that OA can be caused by inflammation elsewhere in the body. Some evidence suggests that molecules released by adipose tissue are involved in triggering OA.[51] For example, oxidized LDL released into the bloodstream may cause oxidative stress throughout the body. Adipose tissue also releases adipokines into the bloodstream. These are signaling molecules like cytokines that modulate overall metabolism of the body and satiety. But they are also thought to be involved in triggering degradation of cartilage in OA by signaling chondrocytes.[52] On the other hand, it is also hypothesized that signals of inflammation that originate in synovitis can initiate or worsen other age-related inflammatory diseases. Overall there are several types of evidence for the influence of inflammation on OA.[53] Thus, to prevent or slow the progression of OA, one should focus on preventing inflammation throughout the body.

The balance of resorption versus regrowth of cartilage is also modulated by the level of nutrients such as glucose (blood sugar). In their normal function, chondrocytes can deal with low or high levels of glucose in the synovial fluid. They merely need to adjust the number of glucose transporters in the cell membrane that provide the cell with glucose from the extracellular fluid. But when glucose levels are very high, such as in diabetes, the chondrocytes can't properly adjust the amount of glucose transporters, so they get too much glucose. This tends to generate reactive oxygen species (ROS), which damages the cells and the extracellular matrix of the cartilage.[54] Further, high levels of glucose upregulate catabolic signaling pathways to cause cartilage resorption.[55] Although a continuous supply of glucose is necessary for life, evidently too much glucose in the synovial fluid can cause OA.

CONTROL OF BODY WEIGHT

Overeating has a cumulative effect on body weight. This is important for arthritis for several reasons. Excess weight can place excessive stress on your knees and hips. Further, obesity can cause inflammation throughout the body, which is a big risk factor for heart disease, cancer, diabetes, and both OA and RA. If you eat just a little more food than your body requires, you will put on weight. The same truth applies to losing weight, for you can lose weight by eating just a little less food. Eating just the right amount of food is extremely important for life and health. If we eat too little, by just a few mouthfuls of food per day, we would get emaciated within a few weeks or months. But eating just a few extra spoonfuls of food per day can build up to several additional pounds over a year. In many people, this weight literally builds up to a huge excess of fat over decades. But there is a reason for this behavior. Eating more food than necessary in the short term is an adaptational behavior specified by evolution over millions of years to guard against scarcity over longer periods.

For many people, keeping track of exactly how much to eat at each meal is a difficult task. We eat when we get hungry. The start of a meal is influenced by several factors, including how much food is available, the time of day, and other learned factors. We stop when we are satiated, but the sense of appetite is complex. Stretch receptors in the stomach, activated by its distention, tell the brain how full the stomach has become. But this does not tell the brain how many calories we've eaten. The body must closely control the process of digestion by sensing the different types of nutrients in the gut as they get digested. The stomach, pancreas, gallbladder, intestines, and liver are coordinated to digest food and break it down into biomolecules that are absorbed in the gut and circulated in the blood to supply energy and nutrients throughout the body.[58] The coordination is largely performed by signaling molecules in the blood that tell the different organs and the brain what type of food is being digested. For example, the pancreas and gallbladder release bile which contains enzymes to assist in digesting and absorbing fat molecules. As the molecules digested from food exit the stomach, they are sensed by specialized cells in the gut that release signaling molecules into the blood, which are sensed by the peripheral nerves and neural centers in the brain to regulate eating behavior.

Many of the satiety signals from digestion function only in the short-term. A temporary loss of appetite after one meal will not keep us from eating the next. As the stomach is emptied, the satiety signals drop and eventually terminate. This raises the question of how the body regulates its weight over the long term. Even after a prolonged period of weight loss the brain remembers its goal in terms of body weight.[59] Although the brain doesn't directly keep track of how many calories we've eaten, it tracks body weight by sensing the amount of body fat. After an extended period during which less food is available and the body has lost weight, the brain will cause behavior to regain weight when food is again readily available. This fact is innately understood by anyone who has successfully lost weight only to regain it later.

To control body weight and fat, the sense of appetite also functions over the long term. This is accomplished by a network of endocrine signals that release hormones, and neural circuits that sense these hormones and also nutrients available from food.[60] It is now known that the brain directly senses the nutrients from the food we eat and integrates this information with signals from fatty tissues to determine when to stop eating. But this computation of satiety is also affected by other psychological and physiological factors, such as sexual activity, depression, anxiety, and amount of sleep. Thus, the amount of food we eat is in some sense a prediction by the brain of the future supply of food.

As everyone knows, the appetite is affected by the taste of food. But it is also affected by the level of fat and essential nutrients, and by the body's ability to utilize sugar and fat. In fact, there is some evidence that diabetes causes a malfunction of the body's ability to sense fat and weight gain.[61] All of these additional factors are influenced by each individual's genetic background. This includes the epigenetic modulation of genes from the parental and fetal environment.

In other studies, restriction of calories has been shown to provide an anti-inflammatory effect.[56] Some types of inflammation are thought to require enhanced glucose intake, and some anti-inflammatory agents are thought to induce a "pseudo-starvation" mode.[57] This suggests that limiting calorie intake to prevent obesity may help to prevent inflammation that can cause arthritis.

Sleep Helps to Prevent Inflammation

Adequate sleep is important in preventing arthritis, because sleep allows the body to recover from stress and inflammation. Sleep is a fundamental biological necessity, affecting many organs in the body. During quiescent periods in deep sleep, the body's cells can repair themselves, and the immune system is also empowered. Several recent studies implicate a lack of sleep as a risk factor for inflammation,[62] obesity,[63] and heart disease.[64] These are important risk factors in arthritis. In one study, after just one week of moderate lack of sleep (six hours per night), the normal circadian (daily cycle of) biochemical rhythms of several hundred genes were modified. These hindered the cellular metabolism and the response to inflammation and stress.[65] A lack of sleep increases the level of inflammatory cytokines, which are thought to be involved in development of arthritis.[66] The body responds to hormonal changes induced by a lack of sleep by increased appetite and resistance to insulin, both of which tend to cause weight gain.[67] Highlighting the problem, some research shows that the circadian rhythms of rheumatoid arthritis patients are disturbed at the molecular level.[68] Although the reason for this symptom is not currently understood, the oxidative stress and inflammation associated with arthritis may be responsible. This would imply that sleep rhythms are disturbed due to the causative factors in arthritis. The disturbed sleep then worsens the body's ability to recover.

Several recent studies suggest that the sleep cycle may be tremendously important in arthritis. One study of sheep showed that removal of the pineal gland, which produces melatonin that regulates the circadian rhythm, causes loss of bone density.[69] Another study showed that there is a circadian clock in chondrocytes that grow and maintain articular cartilage. The clock controls several important aspects of chondrocyte function and cartilage maintenance.[70] This type of clock has daily oscillations in the level of biochemicals inside the chondrocytes. Important extracellular functions of chondrocytes are also regulated by the circadian clock, for example, synthesis of extracellular matrix (collagen, elastin, and others), and the growth of bone. Mice that lack the genes for controlling their circadian clock get ossification of tendons and articular cartilage, abnormal bone formation, and increased susceptibility to inflammatory arthritis.[71] An interesting finding of this study was that the circadian clocks in cartilage can sense small temperature differences. This suggests that by sensing small changes in body temperature from day to night, they can maintain their synchronization with the rest of the body. This may be especially important because cartilage has no nerves or blood vessels to give other reliable clock cues. Changing levels of hormones in the synovial fluid may also be involved in setting the chondrocyte clocks. Evidently the circadian rhythms are attenuated by aging, but the clocks from old and young tissue are similar. This implies that other factors, such as desynchronization by time cues from the rest of the body, are to blame. The authors of the study suggested that to minimize the risk of arthritis, the cartilage clocks could be "retuned" by strengthening the normal circadian clues; for example, scheduled exercise, restricted meal times, or scheduled warming and cooling of joints.[72] This study strongly emphasizes the importance of regular daily activity cycles synchronized with day and night.

In our modern society, people lose sleep for a variety of reasons. Some can't sleep because of pain, anxiety, or sleep apnea. These conditions can wreak havoc for the daily sleep cycle and for recovery from stress and inflammation.[73] Those who work the night shift and then attempt to be active during the daytime may not get adequate sleep. This issue is worsened with our modern lighting and alarm clocks,[74] because these tend to shift our normal cycles of activity away from the daylight hours. Looking at any source of bright light during the night hours, for example, looking at a bright television or computer screen late at night, confuses the circadian rhythms of the brain. The brain's master circadian clock in the suprachiasmatic nucleus (SCN) is set by blue light, and kicks in just before dusk to give us a "second wind" and keep us alert at the end of the day. But exposure to bright bluish light late at night resets the circadian clock, resulting in loss of sleep. Airlines that shine blue light into the cabin at night contribute to the problem. Midnight snacks can also confuse the body's rhythms of activity, and drinks containing caffeine can cause problems with sleep. These effects emphasize that modern technology has decoupled our bodies from the twenty-four hour daily cycle to which they evolved.[75]

As anyone with continual joint pain knows, arthritis is made worse by the lack of sleep induced by the pain. The lack of sleep can prevent the body from accomplishing its natural process of healing the joints, and the resulting pain that builds up can then reduce the amount of deep sleep that is necessary for the healing process.[76] Further, for some with chronic pain, the intensity of the pain signal in the brain is made worse by the lack of sleep.[77] Thus, an adequate amount of sleep (for many people, eight hours or more) is very important.

RHEUMATOID ARTHRITIS

Inflammation in joints is the common feature in rheumatoid arthritis (RA), usually in the hands, wrists, elbows, knees, feet, toes, and neck. It is usually bilateral, that is, it occurs in joints on both the left and right sides of the body. Although rheumatoid arthritis is relatively rare, found in only 1 percent of the general population, it causes major disruption in many peoples' lives. Its onset can be at any age, from young children to old age, but is most often in middle age (twenty-five to fifty-five). It is thought to have a genetic component that increases an individual's susceptibility.[78] Although the specific cause of RA is unknown, it is thought to be an auto-inflammatory or allergic reaction to the tissues of the joints, often the synovial membrane.[79] Evidently, the disease process starts with some sort of stress to the joints, which send out a signal to the immune system. The stress can originate with an injury or infection, or can be due to a genetic predisposition.[80]

One current hypothesis about the origin of RA states that free radicals generated by oxidative stress cause damage to proteins such as type II collagen found in joints. The damage makes the proteins look foreign to the body, which then attacks them with its immune system.[81] If this hypothesis is correct, it suggests that preventing the damage from oxidative stress should prevent RA from developing. Researchers studying RA will measure the level of antibodies that bind to the damaged collagen proteins. This will then be used as an objective metric of RA when testing treatments.[82] A similar hypothesis states that damaged proteins outside the joint are the initial trigger for inflammation, often several years before the symptoms of RA are apparent. This inflammation may cause blood vessels near the synovial membrane to become more permeable, thus allowing antibodies from the bloodstream to reach the inner lining of the synovial membrane.[83] This process worsens the inflammation and initiates RA. This inflammation apparently tips the balance towards resorption of cartilage, because the levels of enzymes that degrade cartilage, collagenase and elastase, are much higher in RA patients.[84] Overall it is clear that oxidative stress is involved in the initial trigger for RA.[85]

Most people who get injuries to their joints heal without any problem. But in a few, the cells from the immune system release signaling molecules (cytokines), that recruit more immune cells and start the inflammation process that becomes RA. The cytokines cause more blood vessels to grow into the synovial membrane and become more porous, so they exude more fluid into the synovial capsule.[86] The cells in the synovial membrane grow too fast (hyperplasia of synovial fibroblasts), and the membrane gets thicker. The immune system then becomes involved. Immune cells attempt to stop the proliferating synovial cells, which starts an inflammation. The extra fluid in the joint increases the pressure in the synovial capsule, which causes it to swell and become warm. These are the telltale signs of joint inflammation. The process continues when cells in the synovial membrane continue to grow as fibrous material, which tends to fill up the space in the joint. But the immune cells also attack the cartilage and underlying bone. This gradually erodes the cartilage, sometimes causing extreme pain. The chondrocytes try to grow more collagen matrix to repair the collagen, and the subchondral plate underneath grows to form new bone. In some RA patients this process is successful, and the pain stops and the joint regrows in a few years.[87] However, in other patients, arthritis occurs in many joints simultaneously (polyarthritis). This is a sign of widespread inflammation. A minority of patients who get polyarthritis recover within a few months. But in other patients, the joint does not grow back correctly and becomes deformed, and the degeneration may progress to get worse.[88] It is thought that RA in any individual is caused by several factors, such as genetic predisposition, some type of injury or infection combined with multiple nutrient deficiencies, food or toxin sensitivities, and dehydration.[89] To optimally lower your risk, you may want to investigate each of these factors.

The genetic predispositions for RA include the "human lymphocyte antigen" (HLA) family of genes, which set how the body recognizes and attacks foreign organisms like bacteria, viruses, and molds. If you have the HLA-DR4 allele, you are considered to have a higher risk for RA. Another gene common in RA patients is HLA-DR1. Another risk factor is a mutation in the gene for glutathione-S-reductase (GSTM1-null allele), which is responsible for assisting glutathione to detoxify free radicals.[90]

However, people with these gene alleles do not necessarily always get RA. Studies of identical twins have shown that when one twin gets RA, the other only has a 20 percent risk of getting it. In other studies, the genetic component has been estimated at 50 percent.[91] This implies that although some genes do not directly cause RA, they may increase the risk for RA. Therefore nutritional therapies are likely to provide some therapeutic benefit.

Many medical doctors advise that diet has no effect on RA. However, nothing could be further from the truth. Tragically, most doctors don't have time to read the nutrition research literature, so they may not be familiar with it. Many studies have shown an effect of diet for RA, and we will discuss this topic in Chapter 5. Although not all studies on RA have shown positive effects of diet, they may not have been performed correctly. For example, some of the clinical trials testing the effect of diet included one or more of the foods likely to trigger episodes of RA. As we will explain below, diet is just one of many factors involved in causing RA, but it can be a big factor in healing RA.

Drugs for RA include analgesics, nonsteroidal anti-inflammatory drugs (NSAIDs), corticosteroids, disease-modifying antirheumatic drugs (DMARDs), biologic response markers, and antibiotics.[92] Each of these drugs has helped some fraction of RA patients, but they all have side effects and they all pose risks. In some cases, NSAIDs or corticosteroids can worsen damage to joints and lengthen the time it takes to heal broken bones.[93] It is possible to select the most appropriate treatment by asking your doctor a series of questions about how each drug may help you. Because RA in each individual may have a different origin, the response to treatment will also differ.[94] Nutritional treatments have helped prevent and reverse RA in many patients and they are much safer, cheaper, and usually more effective than drugs. By strengthening your body with excellent nutrition, including essential nutrients that help the immune system and joints to recover, you can go a long way towards pain-free joints.

Risk Factors for RA

There are several strong risk factors for RA related to lifestyle. Smoking is the biggest. It is responsible for up to 25 percent of the risk for an average individual, and some of the risk continues for several decades after cessation.[95] Obesity and diet are fairly strong risk factors, and coffee intake is a risk factor for some types of RA. Infection is a known risk factor. In fighting off an infection, the body's immune system may be confused and attack the joints. An injury to a joint or a bone is also a risk factor for RA. When a bone breaks, the normal process of healing causes the bone and its surrounding tissue to become inflamed. If the bone takes a long time to heal, the inflammation may trigger RA. About 20 percent of those diagnosed with RA have had such a fracture in the preceding six months.[96] Thus, if you break a bone, it may be particularly helpful to eat an excellent diet with all the nutrients needed by the bone and joint, to minimize the healing time. This may lessen the risk that inflammation from the healing process will trigger RA. And for all arthritis sufferers, and even those who don't have arthritis, it's important to eat an excellent diet to prevent triggering new OA or RA episodes.

Deficiencies of essential nutrients are also a big risk factor for RA. As in OA, the reason is thought to be that the cartilage in articular joints has difficulty getting enough nutrition because it contains no blood vessels. People with deficiencies of antioxidants, the B, D and E vitamins, and minerals such as zinc and selenium are at higher risk.[97] Interestingly, a common cause for such deficiencies is an inability to digest properly because of not enough stomach acid. An inability to digest can be caused by not eating and digesting enough vegetables and fruits, or it can be caused by dehydration, both of which are common in the modern world. Poor digestion can also be caused by not chewing food adequately, or a lack of digestive acid or enzymes secreted in saliva or the stomach. Dehydration can also cause the cartilage of a joint to malfunction, because cartilage depends on water to help cushion the weight of the body. When the body becomes dehydrated, less water is available for the joints. The cartilage will shrink and the surface may become rough, which prevents the joint from articulating properly.[98] We will discuss the topic of nutrition in Chapter 5.

With the advent of genetic testing and powerful statistical methods, researchers hope that the risk factors for RA can be discovered. If those who are genetically predisposed get a disease such as RA without the involvement of any other obvious risk factors, this may allow the genetic factors to be identified.[99] The fact that RA is relatively rare (less than 1 percent of the population) has provided impetus to this effort. The DNA of those who have the disease is analyzed and their mutations are tabulated. The mutations that are most strongly associated with RA then become labeled as risk factors. This process works even in the usual case where the function of the gene is not understood, but eventually it is hoped that the function of the gene and the specific mutation will be determined. This of course is a huge benefit we receive from medical research. In this case, the dysfunction caused by the gene mutation is a relatively straightforward way to determine which gene mutations are involved.

Infection Can Trigger RA

In some cases, the trigger for RA appears to be an inflammatory allergic reaction to the tissues of the joints. For example, if a joint is attacked by an infection, the immune system of the body may attack the synovial membrane. An infection is the trigger for about 20 percent of the cases of early phase RA.[100] The infection is thought to evoke the body's autoimmune response that causes inflammation in the joint. Some strains of bacteria stimulate proinflammatory cytokines and can initiate arthritis. Apparently small differences in biomolecules synthesized by bacteria can make them arthritogenic (able to initiate arthritis) or nonarthritogenic.[101] In some cases, it is thought that the immune system may confuse natural molecules in the joint with the foreign molecules from the infecting organism. Then the immune system attacks the body's own natural molecules and damages the joint. In one type of arthritis, viruses and bacteria can infect the synovial fluid and cartilage. They can "hide out" in joints more readily than in other tissues because the articular cartilage has no blood vessels, and the synovial fluid is to some extent outside the immediate influence of the immune system.

Currently several viruses and bacteria (for instance, hepatitis C and herpes, cytomegalovirus, mycoplasma, staphylococcus, or streptococcus) are being investigated for their possible role in initiating RA. Hepatitis B, hepatitis C, and HIV virus infections often cause RA-like symptoms.[102] Commonly, patients who have previously been infected with hepatitis B, and who are being treated for RA or other immune-mediated inflammatory disease have a reactivation of hepatitis B.[103] In a different type of arthritis, called "reactive arthritis" (ReA, also called Reiter's disease), an infection in the body causes an inflammation in the joint without actually infecting the joint.[104] In a study of people with a salmonella infection in the gut, it was found that the incidence of reactive arthritis was much higher (4.4 percent) than in the general population (0.002 percent).[105] Although this type of study does not show causality, it suggests what RA sufferers already know intuitively: that an infection can trigger pain in joints.

One hypothesis about the cause of RA states that in some individuals it is due to periodontal pathogens (bacteria in the mouth and gums). RA has long been known to be associated with periodontal disease and has on occasion been successfully treated with antibiotics.[106] Higher levels of antibodies to periodontal bacteria have been found in RA, and antibodies in people with certain bacterial infections are also found in patients with RA. Further, the DNA from these bacteria has also been found in the synovial fluid of joints of patients with RA.[107] Of course, these bacteria are also found in many other types of infection. Apparently, in some cases the genetic susceptibility of RA patients allows the infection to take place. The infection may occur in response to a weakened immune system, suggesting that an excellent diet and adequate doses of essential nutrients and antioxidants such as vitamin C may help.

Some patients who have reduced immunoglobulin (a form of immune system disorder) may be at risk for infections such as mycoplasma in their joints. Mycoplasma is a relatively common consequence of pneumonia. An infection of mycoplasma can cause pain and inflammation of the synovial capsule and fluid of several joints simultaneously (polyarthritis), and is commonly misdiagnosed as RA. However, a culture of the synovial fluid may not immediately show the infection, because mycoplasma is slow growing. After a proper diagnosis by a medical doctor, it can be treated with a tetracycline-type antibiotic such as doxycycline.[108]

Smoking and RA

Smoking is a big risk factor for RA, because it introduces many toxins into the body that cause oxidative stress and free radicals. As a result, smoking lowers the level of antioxidants vitamin C and vitamin E in the bloodstream.[109] This causes inflammation throughout the body. Smoking is a known risk factor for heart disease, cancer, and many other diseases such as RA that are related to inflammation. Smoke contains thousands of harmful chemicals, many that can cause oxidative stress in the body. The body attempts to detoxify these chemicals using metabolic pathways involving nicotinamide adenine dinucleotide (NAD), derived from niacin. This suggests that niacin and other B vitamins are important for recovery from exposure to toxic chemicals. Among the toxins contained in smoke are heavy metals such as cadmium and lead that accumulate in the body.[110] The levels of these and other heavy metals are higher in smokers than in nonsmokers, and they are also higher in nonsmoking RA patients. Further, the levels of zinc were inversely proportional to the levels of heavy metals, in smokers and also in RA patients. Zinc is an essential nutrient for many biochemical pathways including the body's immune system. Smoking multiplies the risk for many diseases including RA for the general population by severalfold. The lesson here, of course, is don't smoke, and minimize your exposure to environmental toxins.

Environmental Toxins and RA

Toxins in food and our environment are thought to be a big risk factor for RA.[111] They increase oxidative stress in the body which can cause free radicals. These free radicals can damage cells and their DNA, and can cause inflammation throughout the body. Food allergies are thought to worsen RA. As described above, there are many genetic risk factors for RA, and some of them involve the mutation and functional loss of genes that help to lessen oxidative stress.

A recent book on toxins in our environment explains that our bodies typically contain dozens of chemicals that are known to be harmful and cause disease.[112] They are found throughout the modern environment. Some originate from the petrochemical industry, and others originate from farm runoff, drugs that get into the sewer system, engine exhaust fumes, and smoking. They are especially insidious because they're virtually everywhere in our home and work environment. Some of these chemicals are added to our food and water, and others are in plastic items purchased in the supermarket and stores that sell toys, clothing, hardware, and furnishings.

A common chemical we're all exposed to is phthalates, which are commonly added to plastics to increase their flexibility and transparency.[113] This chemical is volatile and does not remain permanently in its plastic host, but can easily outgas into the surrounding air, especially under high temperatures. The "new car smell" is largely from such plasticizers in the plastic seating and dashboard materials. The phthalates evaporate from the plastic seat covering when the car gets hot, and then tend to condense on the cooler window glass where they are visible as a thin oily film. Phthalates are contained in many household plastic items such as shower curtains, raincoats, water bottles, toys, and foam mattresses. And inevitably, household dust contains phthalates. They are also commonly found in foods, in part because plastic food wraps and containers may contain them. Fatty foods such as meat or cheese can pick up phthalates from stretchy vinyl food wrap. Phthalates are thought to cause developmental defects in humans, and have been associated with obesity, asthma, and cancer. They are also associated with respiratory problems, asthma, and allergy.[114] Although phthalates are eliminated in a few days from the body, most of us have continual exposure that potentially can cause disease.

Another toxic chemical in plastics is bisphenol A (BPA), is used to make polycarbonate plastic (labeled as "type 7: other"), and some epoxy resins, both of which are found in many consumer products.[115] It is also found in cash register thermal printout paper. Its structure is similar to the hormone estradiol, a sex hormone, and it mimics the effect of estrogens. These estrogen effects can affect the development of the fetus, infants, and children, at very low levels that can be caused by BPA leaching from plastics. BPA is considered to be an endocrine disruptor and is now banned in plastics meant for infants. Compounds other than BPA that mimic estrogen can leach from a variety of plastics. The amount of estrogen mimics leached out of plastics is accelerated by UV exposure from sunlight, microwaving, or high temperature washing.[116] Current research on this topic is still in its infancy, and as more is learned about the effects of chemicals leaching from plastics, the public can take better precautions. For now, it appears that glass containers or ceramic plates are best for microwaving.

Another household chemical that causes allergy and other immune problems is triclosan, used as an antimicrobial in hand soaps and detergents.[117] A dangerous persistent chemical that pollutes the environment and the body is polychlorinated biphenyls (PCBs) which were used inside industrial equipment such as power transformers. They can cause oxidative stress and are thought to contribute to arthritis by inducing cell death of chondrocytes.[118] Other prominent sources of pollution in the home are organic solvents, in paints, glues, nail polishes and removers, and dry cleaners. They are also in industrial adhesives, for example in particle board used for cabinetry and house construction, and flame retardants in curtains, rugs, and furniture. These chemicals can cause asthma, allergies, and inflammation. Household water in many communities is polluted by many industrial chemicals, and the purification treatments given to the municipal water don't remove these chemicals.

Another very common set of harmful chemicals comes from the exhaust of cars and trucks. One of the dangerous chemicals in exhaust is benzene and its related compounds, which are aromatic and smell sweet. It is often possible to detect this smell when driving behind a car or truck that doesn't have a properly working catalytic converter in the exhaust system. When you can smell this chemical, it is already at a level considered dangerous, because it is readily absorbed from the air and causes inflammation and cancer. Diesel exhaust particles are very toxic, and can cause allergy and inflammation.[119] Although these chemicals may be present in low levels, many are powerful and can cause harm in low concentrations. Thus the typical household, commuting route, and workplace is heavily polluted with chemicals that over decades can cause disease.[120] You may want to take steps to reduce the pollution in the air you breathe. For example, you can alter your daily commute to work to avoid exhaust fumes, either by commuting in the off-rush hours or by altering the route you take to work. And you may want to take adequate doses of antioxidants such as vitamin C to help the body detoxify the environmental toxins.

Persistent Toxins in the Environment

Persistent chemicals such as DDT and other pesticides get into the soil, ground water, and atmosphere and now pollute every environmental niche on earth. Although normally present in the environment at low levels, once they get into living organisms they tend to get concentrated in the body. Animals at the top of their food chain, such as tuna, tend to concentrate these chemicals and other pollutants. These include the heavy metals lead, arsenic, and mercury. Considering that humans are the top predators, we must be vigilant about the effects of chemicals in the home and workplace. As mentioned above, PCBs are another persistent chemical in the environment that is toxic and causes oxidative stress, potentially leading to arthritis.

Lead is a big problem in the environment for several reasons. For many decades of the twentieth century, lead was added to gasoline used to power cars and trucks. Microscopic particles of lead were emitted by vehicles in their exhaust. For centuries, even before gasoline, lead was added to paint to increase its durability and as a pigment. Further, lead pipes can contaminate drinking water, and many old houses in cities still have lead pipes or copper pipes soldered with lead. The derivation of the word "plumbing" is the Latin word "plumbum," for lead. It was not realized originally that lead is a very toxic element for the body, but once this fact became known it took a long time before medical researchers could determine the extent of the problem in the body. The lead particles from paint and leaded gasoline have contaminated most major cities, settling as fine dust into the soil and water and contaminating virtually all forms of life.[121] Young children especially are prone to lead poisoning, as they tend to ingest lead dust around the house and from contaminated soil. Lead damages the development of the brain in children, and damages the body in many other ways, and therefore it has been a major health problem.[122] Health departments of cities, counties, states, and the federal government all recognize the problem, and lead contamination in the typical household environment has lessened over the past five decades. However, lead contamination is still a problem in most cities and will be for many decades.[123] And, as described above, smoking increases the blood level of heavy metals including lead, arsenic, and cadmium. These are

RACHEL CARSON AND THE ENVIRONMENTAL MOVEMENT

The role of environmental toxins was widely publicized in 1962 by Rachel Carson's famous book *Silent Spring*.[128] She explained how many of the pesticides and herbicides created by the petrochemical industry persist in the environment, even when applied correctly according to standard practice, because they are resistant to breakdown by living organisms. And she correctly foresaw that within a decade or two after their first application pesticides and herbicides in regular use would cause pests and weeds to become resistant to their effects. The poisons kill off most of the pests, but some survive because one or more of the genes in their DNA have changed or mutated. This is a normal process known as natural selection that happens randomly from one generation to the next. Invariably the pests and weeds evolve to make the pesticides and herbicides ineffective. Farmers must then apply higher levels and different combinations of pesticides, which further pollute the environment. This is a continuing problem for agriculture and the entire planet.

Farmers don't want to pollute the environment, and they want their crops to be safe and free of pesticides. Some pesticides are supposed to break down within a few days so they will not persist in the soil, water, and air. But for a variety of reasons they are often not applied correctly to fruits and vegetables in time to allow the residues to degrade before sale.[129] Further, the pesticide residues are typically concentrated in the peel, which contains many of the helpful nutrients.[130] New, "improved" pesticides are being developed, but they are often not thoroughly tested for their effects on humans, wildlife, and soil organisms. For example, over the last several decades, pesticides for spraying on apples have been under continual development to make them less toxic to mammals.[131] Animal products often contain higher levels of persistent toxic chemicals than plants because as the chemicals pass through the food chain, they become concentrated. Although much progress has been made, unfortunately our environment today contains many persistent toxic chemicals at unacceptable levels.[132]

Some chemicals, such as oils, modern detergents, and some pesticides, degrade fairly rapidly in the environment, often with help from bacteria. However, chemicals such as DDT, (dichloro-diphenyl-trichloro-ethane), dieldrin, dioxin, PCBs (polychlorinated biphenyls) and many others are not easily degraded.[133] These chemicals wreak havoc on beneficial insects and wild animals in the natural world. For example, it is thought that several types of pesticides sprayed on crops are a major factor in the large scale loss of honey bee colonies.[134] These pesticides are insidious because they can prevent bees from flourishing and can decimate a hive even at levels far below a lethal dose. The wide use of pesticides and herbicides has decimated populations of butterflies and many other beneficial insects.[135] It seems likely that these and other modern pesticides also have unintended sublethal effects on humans.[136]

Genetically-modified organisms (GMOs) are plants or animals that have been given an artificial gene that can convey a new function or characteristic. Much of the soybean, cotton, maize, canola, alfalfa, and sugar beet crops are now GM. Although similarity exists between some GM crops and varieties created through traditional genetic crossbreeding, many GM crops contain genes completely foreign to the species that are considered potentially dangerous. The reason is that, for a variety of reasons, a foreign gene inserted into a species may cause effects that are unpredictable, based on the content of the foreign gene.

In the GM process, crops are commonly endowed with a gene for resistance to a sprayed herbicide, or a gene to synthesize a pesticide to kill insects. Both of these mechanisms can be dangerous to beneficial plants and insects and to the environment as a whole. A recent study of a GM crop found that a pesticide commonly sprayed on GM crops, and the GM maize that is resistant to it, may increase the risk of cancer.[137] Although the study was quickly criticized by many investigators, including the GMO industry, it remains the only detailed study of the effects of a pesticide at realistic levels on mammals over their life span.[138] A possible mechanism for causing cancer in this case is that at very low levels the pesticide might cause hormonal endocrine disruption.

A current controversy exists about whether genetically modified organisms should be labeled for the consumer.[139] Generous funding from the huge corporations that stand to make a bigger profit from selling GMOs has biased public opinion on this topic. One indication of the controversy is that a large manufacturer of breakfast cereal in the United States has agreed to label and sell one version of the cereal created without GM content.

GM crops are currently regulated in Europe but unregulated in the United States, and new GM crops are currently under review for exclusion from regulation in the United States. A petition for GM apples that lack activation of polyphenol oxidase, so they will not brown when bruised during processing, is currently being by the United States Department of Agriculture.[140] The use and sale of GM crops is currently a controversial topic. It is apparent that more studies by independent laboratories will be necessary to provide assurance that the crops and the pesticides sprayed on them are safe. The memory of the damage done to the environment by DDT and other pesticides and herbicides continues to be very provocative.

In the years after *Silent Spring* was published, it soon became obvious that persistent chemicals and pesticides were dangerous and their use should be limited. This revolutionary book was the start of the modern environmental movement. It led to congressional hearings and then directly to the formation of the Environmental Protection Agency.[141] Although the use of some persistent chemicals has been limited, contamination of our environment and food continues.[142] Because environmental toxins are implicated in oxidative stress and inflammation, sometimes even when present at very low levels, you may want to limit your exposure to them to give your body the best chance of recovery from arthritis.

associated with an increase in risk for RA.[124] You should minimize your exposure to heavy metals.

Another set of triggers for RA is silicon compounds, including silica, asbestos, and silicone.[125] Miners, and agricultural and construction workers are exposed to silica dust in the air and have a higher rate of RA than the general population. Women with silicone breast implants also have a higher rate of RA.

Recently the President's Cancer Panel reported that environmental toxins are a big cause of cancer and other diseases.[126] The doctors on this panel recommended to the president that the previous standards for workplace and home exposure to chemicals are outdated, and they recommended the use of more organic foods, which have fewer chemicals. This and other practical advice can help reduce exposure to toxins.[127] Some RA patients who must remain vigilant against environmental toxins can well take the same advice.

An Orthomolecular Approach to Dealing with Toxins

Toxins can cause inflammation by oxidizing the biochemicals throughout the body. They can impair the immune system, causing inflammation, sterility, cancer, and many other diseases. The industrial chemicals that are found in the body are thought to contribute to triggering RA, because they cause inflammation and impair the immune system. Thus, someone with RA should eliminate as much exposure to environmental toxins as possible.

Antioxidants such as vitamins C and E and glutathione can detoxify many harmful chemicals and toxins.[143] Further, the body can detoxify and metabolize many toxins, drugs, and other synthetic chemicals (xenobiotics). The detoxification is done by enzymes in the liver.[144] Fortunately, the body makes more detoxifying enzymes when exposed to pollutant chemicals. The classical example is PCBs, which are oily polluting molecules that persist in the environment because they are not easily broken down by bacteria. Exposure to PCBs can cause thousandfold increases in the production of the liver enzymes that detoxify them. The enzymes modify the PCB molecule to make it more water soluble, allowing the body to excrete it in the urine. Humans have approximately sixty different enzymes and cofactors that provide some degree of detoxification. But the ability to detoxify chemicals with these enzymes varies among individuals. Therefore, some people are much more prone to their toxic effects. Some of the detoxifying enzymes depend on vitamin cofactors. The cofactor most commonly used by these enzymes is NAD, which is derived from niacin. However, even when levels of the toxin and the detoxifying enzyme are high, a deficiency of the vitamin cofactor can limit the process of detoxification. Taking high doses of niacin along with an excellent diet can increase the detoxification, metabolism, and excretion of many toxic chemicals. This can be achieved by taking high doses of niacin (1,000–3,000 milligrams (mg) per day taken in divided doses). For this purpose, it may be helpful to take a dose high enough to get a niacin flush, and then maintain a high niacin and vitamin C level throughout the day with smaller doses (250–500 mg) every hour.

Oxidative Stress and RA

Many studies have shown that RA patients have elevated levels of oxidative stress, especially from inflammation in the joints.[145] This oxidative stress may originate in several different ways, depending on the individual. Some is caused by the body's normal oxidative metabolic pathways. Indeed, moderate amounts of some reactive oxygen species (ROS) are helpful to prevent infection and signal damage to initiate the body's response.[146] Evidently, some conditions that increase ROS can ameliorate RA.[147] However, severe oxidative stress can cause disease. Infection by bacteria or viruses generates oxidative stress. Eating food that contains polyunsaturated fatty acids that have gone rancid generates oxidative stress. And, as we have seen above, toxins are everywhere in the environment. Smoking is a major one. Toxins such as smoke and heavy metals exert their harmful effects by damaging generating ROS or reactive nitrogen species (RNS) from normal biochemicals in the body.[148] The body attempts to deal with these harmful toxins by detoxifying them; that is, by donating an electron to the free radicals so they cannot cause further damage. The detoxification is accomplished by antioxidants. The liver performs much of this work, but it also takes place in the blood and tissues throughout the body. For example, damage to DNA in synovial cells can contribute to arthritis, and can be prevented with antioxidants.[149] But toxins, and the free radicals they create, are ubiquitous in the environment. This is a serious threat to RA patients susceptible to oxidative stress.

Part of the problem is that it is not known whether many chemicals and environmental pollutants known to be harmful or toxic at high levels are safe at the typical low levels we are exposed to in our everyday lives. Some toxins, such as dioxin, are thought to be unacceptable at any amount or level because they may cause cancer. We know that smoke is bad to breathe, but how about air pollution in a large city? Standards for acceptable environmental levels of many toxins have been set by the government.[150] However, in many cases it is not known how safe these levels really are. In many cases, the acceptable levels have been lowered as more is learned about the effects of environmental toxins on the body. Often the standards are defined for the blood level of a substance, but this doesn't allow ready determination of the source of contamination.[151] Toxins in our food and water are especially important, for we are what we eat.

Many chemicals that we are exposed to, even at very low levels, tend to cause problems with the immune system, such as allergies and asthma and possibly cancer.[152] They can damage the DNA of a cell, preventing it from performing its normal function. In RA, this type of damage can be caused by oxidative stress from the original trigger or the body's immune system. The cells in the synovial lining around the joint try to combat the problem by elevating their DNA repair enzymes severalfold above normal levels.[153] But this is apparently not enough, and damage to DNA occurs and tends to progressively get worse. Beyond their damaging oxidative damage to other molecules, toxins are known to increase the levels of inflammatory cytokines, which signal the immune system inflammatory response. One mechanism for this effect is thought to be the depletion of antioxidants such as glutathione. When this happens, it causes an imbalance in the immune system's cytokine signaling pathways.[154] This can cause inflammation that can lead to disease.

Antioxidants Help Fight Toxins

Antioxidants in the diet can prevent the oxidative stress caused by environmental toxins. Glutathione is often mentioned, because its reduced form, GSH, is used as a measure of oxidative stress.[155] As described in Chapter 2, the antioxidant glutathione is one of the most important antioxidants inside cells. Its reduced (normal) form indicates the amount of oxidative stress in the body's tissues. When inundated with toxins from the environment, the levels of glutathione inside cells go down. In RA patients, the level of glutathione and other antioxidants is lower than normal.[156] This is not thought to be due to a malfunction of the mechanism generating antioxidants. In RA the level of glutathione peroxidase (GSH-Px) differs from normal subjects. In one study, GSH-Px was elevated,[157] and in other studies it was lowered.[158] This enzyme is responsible mediating the reaction with glutathione that removes reactive oxygen radicals. The level of glutathione S-transferase and gamma-glutamyl transpeptidase, enzymes that help recycle gluthathione back to its original form, are also increased.[159] This suggests that in RA the body is trying to increase the level of the antioxidants that have been depleted, but its antioxidant system may be overwhelmed.[160]

If correct, this hypothesis implies that the lower levels of glutathione and other antioxidants such as vitamin C occur in RA patients because of their oxidative stress. This abnormally low level of antioxidants cannot deal with the body's oxidative stress, which may be one of the causes of RA. A supporting bit of evidence comes from a study on mice in which the enzyme superoxide dismutase was overexpressed, causing its level to increase in the synovial tissue. This enzyme is essential in the body's defense against free oxygen radicals. In this study, the increased level of this antioxidant enzyme lowered the amount of inflammation from arthritis.[161] Another piece of supporting evidence comes from a case study in which vitamin C and glutathione were given intravenously to a RA patient. This treatment caused immediate reduction of acute pain.[162] Overall, the evidence that oxidative stress contributes or causes RA is very robust.

As described above in Chapter 2, antioxidants are synergistic, meaning that each one can help combat oxidative stress, preventing depletion of other antioxidants, and also each one can help regenerate the others after they've been depleted. This can happen with antioxidants made by the body, such as glutathione, and other essential antioxidants such as vitamins A, C, and E. A study of oxidative stress in patients with RA showed that the levels of vitamins A, C, and E as well as GSH were lower than in people without RA.[163] This is also true for other antioxidants that are obtained in the diet. Zinc is an essential mineral that is also an antioxidant.[164] In a study on the cause of arthritis, the levels of zinc were measured in relation to the levels of heavy metals.[165] The level of heavy metals was higher in arthritis patients, even in those who didn't smoke. Moreover, the arthritis patients had lower levels of zinc. Since it is already known that zinc is necessary for the body and helps to prevent disease, this finding suggests that heavy metals, which are known toxins for the body, contribute to arthritis, and that zinc and likely other antioxidants can help to prevent this disease.

Finding Allergy Triggers for Your RA

Allergies are another potential trigger for RA. These include food allergies and sensitivities, as well as airborne dust, pollen, and other environmental allergy-causing factors. In her web page on recovery from RA, Dr. Katherine Molnar-Kimber, a professional immunologist, explains that she discovered by chance some things in her daily life that triggered painful RA episodes.[166] She stopped using safflower oil and switched to olive oil, which helped some. After a trip away from home during which her pain went down, she realized that she had become allergic to the chickens her family had been keeping in the back yard. When the chickens were moved farther away from the house, and she changed clothes after collecting the eggs, her allergy got better. Finally, she gave the chickens away and her RA improved even more.

Searching through your daily routine to find the source of an allergy can be difficult. Foods are a common trigger for allergies or food sensitivities. To find which parts of your life cause the allergy can be a difficult path. It can be a lengthy process of elimination that may require trying different foods, different clothes, and different daily routines. Dr. Molnar-Kimber encourages everyone to study their symptoms and potential causes carefully. Make up your own mind about what will help you the most. Many popular books on arthritis advise on how to determine which foods you should avoid.[167] You may find that some of the remedies in these books help, but they may not help everyone, because RA has many different causes.

Food sensitivities can be allergic in nature, due to a problem with the immune system.[168] They can also be due to a metabolic problem such as lactose intolerance causing a problem with dairy products, or a pharmacologic reaction. They are sometimes evident with foods such as bananas, red wine, or Parmesan cheese. They can be "idiopathic," that is, of unknown cause and peculiar to an individual. Food sensitivities, even for foods that you've been eating all your life, can cause lack of sleep, inflammation throughout the body, or depression.

Another relevant aspect of food allergies and sensitivities is that they are generally caused by a weak immune system originating from a poorly nourished body. If you focus on getting excellent nutrition, with plenty of antioxidants and essential nutrients, many of your sensitivities will lessen and may disappear entirely. Further, the gut contains hundreds of different bacteria that are useful in several ways to the body. Different strains of gut bacteria have been shown to lower risk for RA.[169] For anyone taking antibiotics, it is important to take probiotics, either in pill form or as active yogurt once the course of antibiotics is finished. *Bacillus coagulans,* one of the beneficial microorganisms shown to help with RA, is available in many health food stores.[170] And as we describe below, vitamin C empowers the immune system and can prevent many allergies.[171] Vitamin C is a very effective anti-histamine. It lowers the blood level of histamine, so it effectively relieves allergy symptoms that are caused by high levels of histamine in the body.[172]

Everyone with arthritis knows that allergies and food sensitivities typically aren't as severe as the pain from arthritis. These two conditions aren't the same thing, and allergies may not always trigger RA. However, those who have episodes of RA know that allergies can trigger RA and are likely related. RA has many potential triggers, and allergies often play an important role.

The Elimination-Challenge Diet

One way to identify the foods you're sensitive to is to work on an "elimination-challenge" diet.[173] Several food groups are often considered to cause sensitivities, including corn, dairy products of cow's milk, wheat and barley, nightshades (potatoes, tomatoes, eggplant, peppers, and so on). Gluten in wheat and other cereals has been widely implicated in causing food sensitivity. Corn or other food oils can cause allergies depending on the degree of purification that removes the food protein.[174] However, although allergy tests are widely performed, they may not be as relevant for food sensitivities.

You can start by eliminating the food groups that most commonly cause food sensitivities (corn, dairy, wheat, and nightshades).[175] Don't eat one of these food groups at all for two weeks, and if you find no difference, go back to eating it, and then go on to eliminate the next. Many people find that they notice a change within a few days. If your symptoms persist, you can try eliminating more food groups: gluten (found in wheat, spelt, rye and barley), soy products, pork, and eggs. Other common possibilities are citrus, seafood, peanuts, or tree nuts. The idea is to keep a journal throughout this process, in which you write down what you've eliminated and what you've eaten, what symptoms you have or have lost, and your mood and level of energy, so you know exactly which foods are most likely responsible.

When the improvement from eliminating a food group is fairly quick, within a few days or weeks, the problem may be an allergy. Often it is possible to tentatively identify the problem as an allergy because it is accompanied by migraines, canker sores, and runny nose or postnasal drip.[176] Allergies can be greatly reduced with vitamin C taken to bowel tolerance. However, in some cases, improvements from eliminating foods have taken more than six months.[177] These cases may represent a different problem than allergy or food sensitivity. When you identify an improvement from eliminating a food group, you can then move on to try the "challenge" diet. From the culprit food group, add back the foods you've eliminated one at a time, to find specifically which one is causing the problem. This may take several months or more, depending on how many foods you've eliminated.[178]

Abstaining from the foods that cause your RA flare-ups can be more important than any other factor in your diet. Just remember that pain is temporary, but quitting can be longer lasting. Some regimens require that you stick with them in order to give them a chance to work. However, be true to yourself. For example, if you feel miserable when you eat certain foods that are potentially beneficial to treating arthritis, you may have a food sensitivity or allergy. So if a food or supplement makes you feel miserable, then stop taking it, adjust the dosage, or eat it along with a different food.

If you find that abstaining from a food group gives improvement, but only after several weeks or months, the cause may be different than a simple allergy or food sensitivity. For example, abstaining from wheat has been promoted to prevent inflammation, obesity, and a variety of syndromes and diseases. However, those who stop eating large portions of wheat products will be eating larger portions other types of food. Wheat products made primarily from white or enriched flour lack important nutrients, so any reason for not eating them is a good one! If the diet that replaces wheat products includes more fresh vegetables and fruits, and not an excessive amount of meat or fats, it is likely to provide fewer calories and larger amounts of essential nutrients, which will be more healthy. This replacement effect may be a major reason for the healthiness of switching to a restricted vegetarian diet.[179]

Many Causes for RA

Overall it's evident that RA can have many causes. RA in one person may have a different cause or trigger than in someone else, and in some cases RA may have several causes. One hypothesis proposes that there are more than three dozen types of trigger for RA, and that the response to therapy corresponds to the specific trigger.[180] The implication of this hypothesis is that to maximize your recovery from RA, you need to determine its specific cause and adjust the treatment accordingly. A risk factor for one type of RA, such as coffee, may not generate the same level of risk for an individual with a different type of RA.[181] Thus, an individual with RA may need to actively work on several fronts to learn what triggers their RA.[182] For example, you may want to limit your exposure to toxins and allergens in your environment. That includes while commuting to work, at your workplace, and especially in your household. And you may want to stop eating the food groups that give you food sensitivities. You may also want to make sure your diet is excellent, with plenty of green leafy vegetables and essential nutrients and antioxidants.

Discovering the trigger for RA in each individual is a process of searching for likely clues and then evaluating each one. Diet is possibly the easiest and most straightforward. As described above, you can discover RA triggers using an elimination-challenge diet. Lifestyle and environmental toxins may be more difficult, because our daily lives are dependent on many factors that we may not be able to change. Going on a trip where the surroundings and daily routines are different is one way to discover potential RA triggers.[183] For example, you may find that you feel better when traveling to a different city for a few days on business or pleasure. The local environment and daily routine will differ from your usual daily life. If you notice a difference in your RA, either better or worse, this evidence will give clues about the specific trigger. RA can be triggered by the chemicals that evaporate from new house furnishings, and you may find a clue by moving new furniture out of the house for a few days.

Diet can have a big effect on your recovery from RA. First, as explained above, in some individuals flareups of RA are known to be caused by certain foods, and eliminating these will help. Second, the immune system is empowered by an excellent diet, which can help to prevent allergic reactions. Third, an excellent diet along with vitamin supplements can help to prevent RA by lowering the oxidative stress in the body. Antioxidants in the diet and supplements taken in adequate doses can lower oxidative stress which will reduce the risk for RA.

ARTHRITIS-RELATED DISEASES

Although osteoarthritis is the most common form of arthritis, and rheumatoid arthritis is also widely known and feared, many other diseases can cause or be related to arthritis

Arthritis and Heart Disease

In patients with OA and RA, markers of inflammation are often found at high levels in the bloodstream. But inflammation is also a symptom associated with other age-related conditions such as heart disease, diabetes, and cancer.[184] Further, it is known that antioxidants such as vitamin C can reduce inflammation and lower risk of heart disease.[185] This raises the question of whether these diseases are caused by inflammation, or whether the inflammation is a consequence of one disease and initiates another. People with OA are 50 percent more likely than those without OA to have cardiovascular disease, and are twice as likely to have angina.[186] RA is also strongly correlated with heart disease.[187] Smoking is strongly associated with both cardiovascular disease and arthritis.[188] Hand OA is strongly linked to high LDL (low-density lipoprotein) cholesterol, a risk factor in heart disease.[189] Arthritis in the spine is strongly associated with cardiovascular disease.[190] Many lines of evidence point to heart disease being the result of inflammation due to oxidative stress.[191] To maintain blood pressure, the arteries require high strength, which is provided by collagen, the same biomolecule that is essential for the cartilage of joints. When collagen weakens the artery walls lose their strength, and the result is systemic inflammation. The arterial plaques often evident in heart disease are thought to be the result of the body trying to repair the weakened artery walls.[192] Inflammation in the arteries causes oxidative stress on the body and can spread to other areas such as the joints. And as we have explained above, OA is also thought to be the result of systemic inflammation. It is possible that the association of arthritis with cardiovascular disease may be directly causative in some way, but they both seem likely to originate from inflammation. And the causes of these conditions may not always be direct. For example, merely the observation of a spouse's suffering with OA is enough to increase the inflammatory markers for risk of heart disease.[193]

Leaky Gut Syndrome, Food Sensitivities, and Inflammation

There is some evidence that arthritis can be caused by sensitivity to certain foods or drugs such as antibiotics. In some cases, it is thought, the gut becomes more permeable than normal, so the body absorbs large molecules that haven't been fully digested and cause allergies or inflammation. In a recent article, Susannah Meadows, a reporter for a widely read newspaper, wrote that her son got arthritis at the age of three with joint pain and a limp.[194] Drug treatments didn't seem to help much, but a selective diet finally eliminated the arthritis. The diet that worked included no gluten, dairy, or refined sugar. It also eliminated nightshades (the potato, pepper, and tomato family). Her son took a probiotic, sour Montmorency cherry juice, and 2,000 mg or more omega-3 fatty acids from fish oil. These are known to reduce inflammation. The doses of nonsteroidal anti-inflammatory drugs given to the boy were restricted because they damage the gut.

Other studies have shown that lectins, a type of biomolecule that binds to carbohydrates, are likely involved in the inflammation response to foreign molecules that can trigger RA.[195] Some evidence suggests that lectins can cause inflammation of the cells that line the gut, allowing foreign molecules entry into the bloodstream. This can cause inflammation throughout the body, triggering RA. Eliminating the source of lectins in the diet can help some individuals with RA.

Inflammatory bowel disease is a condition in which the cells lining the gut become inflamed, in some cases because they are attacked by the immune system. Leaky gut syndrome may be related to inflammatory bowel disease, and both of these may be involved in or trigger RA. Some evidence suggests that pro-inflammatory cytokines, thought to be involved in inflammatory bowel disease, can be controlled by natural molecules in some foods and herbs.[196] Ginger, tamarind, some species of chrysanthemum, and some mushrooms are widely used as anti-inflammatory agents.

Irritable Bowel Syndrome and FODMAPs

Another related topic, irritable bowel syndrome (IBS), can be caused by FODMAPs, foods that contain certain short-chain sugars such as fructans (wheat, rye, artichoke, asparagus, and onion), fructose in excess of glucose (apples, pears, honey), galactans (beans), and lactose (milk).

These sugars are often poorly absorbed by the gut. Although

WHAT ARE FODMAPS?

FODMAPs is an acronym for a group of foods that can adversely affect some people.

F—Fermentable: carbohydrates that are fermented by bacteria instead of being broken down by digestive enzymes.

O—Oligosaccharides: short-chain carbohydrates, including fructans and galactans.

D—Disaccharides: pairs of sugar molecules. The most problematic is milk sugar (lactose).

M—Monosaccharides: a single sugar molecule. Free fructose is most problematic. Many foods that contain free fructose contain about an equal amount of free glucose. Some fruits have larger proportions of fructose to glucose. Apples and pears contain more than twice as much free fructose as glucose.

P—Polyols: Large amounts of polyols rarely occur in nature, so lots of people have trouble with them. They include sugar alcohols like xylitol, sorbitol, or maltitol.

fructose, a common sugar present in fruit, is not well absorbed by the gut in most individuals, its absorption is increased in the presence of glucose. The short-chain sugars that are not well absorbed remain in the gut and are easily fermented by many types of bacteria. This can cause inflammation, gas, and severe diarrhea.[197] This condition can be diagnosed by testing for breath hydrogen and methane. Irritable bowel syndrome has been successfully treated by strictly reducing or eliminating FODMAPs in the diet, and taking probiotics to encourage beneficial bacterial fauna in the gut.

Crohn's disease is a form of inflammatory bowel disease with a strong genetic component, and is thought to be triggered by a microorganism. It is often associated with ankylosing spondylitis (see below), in which an inflammation of the joints is caused by an autoimmune reaction in the body.[198]

Ankylosing Spondylitis

Ankylosing spondylitis (AS) is an autoimmune disease similar to RA in which the connective tissue in the body degrades, causing damage to the joints and eventually causing bones to fuse together. It is often found in the spine, where degradation of the spinal disks (made of collagen) allows the vertebrae to fuse. AS has a strong genetic component, and is also thought to be initiated by a trigger such as an infection or toxicity from heavy metals. It has been treated successfully with vitamin C.[199] An interesting case history was written by Norman Cousins about the successful treatment of his AS.[200] Although some doubt exists about the diagnosis, Cousins treated his condition by taking high doses of vitamin C. His rationale was that vitamin C is a necessary cofactor for the body in creating and maintaining collagen. Under a doctor's supervision, he took intravenous ascorbate starting with a small daily dose, and gradually increased it over several days to 25 grams (25,000 mg). The pain and stiffness of his joints was much better within a few days, and within weeks he was cured.

Other doctors have treated AS with vitamin C taken orally. Ordinarily, only a relatively moderate dose (2,000–6,000 mg per day, in divided doses) of vitamin C is tolerated, above which it produces a laxative effect in the gut by attracting water. This is known as the "bowel tolerance" for vitamin C. But during an illness, the body's requirement for vitamin C is increased, and much higher doses, up to 50,000–100,000 mg per day, can be tolerated. This treatment has cured ankylosing spondylitis.[201]

One hypothesis about the cause of AS is related to the well-known association between Crohn's Disease (a form of inflammatory bowel disease) and AS.[202] A microorganism, Klebsiella pneumoniae, is thought to cause inflammation in the gut, which spreads throughout the body, causing AS. The inflammation is hypothesized to originate in the similarity between an enzyme created by Klebsiella and normal proteins in the human body. This apparently confuses the body's immune system, which then generates inflammation in the gut. This hypothesis is strengthened by a report that treatment with an antibiotic has in some cases improved the inflammatory symptoms of AS.[203] Moreover, the Klebsiella organism requires a robust amount of starch. Our digestive enzymes cannot digest some forms of starch, so these large molecules normally remain in the gut for excretion. But Klebsiella can easily break down the large starch molecules which give it a ready source of energy. This suggests that those who eat a starchy diet may be encouraging the growth of Klebsiella in their gut. This often happens in young adults, which is the age group in which AS first appears. Thus, it is hypothesized that AS may be improved with a low-starch diet.[204] Ingestion of probiotics in pills or yogurt will tend to displace the Klebsiella and restore health.

Gout

Gout is one of the oldest diseases recognized by medical doctors, traditionally called "the disease of kings."[205] Like rheumatoid arthritis, gout is an inflammatory disease of the joints that is triggered by specific causes often related to diet or lifestyle. In recent decades, gout has become more common, with a prevalence of about 6 percent in men and 2 percent in women in the United States.[206] Typically it starts with a few occasional episodes of severe pain and swelling in the joints that peak within six to twelve hours.[207] These typically become more frequent, and eventually joint damage occurs.

Gout is caused by high levels of urate (hyperuricemia) in the bloodstream. An abnormally high level of urate may not cause gout symptoms for a period of months to years. But eventually as the urate level rises, it forms crystals (monosodium urate) in the joints. The urate crystals trigger inflammatory cytokines in the joint tissues that cause the immune system to generate inflammation.[208] The high levels of urate in the blood may in some cases be related to genetics or trauma such as surgery, but are often related to obesity or hypertension. The most significant risk factors causing gout include use of diuretic medications, alcohol consumption, and excessive meat consumption.[209] Gout can also be triggered by high iron or lead levels, some types of prescribed drugs, or renal failure.[210] High levels of calcium and oxalate in the urine that can cause kidney stones are also associated with gout.[211]

Uric acid is a normal metabolic product of purines that are in the DNA and RNA of all foods. It has a low solubility, so at high levels it tends to precipitate out of solution. Humans and higher primates lack the enzyme that degrades uric acid into a more soluble form. As a result, we tend to have high uric acid levels near to the saturation level.[212] This contributes to the risk for gout.

Lyme Disease

Infections caused by the tick-borne Lyme spirochete (borreliosis) and its associated co-infections can cause a moderate type of arthritis.[213] The Lyme infection is carried by a slow-growing spirochete (helical-shaped bacterium) that sometimes causes a red rash on the skin within a few days or weeks of a tick bite. If this is diagnosed soon enough, it can often be successfully treated by antibiotics taken for thirty days or more in adequate doses. But quite often no obvious rash occurs at the site of the tick bite, or the rash is not noticed. If the skin infection is left untreated, it can progress weeks or months later into secondary "chronic" Lyme disease that manifests as a variety of symptoms, such as blurred vision, numbness, facial nerve paralysis, a "strange headache," fatigue, muscle pains or spasms, a stiff neck, or joint inflammation.[214] Lyme disease, like syphilis, is often known as "the great imitator."

If this secondary infection is left untreated, a Lyme infection can progress over several years to a more serious tertiary stage with a variety of severe neurological problems, such as encephalitis, heart arrhythmias, ALS-, MS- or Parkinson's-like symptoms, epilepsy, marked personality changes, dementia, and death. These Lyme-caused neurological diseases are unfortunately often termed "idiopathic," or peculiar to the individual from an unknown cause, when the Lyme infection hasn't been diagnosed. The Lyme spirochete grows very slowly, with a doubling time of approximately twelve hours.[215] This is much slower than most other bacteria. The consequence of this slow growth is that a Lyme infection develops very slowly and requires antibiotics over a longer time than other types of infection. Also, a Lyme infection can grow in the brain so slowly—over a period of several months to years—that a patient may not notice the gradual increase in symptoms and insidious destruction of his or her life.

Another typical Lyme symptom is an asymmetrical inflammation (on one side of the body) that moves from one joint to another. In addition, many other serious diseases carried by bacteria and other single-celled organisms can be transmitted along with Lyme as co-infections. The deer tick, the tick that carries Lyme, is tiny, about 2 millimeters (mm) in length, about the size of a sesame seed. Its larvae are so small (approximately 0.5 mm, about the size of a speck of black pepper) that they are difficult to see. Both adult ticks and their larvae are commonly infected and can transmit Lyme and co-infections.

Lyme disease can be difficult to diagnose and treat because of the insidious properties of the borrelia spirochete organism. The Lyme spirochete is much more difficult to treat than syphilis, because it can burrow through arterial walls and migrate and encyst throughout the body to hide from antibiotics. When it is attacked by the body's immune system or antibiotics, it can migrate to locations in the body outside easy access from the immune system, such as the joints, which have no blood vessels. Lyme spirochetes are thought to persist in these locations, for example underneath a biofilm or as a cyst, for months or years. Therefore, a regimen of antibiotic treatment longer than the standard three weeks is often necessary. For tertiary or chronic Lyme, treatment with several antibiotics is often necessary for six to twelve months or even one or two years or more.[216] Moreover, several co-infections, including Ehrlichiosis, Babesiosis, Bartonella, and mycoplasma, are commonly carried by the same ticks that carry Lyme disease. And there are many other co-infections that are currently being discovered and studied. In some cases, a patient may have Lyme and one or two other co-infections that get confused with the Lyme infection. Luckily, Ehrlichiosis and Bartonella are stopped by the same antibiotics used for Lyme. However, Babesiosis and several other co-infections are not, and may require more powerful antibiotics. Bartonella is also known as "cat-scratch disease" and is fairly common among those in contact with cats. Although this is usually fairly benign, in some cases it can cause serious neurological symptoms, which can complicate treatment for Lyme disease.

When joint inflammation or pain occurs without any obvious cause, and is associated with other neurological Lyme symptoms such as headache, paralysis or numbness, or severe but transient pain without joint motion, it is best to get a comprehensive set of blood and urine tests for Lyme and its associated co-infections. Lyme can be effectively diagnosed if the proper tests are performed.[217] Generally, immuno-assay tests (ELISA, western blot) are used in the first round of tests. The ELISA tests are sensitive but not very specific, and are not conclusive because they may have a relatively high error rate. The western blot tests are more specific but tend to have a high miss rate. One reason is that several of the bands on the western blots, that indicate antigens from the Lyme organism, can't be tallied because the antigens are also present in the Lyme vaccination. Also, western blot tests can show the presence of antibodies against the Lyme spirochete, but these tests only indicate past exposure to the organism, not necessarily a live infection. The blood and urine PCR tests are helpful because they test for the DNA of the live organism, which is highly specific. The urine PCR test is very sensitive for Lyme because the urine is collected in the early morning which tends to concentrate any DNA from micro-organisms in the blood.

To get the correct tests, you may need to travel to make an appointment with a "Lyme-literate" doctor who has the proper expertise to diagnose the infection. Because Lyme infections often don't show up on tests, the ultimate diagnosis should be based on the clinical signs.[218] Doctors in Connecticut, Rhode Island, Massachusetts, New Hampshire, and Maine generally have seen many cases, and are allowed by their state medical boards to prescribe antibiotics for chronic Lyme disease. An infection with Lyme or mycoplasma is sometimes diagnosed as rheumatoid arthritis because the inflammatory symptoms are similar.[219] Other types of bacterial infections can cause fast degeneration of a joint, but Lyme typically progresses slowly.[220]

To help in fighting off the Lyme infection, several other types of treatment are available besides antibiotics. Several powerful herbs in the repertoire of Chinese herbal medicine are available to combat Lyme disease.[221] The role of nutritional supplements and diet, along with antibiotics, is thought to be very important in aiding the immune system to knock out the spirochete.[222] Large doses of vitamin C (6,000–10,000 mg per day, in divided doses), vitamin D (4,000–10,000 international units (IU) per day, depending on body weight), and vitamin E (400–1200 IU per day, mixed tocopherols), along with other antioxidants in the diet, may help.[223] In fact, the diets recommended for boosting the immune system to combat Lyme disease are excellent and will likely help to prevent and reverse standard osteoarthritis as well!

Although the pain of Lyme arthritis is usually not severe, the Lyme infection is potentially very dangerous and life-threatening. If not stopped it is likely to get worse and slowly destroy the patient's body and life. There is currently a huge epidemic of Lyme disease in the Northeastern United States (about 300,000 per year),[224] but it is spreading to the upper Midwest, to the Rocky Mountain states, and to the West Coast. It also is endemic in Europe, including Austria, Bulgaria, France, Germany, Latvia and Lithuania, Slovenia, Switzerland, the Netherlands, and the United Kingdom.[225] Only a minority of patients have been appropriately treated, for most have not been properly tested and are unaware they have the Lyme infection. Even if the arthritis or other symptoms are mild, it is very important to get properly tested to determine whether it is caused by a Lyme disease infection.[226] If you know or suspect you have been bitten by a tick, you may want to take a "low-risk" antibiotic such as amoxicillin prescribed by your doctor. However, if you have symptoms of chronic Lyme, don't follow the advice of a specialist who, on interpreting one of the (evidently) inadequate tests, explains that you've never been exposed to the disease! Get properly tested and treated, and watch your diet!

CHAPTER 4

What Genetics Can Teach Us about Arthritis

Every year the National Institutes of Health (NIH) spends almost 10 billion dollars performing publicly funded genetics research.[1] The results are available to the public through scientific papers[2] and also through the Online Mendelian Inheritance in Man database, OMIM.[3] The OMIM data provides information about gene function which allows the relationship between genes and vitamins to be readily determined. This data is useful for understanding the cause of arthritis and its prevention and recovery. A genetic mutation can directly cause a disease, or may only generate a tendency for a disease. The human genetic database of OMIM helps to understand the genetic inheritance of a particular individual and what genetic diseases are most likely.[4] Age-related disease may be influenced by genetic differences, but is more generally caused by diet and and lifestyle.

This chapter describes how to apply the fields of genetics and biochemistry to prevent or reverse arthritis, focusing on the specific nutrients involved in joint health. It covers the study of genes involved in osteoarthritis (OA) and gives crucial information about the nutritional requirements for optimizing the biochemical pathways involved in treating arthritis. A summary at the end of the chapter explains that sulfur and vitamin K are essential for preventing and reversing OA. A dietary approach to increasing sulfur and vitamin K is presented in Chapter 7.

THE COMPLEXITY OF NUTRITION TESTING

In order to appreciate the significance of genetics research for arthritis, it's important to understand that nutrition studies on people are very difficult to perform. Nutrition research is an exceptionally challenging scientific endeavor at its best, but it is also urgently needed by those who suffer from age-related disease such as arthritis. Frequently two different studies focused on the same nutritional treatment yield conflicting and opposite results. One study may show that a nutritional treatment works, while another may indicate that it does not. On the other hand, a drug may appear to be of great significance if it produces a desirable therapeutically beneficial effect without any initial apparent toxicity or side effects. When these mixed results are digested by the media (which will always seek novel and startling reports), it can lead to highly questionable or incorrect reports that can have a tragic impact on public health. The resulting confusion often discounts decades of high quality nutritional science.[5] Correctly prescribed drugs are responsible for approximately 100,000 unintentional deaths from side effects each year in the United States alone, while vitamins widely taken in appropriate doses don't cause disease or deaths.[6] Many apparently promising drugs have later been shown to have severe serious side effects requiring them to be taken off the market, while nutritional supplements continue to be safe and effective.

Nutritional Trials

The benefit of just one dietary change may seem obvious when it gives an improvement to a health condition such as arthritis. However, it is difficult for an individual to know for certain whether that specific change was responsible, since every day is different for all of us. We are exposed to different environments, and every one of us has a different lifestyle, including different diets and stresses, and a different genetic inheritance. To be significant, a nutritional effect must be the same for many individuals, and must be repeatable. Testing the same treatment in a population requires organizing at least two groups to be tested. One receives the treatment, and the other does not. It is unethical to give a null treatment (placebo) to test subjects when evidence exists that an existing treatment is effective, which is one of the reasons that animal models are so invaluable. Nutritional trials on animals can be performed in controlled environments, where negative and positive controls can readily be performed and a variety of treatments can be compared. The results can confirm or deny the original hypothesis. This is how the scientific method is ideally performed, but this is rarely done in clinical trials.

Unfortunately, this type of careful testing doesn't always eliminate the chance that two independent studies will reach opposing conclusions for the same nutritional treatment. There are many reasons for this. For example, differences in the dosage tested are common. Even this simple factor can confound the results from several studies. Or it is possible that the most common cause of arthritis in the study's patients is the result of deficiencies unrelated to the treatment. The disease may be the result of a deficiency of some other component of the biosynthetic pathway for cartilage. For example, the afflicted individual may be primarily deficient in magnesium, not calcium. In this case, additional magnesium is really what is needed. Or, worse, there may be multiple deficiencies. Typically, an individual deficient in one vitamin or mineral also has deficiencies of other essential nutrients. After the first deficiency is addressed, the others may still limit the path to recovery. In these cases, testing the effect of other individual nutrients may give unreliable results. This is why apparently well-planned nutritional tests focused on supplements of individual nutrients are often inconclusive.

To get a clear answer, it is often necessary to test multiple nutrients, for arthritis is thought to typically be caused by multiple deficiencies. Most essential nutrients are so safe and nontoxic it is usually best to to test a cocktail containing of all of them. Some essential nutrients, such as vitamin A and minerals such as iron and copper are also safe in appropriate doses, but care should be taken not to exceed these safe doses. After tests have determined the nutrients necessary for healthy pain-free joints, an individual can try a "basket" approach, taking all those supplements along with an excellent diet.

Healthy cartilage, ligaments, bones, and their respective cells are dependent on nutrients. Many different individual molecules and vitamins are required to produce and maintain healthy articular cartilage. The synthetic pathway for cartilage is complex, and deficiencies of any of the precursor molecules can result in an inability to generate or remodel cartilage. For example, this could involve insufficient collagen, carbohydrates, glycosaminoglycans, or nucleotides, or cofactors and enzymes. It could also involve differences in post-translational modifications of proteins and glycosaminoglycans. Deficiencies in other regulatory molecules that control the expression levels of a variety of proteins could be involved. Alternatively, changes in the levels of any of the enzymes involved in the balance of cartilage anabolism versus catabolism could affect OA outcomes. Increased activities of catabolic enzymes such as collagenase and hyaluronase could lead to increased breakdown of cartilage. Moreover, since recovery from arthritis requires cartilage growth it is important to identify hormones or other growth factors that could stimulate the entire synthetic pathway. Thus, in many nutritional tests, there are too many possibilities to get a clear answer, even in tests of animals. In any particular case, it's anybody's guess as to which of these many molecules is (or are) really causing cartilage loss or preventing its regrowth.

Genetics Can Simplify Nutrition Science

In contrast to nutrition science, genetic research can be quite straightforward. It can help identify specific molecular pathways that previously were unknown. The results can be unequivocal and very powerful. Genetics provides an alternative unbiased method for discovering the genes that are critical for preventing arthritis. The function of each gene in cells of cartilage, ligament, and bone is dependent on nutrients. Most genes present in humans have an analogous gene that contains DNA sequences very similar to those in other animals, including mice, fish, and even fruit flies. In fact, basic research using animals is typically twenty to thirty years ahead of clinical practice. This is expected, because these experiments cannot ethically be performed on humans. In most cases where gene function has been determined using animal models the analogous human genetic disease has not yet been discovered. But the animal models provide clues. For example, in cases where entire families of people have heritable osteoarthritis, investigators will sequence the candidate human genes already previously identified from animal model studies.

GENETICS AND GENETIC MUTATIONS

In order to appreciate the science of genetic analysis, it's important to understand what a mutation is, and also how animal models can be utilized to discover the human genes required to maintain healthy cartilage. Genetics is based on the knowledge that DNA sequence molecules are read by the cell machinery to encode for transitory RNA molecules, whose sequence is then used (translated) to make the sequence of amino acids in the resulting protein. This knowledge is called the "central dogma" in biology, and has been well established in many studies over the last sixty years. In essence, genetics is the study of how changes in the gene DNA sequence affect the function of the resulting protein. Ultimately it is the protein that actually performs some kind of biological function. All three of these macromolecules (DNA, RNA, and protein) are organized as chains with a beginning and an end. Proteins consist of strings of twenty different types of linked amino acids, while DNA and RNA consist of just four different types of molecule linked together. Because of this basic organization, changes in the DNA sequence cause a corresponding change in the protein sequence, which usually will affect its specific biological activity. A complication is that many of the possible DNA sequences do not code for valid protein sequences. For example, only part of the protein may be made, or perhaps no protein at all may be made if there is a nonsense mutation in the beginning of the protein-coding region of the DNA. Alternatively, individual amino acids can be substituted with other amino acids. These are considered "loss of function" mutations.

A major advantage of genetic research is its undeniable relevancy and reproducibility. Everyone can agree on the conclusions, and typically there is little equivocation or controversy. This is especially true for "loss of function" gene analysis performed on a mouse or other animal model. The animal with a disrupted gene is monitored by examination as it develops from a young animal to adult. The observations made describe the appearance and behavior of the animal that depend on its genetic makeup. These characteristics are termed the "phenotype." Such loss of gene function tests performed in mice are fairly easy to understand, and usually everyone agrees on the results.

Loss-of-Function Analysis

The function of many genes in mice, zebrafish, or fruit flies have now been tested by genetically engineered mutations that prevent the gene from producing its protein. These "knockout" or "loss-of-function" (LOF) phenotypes have been published and annotated into databases that connect the observations to many genetic human diseases. Loss-of-function analysis has been primarily performed using mice, but also with other organisms, most prominently zebrafish and fruit flies. Each animal model has its own advantage. The advantages of zebrafish for use in genetic research are that it is small (approximately 1 inch in length), easily raised in an aquarium, and transparent in early development, thus enabling the beating heart and other internal organs and cells to be clearly seen and photographed. These advantages allow genetic engineering to effectively create and observe the equivalent of hundreds of millions of years of evolution in the laboratory. In some types of tests, completely random mutations are intentionally created in zebrafish. Then thousands of offspring are raised, and hard-working, energetic graduate students and lab workers screen them for relevant phenotypes. When one is found, for example, with a bone problem, a series of breeding tests can identify the parents that reproducibly generate this phenotype. The researchers then identify exactly which gene was involved, and precisely which mutation is responsible.

This is a truly fundamental scientific method in the sense that it is completely unbiased. Many important discoveries have been made this way, including the categorization of all of the essential genes required to make a vertebrate animal. Similar methods involve eliminating the function of specific candidate genes through deletions of the gene within the DNA or disruption of RNA function. These studies lead to the identification of candidate genes, which are then considered in the context of human genetic diseases that result in phenotypes resembling the animal models. Human families with inherited diseases are examined with respect to mutations in the candidate genes. All the genetic disease associations obtained through human-animal studies are freely available by performing searches at the Online Mendelian Inheritance in Man (OMIM) database, which is accessible indirectly through the National Library of Medicine's website databases.[7] LOF genetic analysis makes it possible to screen all human genes in an unbiased fashion to identify which genes are most important to preventing arthritis. Searches of OMIM are easy to perform for all of the identified arthritis-associated genes, based on LOF or observed human disease phenotypes.

Using the OMIM database, we performed LOF analysis to identify which genes are required for prevention of OA.[8] The gene products listed in Table 4.1 are required for excellent joint health to prevent arthritis. (This is not a comprehensive list, as research is ongoing and early lethal phenotypes preclude analysis of later developing tissues. Nonetheless, it is at least an

TABLE 4.1. WHAT WE CAN LEARN FROM GENETICS ABOUT VITAMINS TO PREVENT OR TREAT ARTHRITIS

NAME (GENE ABBREVIATION; PROTEIN NAMES)	LOSS OF FUNCTION	POST-TRANSLATIONAL MODIFICATIONS	VITAMIN, METALS, AND OTHER REQUIREMENTS
CSPG1: aggrecan 1; chondroitin sulfate proteoglycan protein 1	Early onset OA: Separation of cartilage from subchondral bone	17x disulfide bonds, a very high number! 11x glycosylation sites	B_1, B_2, B_3, and C
HLAN1: hyaluronan and proteoglycan link protein 1	Severe defects in cartilage development; lethal phenotype in animal models only		
COL2A1: alpha 1 type 2 collagen	OA	5x hydroxylations; 9x glycosylations; 2x disulfide bonds 5x glyco	B_1, B_2, B_3, and C
SLC26A2: sulfate transporter	Early onset OA		Sulfur (cysteine, methionine, inorganic sulfate)
CHST3: carbohydrate sulfotransferase	OA		B_3, C, and metals
HS6ST2: heparin sulfate 6-O sulfotransferase 1	OA		
SMA3: Protein named "Mothers against decapentaplegic homolog 3"	Early onset OA; aneurisms-osteoarthritis syndrome	Acetylation	B_3 and zinc

approximation based on the available data.) Prior knowledge about the function of the protein produced by the gene gives clues about the nutrients required for the proper development of joints. For example, this LOF analysis shows how important sulfur is in the pathway for cartilage production. Sulfur cross-links between strands of collagen are required for strength of cartilage. These cross-links are dependent on amino acids containing sulphur (cysteine, methionine, taurine), but also on the cofactors for enzymes that accomplish the cross-links; for example, vitamin C and copper. You can't make stuff you don't have the building blocks for. Starting from this set of gene products, we then search for cofactor/vitamin dependence and potential hydroxylations characteristic of ascorbate dependence as well.

The analysis shown in Table 4.1 was focused on osteoarthritis (OA), and represents our best understanding of the genes whose function must be optimized for preventing or reversing OA. The function is optimized by providing adequate amounts of essential nutrients. For disulfide bonds, vitamins B_1, B_2, B_3, and C are all involved. Some cartilage proteins, particularly aggrecan, have exceptionally large numbers of disulfide bonds. Hence these cartilage proteins have a greater dependence on sulfur-containing amino acids. Other types of arthritis such as rheumatoid arthritis (RA), that are immunologic in nature are thought to be much more complex, and may be dependent on many other gene products.

Aggrecan core protein is one of the most important proteins involved in the formation of cartilage, yet it is sorely underappreciated and understudied. Loss of function of aggrecan leads to early onset osteoarthritis. It has over 100 chondroitin sulfate chains and it also has keratin sulfates. That is a lot of sulfate and glycosaminoglycan! No other protein comes close to these numbers, not by an order of magnitude. These carbohydrate groups provide essential strength in the cartilage. Aggrecan also has a tremendous number of disulfide bonds (seventeen), an unusually high number for a protein! Several vitamins are involved in establishing these disulfide bonds. In the final assembly of the aggrecan matrix, these disulfide bonds are "shuffled" or redirected to new locations within the molecules. The vitamins most involved in this disufide shuffling are niacin, riboflavin, and ascorbate. Niacin works through thioredoxin pathways, riboflavin through disulfide isomerase pathways, and ascorbate through glutathione pathways. Another protein identified in the genetics search, and related by its association with aggrecan, is the hyaluronan and proteoglycan link protein encoded by the HLAN gene. Loss of HLAN gene product function results in dramatic cartilage deficits with early death in knockout mice (mice that have been genetically engineered to have specific genes inactivated, or "knocked out"). Both aggrecan and HLAN proteins also bind to chains of hyaluronic acid.

Another protein required to prevent arthritis is collagen type II. Collagen is the most abundant protein in the human body. As explained in Chapter 2, collagen has long been known to require ascorbate (vitamin C) for its cross-linking into the extracellular matrix. This cross-linking involves a hydroxylation reaction of lysine and proline amino acids that requires iron and vitamin C as cofactors.[9] The symptoms of scurvy are in large part due to the catastrophic loss of strength of collagen in connective tissue due to the missing cross-links. There are several types of collagens. Alpha 1 type 2 collagens are required for preventing OA. The amount of collagen that is made by the body is controlled by Smad3, another protein identified in our screen as critical to preventing arthritis (Table 4.1). Loss of function of Smad3 also results in a syndrome with osteoarthritis symptoms because there is increased production of collagenase enzymes that break down collagen.[10] Smad3 activity is modulated by NAD, and therefore is limited by the availability of niacin.[11]

Another example is that of transporters, or "carrier proteins," a class of proteins that sit in the cell membrane and transport molecules in or out of the cell. Whenever a loss of function occurs for a transporter and results in a phenotype, this implies a function for the transported molecule. Usually such a transported molecule is obtained from the diet. This is a very practical application of genetic analysis. A loss of function in the gene product encoded by SLC26A2, a solute carrier protein, causes a problem in transporting sulfates. This is particularly interesting because the role of sulfate in nutrition has not been well studied.[12] It is unfortunate that the effect of increasing sulfate intake has not been carefully studied in patients with problems in the SLC26A2 gene. Nonetheless, the disease called "achondrogenesis" (lack of articular cartilage) is one of the outcomes of a SLC26A2 mutation. There is currently no known commonly accepted treatment. A straightforward test might be to simply increase the patient's amount of dietary sulfate in an attempt to make up for decreased sulfate transport. But such a test would not be obvious without a basic understanding of the pathway.

NUTRIGENOMICS: FAMINE AND EPIGENETIC CONTROL OF CELLULAR FUNCTION

In recent decades it has been discovered that, during development, the fetus adapts to the levels of nutrients provided by the mother. An "epigenetic" mechanism (a change in heritable cellular function not due to the DNA sequence) is thought to be responsible for setting up long-lasting or permanent changes in the developing fetus due to its nutrition.[13] A study of people born in Netherlands during the famine of 1944–1945 found that they developed a lower glucose tolerance and had a higher risk of heart disease and obesity as they grew into old age.[14] It is now thought that people who were either undernourished or overnourished as a fetus may be affected throughout their life. This implies that body chemistry is controlled over many years by the nutritional environment of the fetus. Many such epigenetic mechanisms have been identified. They are an important part of the development of the fetus, allowing long-lasting adaptive changes to the environment. Epigenetic mechanisms can regulate cells over a lifetime, similar to the genetic heritage that we know as DNA, except that the epigenetic mechanisms are modulated but not always inherited from one generation to the next. They are set by a variety of molecular signals.

Recently it has been shown that the body adapts to the available levels of different nutrients throughout life. Even in old age, metabolic byproducts and vitamins help to regulate the epigenetic control of the genes that direct cell function. These metabolic products act as cofactors for the enzymes that regulate the epigenetic control of genes to maintain health.[15] The implication of this is that what we eat determines how the body functions at a very deep level. Our genes can sense the stresses on the body and the nutrients available for maintenance. These genes can then up-regulate different cellular functions, dependent on the nutrients and tasks on hand.

For example, when fasting the body must utilize fats for energy. This releases ketone bodies, which can smell like acetone in the fasting person's breath. But the ketone bodies then up-regulate an epigenetic mechanism to deal with oxidative stress. Another example comes from diabetes. Even though an individual with diabetes controls the diet and keeps the level of blood sugar in check, the risk for diabetic organ damage remains high for years after the initial diagnosis.[16] As explained in Chapter 6, vitamin C strongly enhances the efficiency of reprogramming stem cells, acting as a cofactor in regulation of epigenetic control of genes.[17] NAD, derived from niacin, is one of the molecules known to modulate the epigenetic control of genes.[18] It is one of the most important molecules for energy metabolism, and as we have learned, is important for the health of joints. Also, the level of molecules such as NAD, so important for providing health in one generation, may also regulate health in descendants.[19] Some of this epigenetic information set by exposure to the dietary environment is passed on to children. How obesity or other effects of nutrition in adults will affect their children through epigenetic modulation is not understood.

The medical discipline of nutrigenomics attempts to discover how the levels of nutrients available to cells regulate the genes and the body's response to disease.[20] The discipline of metabolic phenotyping attempts to discover which particular metabolic pathways in an individual are most affected by their genetic background.[21] The field of genetics is very wide with many subdisciplines, and is proceeding rapidly, but is still in its infancy. We only know the functions of a small fraction of the 23,000 genes in the human genome.[22] It seems likely that the nutrition given to the fetus and young children can affect their growth into adults. The nutritional stresses that adults receive throughout their life can be programmed into epigenetic modulation of their childrens' genes. Likely these mechanisms are involved in arthritis.

Ways to Increase Sulfate

Adequate sulfate is required to make cartilage, and this can be obtained with extra dietary cysteine along with methionine.[23] For example, the diets of poultry are always supplemented with extra cysteine and methionine to increase growth. Other nonamino acid sulfate containing molecules are commonly appreciated as treatments for OA. The tolerable upper limit of dietary sulfate is not known, but as anyone who has taken magnesium hydroxide or magnesium sulfate knows, an excess causes diarrhea.[24]

Methylsulfonylmethane (MSM) is a natural molecule that contains sulfur, and it can be helpful in preventing symptoms of OA. In some studies it has reduced pain, increased function, or reduced the need for painkillers.[25] S-adenosyl methionine (SAM), another natural molecule found in the body, has been consistently shown to help in the treatment of OA[26] by helping chondrocytes to generate proteoglycans. It is as effective as NSAIDs but has fewer side effects.[27] SAM and MSM are often included in food supplements for OA. Most interestingly, MSM does not contain an amino acid, suggesting that the sulfate portion of the molecule is important.

Sulfate can be obtained from cruciferous vegetables such as broccoli, cauliflower, Brussels sprouts, or cabbage, and also from onions or garlic. Sulforafane sulfates present in these plants are thought to have potent anticancer activities. This is being explored currently in clinical trials. However, most dietary sulfate is derived from breakdown of cysteine or methionine. Sulfate available in the bloodstream is utilized to form the cofactor 3'-phosphoadenosine-5'-phosphosulfate (PAPS), which is necessary to make chondroitin sulfate. PAPS is also necessary for the sulfotransferases, whose loss of function results in OA as listed in Table 4.1. The sulfotransferases are encoded by the genes CHST3 and HS6ST2. Thiamine, vitamin B_1, is essential for synthesizing PAPS and utilizing the sulfur in aggrecan for preventing OA. Articular cartilage containing aggrecan is chock full of chondroitin and keratin sulfate. Overall, this analysis reveals how critically important sulfate is for cartilage formation.

This suggests that high doses of thiamine, the only sulfur-containing vitamin, may be helpful for the treatment of arthritis. Thiamine is nontoxic even at high doses (1,000–5,000 milligrams (mg) per day).[28] The RDA for thiamine is approximately 1 mg, but it has been used very effectively at doses of 1,000 mg or more for treating nutritional deficiencies that cause diseases (multiple sclerosis and alcoholism). The effect of these high doses can be dramatic.[29] Alternatively, taking 100 mg every hour is another possibility.

Vitamin K

Vitamin K is another example of an essential nutrient linked to arthritis by genetic studies. Several decades after the role of vitamin K in blood clotting was discovered, several other functions of vitamin K were also found. These other functions involve controlling calcification. Loss of function in the genes associated with these other functions is prematurely lethal, so these other functions are difficult to study. Vitamin K is thought to be involved as a cofactor with only one enzyme, gamma-glutamyl carboxylase.[30] This enzyme is necessary for adding a second carboxyl group to glutamate, thus creating gamma carboxylglutamate (gla) on at least seventeen known proteins. Three of these are intimately involved in limiting over-calcification of articular cartilage typically found in OA.[31] These include the vitamin K-dependent gene products, osteocalcin/bone gla protein (BGLAP; made in bones), Matrix Gla-protein (MGP; made in cartilage and bones) and the Gla-rich proteins (cartilage).

The Gla structure in these molecules can "chelate" (grab and remove) calcium. It functions like the end of the chelation therapy molecule, ethylene diamine tetraacetic acid (EDTA). In both EDTA and the Gla amino acid, two closely spaced carboxyl groups are involved in binding to divalent cations such as calcium. EDTA is injected in people to clean out their hardened vascular calcifications by a treatment known as chelation therapy. This vitamin K-dependent modification is required in order for these Gla proteins to function correctly. For example, loss of function of MGP in mice results in excessive calcification of the arteries, which invariably lead to arterial rupture.

Several forms of vitamin K exist, including K_1, phylloquinone or "plant vitamin K," and K_2, or "animal vitamin K." To know which form to take, it is important to understand the similarities and differences in their roles. Some of these are available only from the diet. The K_1 form is used by plants in photosynthesis, but in the body it is used for clotting, and is preferentially distributed to the liver. However, it is also converted in the body to the K_2 form.[32] Several subtypes of vitamin K_2 exist, and originate from different dietary sources. They are termed MK (menaquinone) followed by a number, which reflects the length of the side chain.[33] One form of K_2, menaquinone-4 (MK-4, also called menatetranone), is created in the body by conversion from vitamin K_1.[34] Another form of K_2 (MK-7) is made by bacteria in the gut, and in some fermented foods such as natto.[35] Other forms of menaquinone include MK-8 and MK-9, found in cheeses.[36] A synthetic form of K_2 called menadione, sometimes used in animal feeds, can be converted in the body to MK-4.[37] Vitamin K_2 in any of its forms (including MK-4 and MK-7) helps to control calcium storage and calcification in the body. The relative amount of K_1 and K_2 varies in organs throughout the body. Vitamin K is mainly found in an oxidized form because of the presence of oxygen.[38] However, it is actively recycled back into its active reduced form by a sequence of enzymes. This lowers the body's need to acquire it from the diet. The body utilizes K_2 for many of its functions outside of the liver, including its bone and joint biochemistry, and a deficiency in K_2 can occur within seven days. The K_2 form is preferentially distributed to other tissues outside of the liver, such as the pancreas and bone.[39] Although some clinical trials have focused on the effects of ingesting plant vitamin K_1, when taken in supplement form, K_2 is better absorbed than K_1.[40] One study showed that a high dietary intake of vitamin K_2, but not K_1, reduces coronary heart disease.[41]Since bones generally contain more K_2 than K_1, the K_2 form is thought to be most relevant to bone health.[42]

Arterial calcifications are a better indicator of cardiovascular disease risk than measures of cholesterol.[43] As one would predict, based on the knowledge that vitamin K helps to reduce arterial calcification, vitamin K levels are inversely correlated with coronary artery disease. Increased intake of vitamin K is associated with a 56 percent reduction in coronary artery disease, a 52 percent reduction in aorta calcification, and a 26 percent reduction in all cause mortality.[44] Unfortunately, vitamin K is blocked by drugs such as warfarin that are given to prevent clotting.[45]

As described in Chapter 3, calcification is intimately involved in the health of joints, because the basal layer of articular cartilage is naturally calcified where it contacts the underlying bone. In late OA, there is increased bone formation around the joint. Low vitamin K levels have been detected in knee osteoarthritis.[46] Although a clinical trial involving administration of 1 mg of vitamin K_1 for three years failed to detect benefits for hand OA,[47] it is known that the function of K_1 is mainly for blood coagulation and only to a lesser degree for calcium metabolism. This is because only some of the ingested K_1 is converted to K_2 in the body. Morever, vitamins A, D, and B_2 are all required for vitamin K to work ideally and this was not taken into account. Vitamin A and D regulate the production of MGP and osteocalcin/BGLAP, which are then modified by a vitamin K dependent process (in other words, carboxylation of the glutamate residues on the matrix gla protein in cartilage). Vitamin B_2 is required for the recycling of vitamin K. To get the benefit of vitamin K, it is necessary to take high levels of both vitamin D and K.

Vitamin K also increases sulfatide production in myelin sheaths surrounding neurons. This was discovered when it was observed that warfarin, which blocks the function of vitamin K, decreases sulfotransferase activities in myelin. As shown in Table

4.1, sulfotransferase is implicated by the LOF results in OA. How vitamin K may impact on the sulfotransferases working joint health remains completely unexplored.

In summary, vitamin K is an important nutrient and is essential for preventing and reversing OA. Several studies show positive results for vitamin K in arthritis, and overall the data indicate that vitamin K represents a "nothing to lose, possibly everything to gain" treatment for arthritis. Vitamin K_2 is also being explored as a treatment for RA,[48] and results clearly indicate that it works in animal models of arthritis.[49] As a bonus, vitamin K also dramatically whitens some people's teeth, as it limits buildup of plaque. Vitamin K may turn out to be the most dramatic contribution to newly recognized nutritional treatments for osteoarthritis.

In summary, genetic analysis indicates that the body requires at least the following essential nutrients to insure the correct function of genes known to be involved in OA:

- Vitamin B_1, thiamine
- Vitamin B_2, riboflavin
- Vitamin B_3, niacin (or niacinamide, but the former has a longer record)
- Vitamin C, ascorbate
- Vitamin K, as K_2/menaquinone, obtainable through Japanese natto or grass-fed butter and eggs, but preferably supplements for more effective therapeutic concentrations
- Sulfur (cysteine, methionine, and other sulfur-containing compounds)
- Zinc

These essential nutrients are required for building up cartilage in the joint and the bone underlying the joint. The evidence from the science of genetics indicates that even a slight a deficiency of any of these essential nutrients will increase the risk for OA. The triage theory of nutrients (described in Chapter 2) explains why. All of these nutrients are required throughout the body and are assigned to many important metabolic functions. But their involvement in maintenance functions are often given lower priority because the gene products that use them have lower affinity for the essential nutrient cofactors. Because many people with OA are deficient in these nutrients, it stands to reason that providing them at higher doses than the minimum will help prevent and reverse OA.

CHAPTER 5

NUTRITIONAL TREATMENTS FOR ARTHRITIS: THE EVIDENCE

This chapter describes how foods and supplements can prevent and reverse arthritis. As we have seen in the previous chapters, osteoarthritis (OA) and rheumatoid arthritis (RA) are progressive conditions in which the cartilage in a joint gets damaged and does not readily regrow. Long-term nutritional deficiencies are thought to contribute to the damage for several reasons. Articular cartilage in joints has no blood vessels and so has a restricted supply of nutrients. This limits the ability of the cartilage to regrow after damage. Exercise with joint motion under moderate load is known to promote healing. This is thought to provide better distribution of nutrients into the articular cartilage, and also better cleansing of metabolic waste products from the joint. Moderate exercise also inhibits inflammatory biochemical pathways and promotes regrowth of cartilage.[1]

ARTHRITIS, NUTRITION, AND LIFESTYLE

Arthritis is associated with an increased risk for other chronic diseases such as heart disease and cancer. This phenomenon of several simultaneous chronic diseases is known as "multiple chronic conditions" (MCC) or "multi-morbidity." In recent years, the prevalence of MCC has increased.[2] This is likely due to the large component of processed foods in the modern diet. An excellent diet containing a variety of beneficial fruits and vegetables that avoids refined grains such as white or enriched wheat flour, white rice, and refined sugar and oils, can reduce the risk for such age-related diseases.[3]

Currently, modern medicine offers no therapy that can modify the progression of arthritis. Instead it consists of a course of disease management therapies, involving corticosteroid injections or NSAIDs. This therapy is generally given with the understanding that the patient will eventually need a joint replacement, which consists of cutting out and discarding the entire joint and replacing it with a metal ball and plastic. If the artificial joint ever becomes loose or causes other problems, as it quite commonly does, the only therapy is to have another surgery. Yet, an excellent alternative to standard drug and surgical treatment is nutritional therapy. The nutritional approach is gaining favor because recent research shows it is usually more effective.

To prevent or recover from OA, it is important to get on an excellent diet that includes robust servings of fresh vegetables and fruits. Especially important for joint health are green leafy vegetables. You can benefit by making sure the food you eat contains adequate amounts of vitamins. If it doesn't, as is so common in our modern world with processed foods, you can benefit by taking vitamin supplements, especially the B vitamins, vitamins A, C, D, E, and K, the essential minerals calcium, magnesium, and phosphorus, micronutrients such as selenium and iron when needed, and omega-3 polyunsaturated fatty acids. A deficiency in any of these essential nutrients, or others not yet even discovered, can cause inflammation and joint disease. When the deficiency and associated inflammation is removed with an excellent diet, recovery can occur.

It's helpful to consider the time scale of the healing process. After an acute injury, time is of the essence for a smooth recovery. In the short run, you can get pain relief by taking 1,000–4,000 milligrams (mg) of niacinamide and 3,000–10,000 mg or more of vitamin C, taken in small divided doses throughout the day, along with 100 mg of vitamins B_1, B_2, B_5, and B_6.

These megadoses are very safe for most individuals and will help the tissues deal with injury and acute pain quickly. High doses of vitamins will also help with another option, stem cell therapy, in which live stem cells are injected into the afflicted joint. This is discussed further in Chapter 6. But with chronic pain, the healing process may take many months in any case. During this long-term recovery period, a full palette of vitamins and minerals, taken along with an excellent diet, is helpful. We will discuss foods and doses of supplements further in Chapter 7.

Exercise

One of the first points about the natural way of treating arthritis is to remember that joint motion under moderate load will help the joint recover.[4] Moderate exercise can help by exchanging waste products from the chondrocytes in cartilage with the nutrition in the synovial fluid. Moderate exercise also helps to downregulate inflammatory biochemical pathways in chondrocytes and upregulate the pathways that promote regrowth of cartilage.[5] Adherence to a regular program of moderate exercise takes time, but it is associated with improvement in OA and RA symptoms.[6] It also is associated with many other health benefits, including a reduced risk of breast cancer in older women.[7] As long as you don't damage your joints with too much weight or stress, adequate exercise can help to keep you more healthy.

Running typically generates a higher (3x) peak force on the knee joint than walking. Yet, interestingly, most runners don't get OA in their knees any more than walkers do. One reason is that the length of the running stride is longer and requires fewer steps to go the same distance, compared to walking. Also, the duration of ground contact is less during running. These factors reduce the overall load on the knees per unit of distance, equalizing its damaging effects compared with walking.[8]

Doing the right type of exercise is important.[9] For some, this is walking, dancing, swimming, or bicycling. These exercises help you to maintain strong muscles, reduce stress, and get more sleep and a good mental outlook.[10] Doing yoga, tai chi, and other breathing exercises will help you stretch your joints and get fresh air into your lungs. The Arthritis Foundation recommends regular aerobic exercises for rheumatoid arthritis patients to build up stamina. Stretching your muscles and joints will also help. But it's important to warm them up first, and not to damage them by stretching too much when using weights. It's best to get the joint and muscles surrounding it relaxed before stretching, usually at the end of an exercise period, not before.[11] The stretching should be done gradually, holding the maximum position at first for only a few seconds, and working up to thirty or forty seconds. It will help to breathe deeply during this process, because this provides oxygen to the body, allowing the tissues of the muscles and joints to recover faster.

However, exercise can be a dual-edged sword for recovery from OA and RA. As explained above, mild exercise is helpful for providing nutrition to and flushing wastes from the cartilage in the joint. Any exercise generates reactive oxygen species (ROS), or free radicals, as a normal consequence of damage to the tissue. Moderate exercise can generate low to moderate levels of ROS. A low level of ROS is thought to have a beneficial effect as a signal that damage has occurred.[12] This signal helps the tissue to recover from the damage. But at high levels, the ROS molecules can overpower the antioxidants normally present in cells, which will further damage tissues, especially those in the joint that do not have direct access to blood circulation. This is what happens in OA and RA, in which low levels of antioxidants and high levels of ROS are evident. Therefore, moderate exercise is thought to be helpful.

Commuting to Work

Many people spend an hour or two each day commuting to and from work. Although some may feel that the time spent commuting is necessary, it contributes to many health problems, including arthritis. In terms of the body's health, the time could be better spent in activities such as walking or riding a bicycle, or even socializing with friends and family.[13] Those who exercise are on average more healthy, and as long as the exercise is moderate their joints and entire body will derive a benefit. As explained above, joints need motion under load in order to tip the balance from resorption of bone and cartilage towards regrowth. Even when it is easy to walk or ride a bicycle, many people prefer to take a car or public transportation. The effect of this preference for less exercise is less healthy activity. Over decades this inactivity causes damage to build up within the body. This effect of relying on powered vehicles for commuting and errands is insidious. Over decades it leads to a major loss of exercise, which causes problems with mental and physical health.[14] A recent study showed that commuting a long distance is associated with less activity, lower cardio-respiratory fitness, and more obesity.[15] Both of these are associated with damage to joints, often over several decades. If a commuter could instead spend the hour doing exercise instead, the joints would be most grateful.

Sleep

To prevent and recover from the inflammation that causes arthritis, it is essential to get adequate sleep on a regular basis. Adequate exercise will help, as it's easier to get to sleep when tired. Napping for fifteen minutes after lunch, when needed, can also help. Setting your daily activity cycle by the sun will help keep your internal circadian (daily) rhythms correctly synchronized for the best health. For example, it is best to schedule exercise and meals at regular times to allow the body to fully synchronize its circadian clocks.[16] During sleep the weight is off the knees and hips, which allows their articular cartilage to regenerate. To tip the balance away from resorption of cartilage further towards regrowth, it is helpful to take part of your daily dose of essential nutrients just before bedtime. We will discuss these nutrients below.

To help prevent insomnia and improve the daily activity-sleep cycle, it helps to look at bright light for a few minutes in the early morning.[17] Going outside in the morning after sunrise is the natural way to synchronize the internal clock. Blue light is most effective at setting the circadian rhythm because the rod-melanopsin photoreceptor system in the retina, which controls the circadian rhythm, is most sensitive to light at 480–500 nm.[18] However, any very bright light viewed for a few minutes will tend to synchronize your activity cycle; that is, it will wake you up!

Another way to synchronize the activity-sleep cycle is to take melatonin in the evening. This biochemical is a natural hormone that the body uses to regulate the daily sleep cycle, and it is widely taken to to prevent insomnia and get better sleep. It is available over-the-counter in some countries. Interestingly, cherries contain high levels of melatonin and also have antioxidant and anti-inflammatory properties.[19] You can use bright light in the morning and melatonin in the evening to help synchronize your circadian rhythm, allowing more and higher quality sleep.

It's also useful to remember that if you do the opposite, that is, look at bright light at night, such as a bright computer screen (white or blue light), or bright bathroom lights, or take melatonin in the morning, this will likely desynchronize your activity cycle so that it's opposite to daylight. For example, workers on the night shift need to be attentive during a time when their circadian rhythms set by the sun would normally be in the sleep phase. In one study, nurses on the night shift, who had insomnia, were exposed to bright light in the beginning of their night shift, and used dark glasses to prevent exposure to bright light in the day. Over several weeks this treatment helped their circadian rhythms to synchronize their activity with their night shift, improving their insomnia and lessening depression.[20] Obviously, this is a special case that should be avoided by most people, who are active in the day and just want to sleep well at night.

To avoid confusing your activity-sleep cycle, you may want to set up your bathroom or other late-night lighting to be a moderate intensity of yellow-orange. It's best to avoid viewing a computer or television screen just before going to bed. If you must use your computer late at night, try to reduce the intensity of the screen. The easiest way is to reduce the intensity and contrast settings. Those who already wear glasses can purchase amber colored wraparounds or clip-ons. Amber glasses that block blue light worn three hours before bedtime have been shown to increase the quality of sleep.[21] Avoid exercise at least two hours before going to bed. Avoid caffeine or sugar in the afternoon, and limit eating cherries to dinner, or lunch if you can have a nap afterwards.

As any arthritis patient knows, the quality and amount of sleep is lessened by pain. Vitamin D is a hormone that modulates many body functions, including the immune system and recovery from injury. In one study, chronic pain patients who were deficient in vitamin D were given supplements for three months. Their pain was significantly improved, as was the time it took to get to sleep and their sleep duration.[22] This highlights the importance of getting adequate doses of essential nutrients, for many people suffer from vitamin deficiencies.

It's widely appreciated that a good mattress is important for sleep, especially as we get older with various aches and pains.[23] However, it's not so widely understood that modern foam mattresses can exude harmful chemicals, such as formaldehyde, plasticizers, and flame retardants, that can contribute to inflammation.[24] Mattress foams typically release the chemicals at a higher level in the first several months after they're purchased, but this can continue for several years. When you sleep on a new foam pillow or mattress, you are exposed to much higher levels of these chemicals than in the rest of the air in your house. The same is true of clothes and bed linens. Therefore, it's important to be aware of the problem. Individuals with RA who have sensitivities to the chemicals in mattresses and linens should consider purchasing a mattress and sheets made out of natural materials such as cotton, wool, and wood.[25] Wash clothes and bed linens thoroughly before use to remove chemicals.

ARTHRITIS RECOVERY DEPENDS ON EXCELLENT NUTRITION

Osteoarthritis is typically caused as a result of damage to cartilage. In many cases this is caused or worsened by a deficient diet. But just one essential biochemical taken as a supplement does not cure arthritis. An excellent diet including plenty of green leafy vegetables is a necessary first step. However, looking more closely, we know that to produce and maintain healthy articular cartilage, the chondrocyte cells must have robust and productive biochemical pathways. The health of these pathways involves hundreds of biochemical reactions, most of which rely on vitamin cofactors. These, in turn, depend on the supply of nutrients in the synovial fluid, generated by the surrounding tissues, that bathes the articular cartilage. All of the vitamin cofactors and other essential nutrients must be present in order for a biochemical pathway to be fully productive. The necessary nutrients can be obtained from the diet or from supplements. Any deficiency of these ingredients of food will limit the rate of the biochemical pathway, slowing the healing process. For example, deficiencies of vitamin A are very common in the modern world. But an adequate dose of vitamin A helps to suppress the inflammation in RA.[26]

Although the essential vitamin cofactors such as the B vitamins are widely considered to be necessary for a healthy individual only in small amounts (less than 10 mg per day), the biochemical pathways they are involved in can be enhanced by much larger doses.[27] The reason is that all of the precursor molecules of a pathway must be present in abundance to allow the pathway to perform its function. The most critical molecular component of a biochemical pathway for any individual is the one most deficient relative to the pathway's requirement. This specific molecule is said to be "rate-limiting," because it will be the factor that slows usage of all of the other required components, even if they are present in abundance. In modern societies we are particularly prone to become deficient in vitamins and other essential nutrients because they are often removed from our food by so-called "modern" food processing. Other factors that are potentially rate-limiting for the optimal production of cartilage include: the levels of the substrates (such as protein and glycosoaminoglycans) for the enzymes that make cartilage, the levels of other enzyme cofactors such as vitamins and essential trace minerals, the levels of the enzymes themselves, and finally the acidity requirements for the reactions. The level of the essential nutrients is limited by absorption from the diet. If we do not have proper absorption of materials into the bloodstream, we cannot expect our biochemical pathways to do their proper job. That is why an excellent diet and the supplement dose are all-important.

REGULATION OF FOOD SUPPLEMENTS DUE TO MISINFORMATION

A recent lobbying movement is pressuring governments to regulate foods and food supplements, including vitamins and essential nutrients, as if they were drugs. This action would benefit industrial farmers, large food corporations, and the pharmaceutical industry, but would limit the ability of small farmers to produce and sell food. It would also limit the ability of the public to purchase foods and food supplements they need for health. In Europe, laws are now in place to regulate the maximum permissible doses of food supplements and prevent undocumented claims in labeling.[28] In one case, bottles of water were blocked from sale because they made the unsubstantiated claim that the contents could prevent dehydration![29] Although this judgment was obviously flawed, the push to treat food supplements as unregulated drugs seems relentless. While everyone would agree that foods and food supplements should be safe and of high quality, the effect of the legislation in Europe is to stifle freedom to choose and purchase food supplements.

The European food legislation also regulates the labeling and doses of vitamin and mineral supplements. Many of the regulations are based on the potential interaction with drugs. This has the effect of "drug-ifying" essential vitamins and minerals. Unfortunately, the concern about the safety of drugs is misplaced when applied to essential nutrients. For example, magnesium is an essential nutrient required for health. As described in Chapter 2, many people are deficient in magnesium. Many drugs interact with magnesium, and it is common to find warnings to avoid magnesium in foods and supplements on the labels of these drugs.[30] But magnesium is usually not the problem — it is the solution to the problem. Many drugs deplete the body's magnesium, leading to magnesium deficiency.[31] But in some of these cases, adequate magnesium obviates the need for prescription drugs. Eating a poor diet that lacks magnesium, and taking prescription drugs that interact with magnesium and cause it to be excreted is the problem.[32] The situation is similar for the other essential nutrients such as niacin, and vitamins C, E, and K. Those taking prescription drugs are often advised not to take supplements of these essential nutrients. In fact, many age-related diseases can be prevented or reversed with adequate doses of vitamins and minerals, so they obviate the need for drugs. The optimal doses vary according to the individual, and should not be dictated by an expert panel. Thus, the food legislation in Europe that limits doses of vitamin supplements is doing a disservice to the health of the consumer.

In the United States, there is also movement towards this unfortunate goal.[33] Evidently there are wide misconceptions about the safety and efficacy of vitamins and food supplements compared to drugs. This is due at least in part to the media that present controversial articles about supplement safety. The articles attract wide attention, because most people (including doctors) who are concerned about their health know that vitamins are safe and prevent disease, so they take supplements every day. In contrast, most drugs are artificial synthetic molecules that have side effects, and many are potentially extremely dangerous. For example, a twofold overdose of acetaminophen, a widely-taken over-the counter painkiller, can cause liver damage. Acetaminophen and other similar painkillers cause many deaths every year.[34] Indeed, properly prescribed drugs cause many tens of thousands of deaths in the

United States every year, and errors in medications cause tens of thousands more.[35] Unintentional overdoses of painkillers are a major source of these deaths.[36] Fatal adverse reactions from drugs properly prescribed and taken in American hospitals have killed more than 100,000 people per year.[37] Worse, for every death from prescription painkillers, there are 10 admissions to hospitals for treatment of overdoses, 32 emergency department admissions for misuse or abuse, and 825 people who take prescription painkillers for nonmedical use.[38] Thus, it's not surprising that drug safety is of wide concern.

However, foods and food supplements, including vitamins and other beneficial nutrients, are not drugs. They are natural biomolecules that life on earth has evolved with over millions of years, and should not require the same stringent testing for "efficacy." Many foods contain powerful molecules, such as caffeine in tea and coffee. Although these ingredients are natural they can cause harm to some people if taken in large doses. Thus, the reaction to reports of food supplements causing harm is likely to be pressure to regulate all food supplements, including doses of essential nutrients as drugs. Recent media coverage has misinformed the public, placing vitamins in the category of drugs by stating that vitamins are dangerous and unregulated.[39] In fact, vitamins and supplements of essential nutrients are already regulated, and when taken in appropriate doses they are very safe, much safer (by 1,000,000-fold) than many commonly used drugs.[40] Further, supplements of essential nutrients are very effective in lowering the risk of age-related diseases such as cancer and heart disease.[41] As described above, essential nutrients can often obviate or prevent problems caused by drugs.[42] Niacin can prevent acute liver damage from overdoses of acetaminophen, a drug widely used to prevent pain in OA.[43] The cure for ignorance about essential nutrients is not legislation designed to regulate food and vitamin supplements. Instead, what is needed is widely disseminated knowledge about the benefits of essential nutrients and their proper doses. As we explain in this book, supplements are effective for preventing many types of arthritis when taken in appropriate doses along with an excellent diet.

B Vitamins

The balance between resorption and formation of cartilage depends on adequate nutrition. Blood vessels don't reach the cartilage directly, so the synovial fluid is responsible for providing nutrients to the chondrocytes that make new cartilage. As explained in Chapter 2, the B vitamins are necessary for the metabolism of all cells, including the chondrocytes that generate new articular cartilage in joints.[44] A continuous supply of all the vitamins, including the B vitamins, is essential for the health of synovial membrane and articular cartilage. There is considerable evidence that vitamins B_1, B_2, B_3, and B_5 can help prevent OA.[45] Patients with OA are commonly obese and have vitamin deficiencies.[46] Deficiencies of B vitamins contribute to joint disease, and adequate doses of these important vitamins may help reduce joint pain and recovery from OA and RA.[47] The enzyme that recycles glutathione in cells back to its normal reduced form is dependent on B vitamins, especially riboflavin (vitamin B_2). Because glutathione is crucial in preventing the oxidative stress inside cells that contributes to RA, a riboflavin deficiency can contribute to RA. And indeed, a riboflavin deficiency is common among patients with active RA.[48] Folate (B_9) and vitamin B_{12} are important for regrowth of bone, and older people are often deficient. Supplements of these B vitamins can improve pain, balance, and hand strength, in some cases more than NSAIDs.[49]

Biotin is important for the metabolism of fatty acids, amino acids, and glucose.[50] Low levels of biotin (B_7) are associated with oxidative stress and lameness in animals.[51] Biotin and folate are synergistic in suppressing inflammatory pathways.[52] A deficiency of biotin is rare, because it is usually made in adequate amounts by bacteria in the gut,[53] but the optimal level of biotin is unknown and there is no RDA for it.[54] It is widely distributed in foods such as liver, yogurt, whole grains, beans and legumes, nuts, and egg yolk. However, some individuals are deficient, either because of genetic differences, problems with composition of microbiota or absorption in the gut, or consumption of raw egg white.[55]

Niacinamide at high doses has been shown to reduce the pain and inflammation of OA, even in patients with severe symptoms.[56] Niacin or niacinamide is an excellent first-line treatment for OA for doctors using nutritional treatments.[57] The disappearance of pain in response to niacinamide treatment is evidently not due to an analgesic effect. Instead it appears due to a gradual physiological improvement in the tissues of the joint, allowing greater joint motion without pain.[58] A randomized controlled trial (RCT) tested the effect of 3,000 mg per day of niacinamide taken in divided doses throughout the day over twelve weeks and found reduced markers of inflammation and increased joint mobility.[59] Although niacin and niacinamide are both vitamin B_3, and both will give the same relief from arthritis symptoms, niacinamide (250 mg, 16 times per day) is often given because it does not cause a flush.[60]

This beneficial effect of niacinamide may in part be related to its action of downregulating cytokines released by the synovial membrane, including interleukin-1 (IL-1), that inhibit the production of chondroitin sulfate and collagen required for formation of the extracellular matrix of cartilage.[61] The inhibition of the extracellular matrix collagen by this molecular pathway is mediated by the signaling molecule nitric oxide (NO), which is released by chondrocytes in response to cytokines such as interleukin-1 in the synovial fluid.[62] Another bit of evidence is that niacin cream applied to the skin of patients with RA does not cause the usual niacin flush. This method was described as a way to diagnose RA, but at the time the mechanism was unknown.[63] This suggests that in the presence of systemwide inflammation, such as in RA or OA, the body has a deficiency of niacin, which prevents the usual niacin flush. Thus, niacin or niacinamide may be beneficial in preventing inflammation throughout the body and especially in the joints. Interestingly, niacinamide can prevent acute liver damage from overdoses of acetaminophen, a drug widely used to prevent pain in OA.[64]

B Vitamins for RA

The B vitamins are also helpful reducing pain and inflammation in RA. High-dose niacinamide (nonflush niacin) has been shown to relieve the symptoms of OA,[65] and it will also help to relieve RA symptoms. A deficiency of vitamin B_6 (pyridoxine) as well as other nutrients is common in rheumatoid arthritis and in atherosclerosis.[66] Such deficiencies are associated with immune system problems and inflammation.[67] In one study, vitamin B_6 supplements decreased inflammatory markers in RA.[68] One hypothesis is that the connection between low vitamin B_6, RA, and heart disease is inflammation.[69]Anemia is very common among RA patients. One study concluded that several types of anemia are often present simultaneously in RA.[70] Folate and vitamin B_{12} were low in 25 to 30 percent of RA patients, and over half were low in iron. Adequate iron, folate, and vitamin B_{12} levels are critically important, for without these essential nutrients, cells cannot grow, and the joints suffer. These essential nutrients are easy to get from an excellent diet. Folate and most of the other B vitamins are available in many vegetables including beans, nuts, and dark green leafy vegetables. Vitamin C helps the gut to absorb iron from vegetables. Vitamin B_{12} is available in clams, liver, fish, meat, eggs, poultry, and supplements.

It's important to point out that methotrexate, a drug commonly used to treat RA, interacts with folate from the diet.[71] This drug inhibits the action of folate in the body (biosynthesis of purine nucleotides), which helps to prevent proliferation of cells in the synovial membrane in RA. However, at high doses this drug can be toxic if not managed carefully. That problem can be prevented by supplementing with folinic acid as opposed to folic acid.[72] Of course, with an excellent diet along with adequate doses of supplements, RA flareups can be prevented without drugs.[73]

BIOTIN AND AVIDIN

Biotin (vitamin B_7) is an essential nutrient for all living organisms, from bacteria to reptiles and mammals, but is only made by plants and some bacteria and fungi.[74] Like the other B vitamins, biotin is required for basic functioning of cells, and some bacteria and fungi and all animals including humans must obtain it from their diet. The eggs of reptiles and birds contain all the essential nutrients for life including biotin. If its outer membrane is broken, however, the egg is at risk for a bacterial or fungal infection. Remarkably and notably, eggs contain powerful mechanisms to prevent microbial infections.

The egg white that surrounds the yolk is protected by several special molecules that act as antibiotics.[75] One of them, called avidin, has a unique property. Avidin is a large protein that binds to biotin very strongly. The bond is similar to the very specific bond formed between an antibody and an antigen. This type of electrostatic bond is called "noncovalent" because the molecules it joins remain separate. But the bond between avidin and biotin is far stronger than achievable by antibodies. In fact, the avidin-biotin bond is the strongest noncovalent bond known in nature. This bond is rapidly formed and under most conditions is essentially permanent.[76] Its chemical dissociation constant, Kd, which measures the tendency of the bond to break apart, is very small, ($\sim 10^{-15}$ M). It is not affected by acids, high temperature ionic solvents, or organic solvents. Further, the avidin-biotin complex is indigestible and cannot be absorbed by the gut or by microorganisms.[77] Yet, the avidin molecule is denatured by cooking, which prevents it from binding biotin, and allows cooked egg white to be digested without causing loss of biotin.

Interestingly, the vitamin biotin was discovered through its tight bond to avidin. When animals on a healthy diet were given uncooked egg white, they developed a disease syndrome similar to other vitamin B deficiencies.[78] But when these animals were given a sufficient dose of foods containing other essential nutrients, the syndrome caused by raw egg white disappeared. It was then possible to determine which component of food corrected the "raw egg white syndrome." This led to the discovery of biotin as an essential vitamin. Biotin is found in a variety of foods including liver, wheat germ, dairy products, beans, legumes and nuts, and egg yolk.

After the discovery of biotin, the molecule that caused the deficiency was isolated and named avidin (from "avid albumin," literally "craving albumin"), and its role in the deficiency of biotin was determined.[79] Avidin is now known to bind four biotin molecules. In chemistry, this property of binding to a specific number of molecules is called "stoichiometric." When more than four molecules of biotin are present, an avidin molecule cannot bind to all of them. But when the level of avidin is in excess, it becomes a very effective antibiotic. Egg white contains enough avidin to bind and sequester the biotin from microorganisms so they cannot flourish. Moreover, some bacteria make a protein similar to avidin called streptavidin, which is thought to slow the growth of competing bacteria.

However, the antibiotic property of avidin can readily cause a deficiency of biotin in people who eat raw egg white. When eaten with other foods, a large serving of raw egg white can very effectively bind and sequester all the biotin they contain. This can happen, for instance, when a large amount of whole-egg mayonnaise or other foods containing raw egg white are consumed. If mayonnaise is used sparingly as a spread on a sandwich containing meat or cheese, the biotin present in these foods is adequate to overwhelm the avidin present in the raw egg white. There is little risk for a biotin deficiency when only moderate amounts of mayonnaise are eaten.

The strong bond between avidin and biotin is widely utilized in the biological sciences.[80] Biotin is a small natural molecule that can spread throughout the cytoplasm (the inside of) cells. It can also be readily attached to other molecules. These properties allow biotin to be utilized as a tracer molecule. For example, when injected into a cell the biotin will diffuse throughout the cell, even in cells such as neurons of the brain that have an extensive network of cell branches and dendrites. Then avidin coupled to a fluorescent dye is added to the preparation. A fluorescent microscope is then used to see where the biotin has spread by visualizing the avidin bound to the biotin. The strong bond of avidin with biotin makes this process of visualization uniquely specific. Avidin is also used to study the role of biotin as a cofactor in metabolic pathways.

Biology goes to great lengths to protect the body from harm. Because biotin is an essential nutrient for all species that is only made by a few, the egg has developed a remarkably robust defense that makes use of this wide dependency.

Vitamin C

Vitamin C is one of the most important water-soluble antioxidants in the body.[81] It is required for the body to make collagen, and it stimulates the production of collagen and other extracellular matrix molecules in cartilage.[82] When vitamin C is deficient in the diet, even when symptoms of scurvy are not apparent, joints will take longer to heal, and the balance between resorption and reformation will tend to shift towards resorption. Vitamin C is required for healthy articular and meniscal cartilage, for the synovial capsule and arteries around the joint, and for the ligaments and tendons that hold the joint together. It is essential for the formation of the extracellular collagen matrix of cartilage.[83] Sufficient vitamin C increases the synthesis of collagen and aggrecan, shifting the balance towards regeneration of cartilage.[84]

Vitamin C is also essential in preventing systemic inflammation. It increases the elasticity of arteries,[85] and along with adequate magnesium supplements can prevent high blood pressure that is associated with inflammation in arteries and heart disease.[86] The antioxidant capacity of vitamin C is also essential for reducing oxidative stress due to damage in the joint and the surrounding tissues. Inflammation is associated with OA, and lessening systemic inflammation can prevent OA.[87] Inflammation is thought to be caused by oxidative stress, which is prevented very effectively by antioxidants such as vitamin C. It is transported into chondrocytes[88] and effectively reduces the concentration of free radicals. Interestingly, one cause of arthritis is scurvy, which in recent years has been diagnosed in emergency wards in patients who had a very low intake of vitamin C in their diet.[89] Joint and muscle pain from acute hemarthrosis (bleeding in joints) of scurvy was cured in a few days with 1,000 mg per day of vitamin C.[90] After surgery for thumb arthritis or wrist fractures, vitamin C reduced pain very effectively and is recommended by surgeons.[91] Significantly, oxidative stress is increased and vitamin C levels are reduced in OA.[92] Further, antioxidants in the synovial fluid of late-stage OA are decreased compared with early stage OA with intact cartilage. Apparently, even when joint tissues are painful, as long as they are healthy, they can release antioxidants into the synovial fluid, a sign that recovery is taking place. But with increased oxidative stress and damage in late-stage OA this process slows.[93] This is a compelling reason why vitamin C and other antioxidants and essential nutrients are helpful to prevent progression of age-related diseases such as OA.[94]

Interestingly, vitamin C attenuates the degradation of hyaluronic acid (HA), which is a molecule in the synovial fluid important for its lubrication qualities. HA helps to prevent physical damage to cartilage and is also thought to be anti-inflammatory. Vitamin C inhibits the reaction of the enzymes in the synovial fluid (hyaluronidase and associated lysates) that degrade HA.[95] This suggests that high doses of vitamin C will help to increase the level of HA in synovial fluid, and tip the balance towards regrowth of cartilage.

In many studies, vitamin C has reduced the risk and pain of OA, whether in supplements[96] or from fruit and vegetables in the daily diet.[97] Vitamin C reduced the risk of bone marrow lesions in OA by 50 percent and its level in the body was inversely proportional to the area of damaged bone.[98] In a carefully performed observational study, vitamin C in the diet reduced the progression and pain of OA by 70 percent.[99] The same study also found a benefit of beta-carotene and vitamin E. In female mice lacking ovaries and thus at risk for bone loss, vitamin C increased bone regeneration, establishing its role as a skeletal anabolic agent.[100] In a study of induced arthritis in rats, vitamin C (equivalent to approximately 20 grams (gm) per day for a 150 pound human) suppressed the development of arthritis.[101] Rats and mice can make their own ascorbate, so for them it is not a vitamin. But evidently a higher level of ascorbate than normal is helpful for their bodies to repair damage when oxidative stress is present. One likely mechanism is that in damaged cartilage, the chondrocytes generate copious free radicals, and vitamin C effectively neutralizes them.[102] This reduces oxidative stress and telomere shortening (aging) in chondrocytes.[103] Besides its antioxidant effects, vitamin C increased the synthesis of type II collagen and aggrecan in cartilage.[104] Rose hip powder, which contains vitamin C and many other antioxidants has been shown effective in preventing pain and inflammation from arthritis.[105] One of the biochemicals associated with vitamin C, a bioflavonoid called hesperidin, reduced inflammation from arthritis in a mouse model of RA.[106]

In most of these studies the doses were small by orthomolecular standards (100–1,000mg per day). Higher doses are likely to be more effective, especially when the level of vitamin C in the blood is low.[107] This is especially true for smokers, because the toxins in smoke cause oxidative stress and lower the level of antioxidants such as vitamin C and E in the bloodstream.[108] It is also true for individuals who are sick with flu or other diseases, or under physical stress such as athletics or exposure to severe cold. These can cause oxidative stress, reducing antioxidant levels. Because antioxidants are so important in the body's ability to recover from bone and joint damage, it is doubly important to take additional antioxidants when you're under stress.

Vitamin C Improves Mood

In a recent RCT, typically malnourished hospital patients who were given vitamin C for eight weeks had significant improvements in mood and a reduction in distress.[109] It is important to note that it is unethical to perform trials of vitamins and other essential nutrients if a "control group" of participants is given a placebo. The reason is that these essential natural substances are known to be effective, and all patients deserve the most effective treatment.[110] This "ethical criterion" is one of the factors that have limited the proper testing of vitamins, for they cannot ethically be withheld. However, this trial had an "active control" of vitamin D. Instead of a placebo, vitamin D was given to the control group who were not assigned vitamin C. Vitamin D is already known to improve mood,[111] but because it was given at a normal dose of 5,000 international units (IU) for only a few weeks, the level in the control group hardly increased. Although it was an "active control", vitamin D in this short term trial could not have much effect. Thus, the vitamin D given to the active control group was essentially a placebo without the ethical limitation. This trial clearly showed that vitamin C quickly improves the mood and reduces psychological distress.[112] This can be an important factor in getting better sleep, reducing inflammation, and improving recovery from any type of arthritis.

Vitamin C for RA

Diet has a big effect on recovery from RA. Vitamin deficiencies directly limit the ability of joints to recover. Deficiencies also cause inflammation and prevent the body's immune system from functioning properly. A deficiency of vitamin C can halt the regrowth of cartilage because the synthesis of collagen requires vitamin C. As explained in Chapter 3, during stress that can cause RA or with inflammation caused by RA, the body's requirement for antioxidants such as vitamin C increases. In a study of older people, those with reduced vitamin C intake were threefold more likely to get RA.[113] Even before RA was evident, when comparing those with higher levels of vitamins in their bloodstream with those having lower levels of vitamins, those with higher vitamin levels had a lower risk of developing RA. In an early clinical study of rheumatic fever, vitamin C relieved symptoms of fever and pain in a few days, but high doses (for the time) of 4,000 mg per day were necessary to achieve the effect.[114]

Antioxidants and other essential nutrients and beneficial biochemicals in foods are known to be beneficial in managing RA.[115] There are several ways that antioxidants can help. First, damage to DNA is thought to be a big risk factor for RA.[116] Those with RA have higher levels of DNA damage. Antioxidants such as vitamins C and E, glutathione, and alpha-lipoic acid are known to help prevent DNA damage by neutralizing free radicals such as reactive oxygen species (ROS). Recent evidence also suggests that antioxidants can prevent the proteins in the joint from being damaged by oxidative stress. In this type of damage, the immune system may confuse damaged joint proteins with an external antigen, and thus may attack them. This is thought to be the trigger that causes autoimmunity in some types of RA.[117] Further, antioxidants such as beta-carotene and vitamins C and E are known to downregulate inflammatory signaling pathways.[118]

Vitamin C is helpful in preventing and recovering from a wide variety of bacterial and viral infections.[119] Because infection is a common trigger for RA, adequate doses of vitamin C when taken early in an infection can prevent or reduce the intensity of the infection and thus prevent it from triggering RA. Vitamin C is also effective at preventing toxicity from a wide variety of environmental toxins and drugs.[120]

Moreover, antioxidants in the body are synergistic, meaning that each antioxidant, such as vitamin C, helps all the others such as vitamin E, beta-carotene, and flavonoids, to neutralize free radicals. Most of these antioxidants have other functions in the body besides their antioxidant properties. Therefore, a combination of antioxidants in an excellent diet of fresh vegetables and fruits will be helpful. Although some RCTs of vitamin supplements have not shown a large benefit for RA, it is likely they will show more positive benefits as more studies are performed with better controls and higher doses of supplements. Dozens of observational studies have shown the importance of an excellent diet in RA.

In a study of the Mediterranean diet, the level of vitamin C and other antioxidants in the blood was inversely related to RA severity.[121] Patients report that antioxidants lower their level of pain. Several studies have tested high-dose intravenous vitamin C on RA. In one case, an intravenous injection of vitamin C and glutathione immediately reduced acute pain after an RA flare-up for several pain-free hours.[122] In another study, intravenous vitamin C given to RA patients significantly reduced levels of C-reactive protein (CRP), a marker of inflammation.[123] Vitamin C given intravenously decreases histamine levels in the bloodstream, which can prevent or largely alleviate allergic reactions.[124]

Vitamin D

Vitamin D was originally discovered as the essential nutrient that prevents rickets, and it is essential for the body's utilization of calcium in the bones.[125] You may already know that a deficiency of vitamin D can cause osteomalacia or osteoporosis in older people.[126] But, from recent research, vitamin D is known to be a hormone that affects many other tissues of the body.[127] A deficiency of vitamin D is thought to impair the ability of bone and cartilage to respond to damage that occurs in OA.[128] Further, the bloodstream level of 25-hydroxy vitamin D (the form measured in blood tests) is not directly associated with the amount of vitamin D intake. Moreover, people with more body fat require a larger dose of vitamin D to maintain an adequate blood leve.[129]

In a study on the risk of incidence and progression of OA, those with adequate vitamin D levels had a 70 percent reduction in risk for OA progression.[130] Recent studies have shown that chondrocytes have vitamin D receptors, and that vitamin D may help them to regulate cartilage remodeling. In a study on different stages of OA in rats, it was found that vitamin D protected against disease progression during the early stages of OA, but less so in later stages of OA.[131] Evidently the protective effect is due to the ability of vitamin D to downregulate an inflammatory pathway that causes cartilage to be degraded. A study of older women found that those with the lowest vitamin D levels in the bloodstream had the most joint pain.[132] In one study, vitamin D improved the pain and quality of sleep in chronic pain patients.[133] Another study of men and women performed over six and a half years found that those with low vitamin D levels and low bone mineral density had a higher risk of incidence and progression of OA.[134]

Many studies of vitamin D deficiency have found no consistent association with incidence or with progression of OA. However, it seems likely that negative results can be reconciled with studies showing a positive association. For example, the results likely depend on the levels and intakes of vitamin D involved, and on the pre-existing conditions of the participants. One study found a significant association between OA and low levels of vitamin D, but the effect was mainly in patients younger than sixty.[135] This again suggests that vitamin D may be important in the early stages of OA. Studies that show a range of 25-hydroxy vitamin D blood serum levels below 30 ng/ml may not show a significant difference in OA simply because that range of levels may be too low to have a beneficial effect. Further, to initiate OA may take one or more other factors that may not be directly associated with vitamin D levels, such as systemic inflammation or joint damage. Given that many studies have found inverse associations of vitamin D intake and blood levels with OA, and there is a likely mechanism that can explain these results, the conclusion that vitamin D can help to prevent OA seems robust.

Interestingly, vitamin D is made from skin exposure to midday summer sunlight. It is made from a derivative of cholesterol by UVB (short-wave ultraviolet) light. Therefore some rare individuals with genetic mutations affecting the synthesis of cholesterol have a greater risk of low vitamin D levels.[136] This emphasizes that individuals differ in their absorption and biological utilization of essential nutrients. Learning how the essential nutrients are supplied by lifestyle and diet is important, for some people may need them in much larger amounts than others. We must all attempt to determine our individual needs.

A study of OA pain in older people with differing skin color found that African Americans with dark skin had lower blood levels of vitamin D. These lower levels were associated with worse OA pain in an experimental test.[137] Low vitamin D levels are very common among people living in North America and Europe, because for much of the year (October through March) the sun is too low in the sky to provide enough UVB radiation to generate adequate vitamin D. A study of veiled older Egyptian women in a clinical exam found that those with low vitamin D levels were more likely to have OA.[138] These results suggest that older people who have low vitamin D levels, especially those with dark skin, or who wear a veil, or stay indoors, could prevent or relieve pain and OA symptoms with an adequate dose of vitamin D (2,000–5,000 IU per day or more, depending on body weight), along with an excellent diet that supplies adequate calcium, magnesium, and other essential nutrients.

Vitamin D for RA

It has become clear in recent years that vitamin D has an important role in preventing RA. Besides its role in bone and joint health, vitamin D has a powerful modulatory effect on the immune system, downregulating pro-inflammatory cytokines.[139] It also inhibits cell proliferation, for example, in the synovial membrane.[140] Patients with RA are often deficient in vitamin D, and the patients with the most severe cases are the ones most deficient.[141] Further, RA patients have a decreased expression of vitamin D binding protein in their synovial membranes, which tends to prevent vitamin D from performing its anti-inflammatory role.[142] Disability and NSAID use in RA is associated with a deficiency of vitamin D.[143] Thus, a deficiency of vitamin D is thought to have an important role in RA.[144] This suggests an adequate dose of vitamin D is crucial in preventing RA.[145] For example, in cell cultures, vitamin D lowered the expression of inflammatory cytokines.[146] This is thought to be one of the causes of the inflammation in joints that initiates RA. In another recent study, vitamin D reduced nitric oxide (NO) levels and downregulated inflammatory signal pathways in macrophages.[147] Moreover, in RA patients a deficiency of vitamin D carries an especially high risk of cardiovascular disease.[148] Vitamin D is also important in preventing other autoimmune diseases.[149] Thus, although it has been known for decades that vitamin D is essential for bone health, we now know that it is also essential in preventing and reversing joint damage, including inflammatory disease such as RA.

SUNLIGHT, SKIN COLOR, AND VITAMIN D

An acquaintance who is apparently a sun worshipper often sits out in the sunlight for several hours, even on a cold winter day. Although he is light-skinned, he maintains a dark tan on his exposed skin year-round. Tanning is an adaptation to seasonal changes in sunlight. Darker skin protects against disease caused by strong overhead sunlight, but lighter skin allows greater production of vitamin D from the sun in the early spring and late fall.[150] For this reason, vitamin D is thought to be responsible for the evolution of light skin in populations living at latitudes far from the equator.[151]

Modern humans originated in Africa 200,000 years ago, with dark skin. They migrated from Africa in the period from 50,000 to 100,000 years ago.[152] When they moved northward into the Middle East, Asia, and Europe, their skin generated much less vitamin D, so they became deficient, especially in the long winters. The resulting deficiency of vitamin D caused disease and early death. But their descendants who had lighter skin survived better. Their skin could make more vitamin D from the scarce UVB in the fall, winter, and early spring. As a result, these populations evolved by natural selection to have lighter skin.[153] The same change to lighter skin color also occurred in southern Africa. The farther away people migrated from the equator, the lower the sun was in the sky, and the lighter their skin became.

Around 50,000 years ago, some modern humans interbred with Neanderthals, who were archaic hominins (primitive humans) that shared much of our genetic heritage. Neanderthals originally diverged from our line 800,000 years ago, and had emigrated from Africa to southern Europe 230,000 years ago.[154] They had about 100,000 years more than modern humans to evolve to fit their northern environment. The skin color of Neanderthals is unknown, but was probably light to maximize generation of vitamin D.[155] The reverse effect happened when some lighter skinned modern humans migrated to what is now southern India. They regained the original dark skin through natural selection under the strong hot sun. In regions with a lot of strong midday sunlight, natural selection evidently drives evolution towards dark skin by preventing skin cancer and degradation of folate (vitamin B_9) in the bloodstream. A dramatic change of skin color in a naturally evolving human population takes only 50 to 100 generations (approximately 2,000 years). Thus skin color is mostly a matter of sunlight and vitamins![156]

In the northern United States, Canada, and Europe, the UVA (long-wavelength ultraviolet) rays of the winter sun can give a tan. Window glass transmits much of the UVA in sunlight falling on them, but windows block most of the UVB (short-wavelength ultraviolet) that produces vitamin D. Alas for the winter sun worshiper, for although winter sunlight in North America or Europe can maintain a tan, it gives almost no UVB nor vitamin D when the sun is lower than forty-five degrees above the horizon. Worse, a winter tan will hinder absorption of UVB, further lessening the small amount of vitamin D made from the midday sunlight of late winter, when it is typically needed the most. And prolonged exposure to sunlight, even in those who have naturally dark skin or a tan, increases the risk of skin cancer. Regular moderate exposure to direct summer midday sunlight reduces cancer risk because it provides vitamin D. But heavier exposure, including sunburn, increases risk.[157] Further, exposure to UVA without UVB may be harmful. One theory suggests that UVA from sunshine through windows is responsible for degrading vitamin D in the skin and contributing to the recent increase in skin cancer.[158]

The moral of the story is, the amount of vitamin D made in the skin from exposure to sunlight is not directly related to the darkness of the resulting tan. To get an adequate amount of vitamin D, get moderate regular exposure to the UVB rays in direct summer midday sunlight, and take supplements in the fall, winter, and spring when the sun is low in the sky.

Vitamin E

As one of the main fat-soluble antioxidants in the body, vitamin E is important in preventing oxidative stress, which is thought to trigger OA and RA. The form (isomer) of vitamin E most commonly sold is d-alpha-tocopherol, because it is actively absorbed by the body. When patients with OA were given vitamin E, either alone or in combination with fish oil, their pain and joint mobility improved.[159] In another study, 600 IU of vitamin E per day, given for ten days reduced pain in OA.[160]

Yet the other active forms of vitamin E also have important distinct roles. The d-gamma-tocopherol form of vitamin E is thought to help regeneration of bone.[161] This form is has greater anti-inflammatory properties than d-alpha tocopherol, and is the most common form available in the typical diet in the United States. It is available in nuts and seeds, including oils such as soybean oil. Vitamin E is known to reduce inflammatory pathways, and may be involved in tipping the balance in cartilage towards regrowth.[162]

Although the body actively absorbs d-alpha-tocopherol, it is thought to compete with the d-gamma-tocopherol in the body. In one study, those who took d-alpha-tocopherol had a lower level of d-gamma-tocopherol, which appeared to lower their rate of bone repair.[163] Evidently a high level of the d-alpha form depletes the d-gamma-tocopherol in the body. This may be the reason why some interventional studies of d-alpha-tocopherol showed negative results, whereas observational studies that measure blood levels of d-alpha-tocopherol generally show positive results. Thus it may be best not to take the pure d-alpha-tocopherol form, but to take a balanced mixture of all the alpha-, beta-, delta-, and gamma- forms of vitamin E.

The tocotrienols, also considered to be vitamin E, are antioxidants and signaling modulators with roles distinct from the tocopherols. They have numerous effects in preventing cancer and heart disease, because they are powerful inhibitors of inflammatory pathways.[164] This suggests that a mixture of the different forms of vitamin E, including both tocopherols and tocotrienols, will help to prevent oxidative stress that is a risk factor for both OA and RA, and will also lessen inflammation.

Vitamin K

In addition to its role in blood clotting, vitamin K is involved in controlling cartilage and bone formation, and vascular calcification. Like vitamin D, vitamin K is important in bone remodeling and in maintaining proper blood levels of calcium. A deficiency of vitamin K is widespread in modern societies today.[165] But in the long term, even a slight deficiency of vitamin K will tend to cause problems with bone and joint health. The triage theory of essential nutrients explains why. Coagulation of blood is critical for life. Accordingly, the enzymes in the liver that utilize vitamin K to generate coagulation proteins have a higher affinity for vitamin K than enzymes outside the liver that regulate calcium. When the body has a mild deficiency of vitamin K, the liver can still generate coagulation proteins to prevent uncontrolled bleeding. But the same mild deficiency of vitamin K wreaks havoc in the long run with bone and joint health.[166] Vitamin K is widely used to treat osteoporosis, but it is burgeoning as a treatment for arthritis.[167] As a bonus it also will reduce your risk of heart attack.

As described in Chapter 4, vitamin K is essential for bone and joint health, and helps to tip the balance from bone resorption towards bone regrowth. It is thought to be so essential for bone health that blood levels of vitamin K are used as a diagnostic measure for osteoporosis.[168] A recent study of vitamin K found that a deficiency was associated with an increased risk of knee OA.[169] Thus vitamin K is an excellent candidate for supplementation. However, as is the case for many promising nutritional treatments, not all studies have found supplements of vitamin K to be effective in preventing loss of bone density. This may be due to the duration of the study being too short, the use of the wrong doses, or it could be linked to a deficiency of other associated essential nutrients such as vitamin D, calcium, and magnesium.[170]

A deficiency of vitamin K is directly linked to the level of circulating incompletely synthesized osteocalcin, an important bone building protein.[171] This is true for both K_1 and K_2 forms.[172] Interestingly, a problem related to the function of vitamin K highlights its function in the body. The long-term use of anticoagulant drugs such as warfarin that block the action of vitamin K can cause loss of bone density, which can trigger or worsen OA.[173] This further emphasizes the important function of vitamin K in bone and joint health. Vitamin K_2 is of particular interest in OA because it is thought to be the active form for regulating calcium. A recent study showed that in bones from people who had knee replacements, the medial condyles of the knee, which had more severe OA, also had lower levels of vitamin K_2 than the lateral condyles, which had higher K_2 levels.[174] Another recent study found that supplements of the bacterial form of vitamin K_2 (MK-7), taken over a year, improved bone density.[175] Vitamin K_2 prevented inflammation and lessened the disease activity in RA in yet another study.[176] Vitamin K_2 as the MK-4 form helps to reverse osteoporosis.[177]

Unfortunately, the importance of vitamin K is still underappreciated today. Interested readers are strongly encouraged to read Dr. Kate Rheaume-Bleue's book, *Vitamin K_2 and the Calcium Paradox.*[178] She explains that death from cardiovascular disease is mostly due to excessive calcification. The plaques found in atherosclerosis and strokes begin with calcifications on the arterial wall, and the fatty cholesterol component builds on this. Vitamin K is necessary to regulate calcification, but the other fat-soluble vitamins A and D are necessary in order for the body to utilize vitamin K in this role. A patient who was advised to get an aortic valve replacement due to excessive stenosis and calcification started taking a dose of 8,000 IU vitamin D daily, because this had been shown to halt the progression of aortic valve stenosis. Next this patient tried vitamin K. After ten months the valve cross-sectional area had nearly doubled in size.[179] This was remarkable, but suggests that vitamin K can accomplish similar miracles for arthritis. Other patients have had their hypertension dramatically reduced by vitamin K, again presumably due to removal of calcification blockages. This clearly shows that vitamin K helps to prevent and reverse calcifications in blood vessels. Calcification (ossification) of cartilage is an established hallmark feature defining osteoarthritis.[180] Because many individuals are deficient in vitamin K, its critical role in controlling ossification and improving circulation strongly suggests that adequate vitamin K can prevent and reverse arthritis.

Omega-3 Fatty Acids

The body requires a dietary source of both omega-3 and omega-6 fatty acids because they are essential for health. Although they are not considered vitamins, the body cannot make them and must get them from the diet. The balance or ratio of these two essential nutrients is thought to be important, because they are to some extent antagonistic in their effect on inflammatory pathways in the body.[181] Omega-6 fatty acids are considered inflammatory, while omega-3 fatty acids are considered anti-inflammatory. Although with modern diets the ratio is typically 20:1 (omega-6: omega3), it historically was and should be closer to 1:1 for best health.[182]

Several RCTs have shown that fish oil containing omega-3 poly-unsaturated fatty acids (PUFAs) is effective in reducing pain and increasing function in OA and RA.[183] In an RCT studying frailty and physical mobility of older women with OA, a dietary supplement of long-chain omega-3 fatty acids for six months allowed the participants to walk faster, likely because of a reduction in pain and an increase in joint mobility. They were given daily supplements of 1,200 mg of both eicosapentaenoic acid (EPA) and docosahexaenoic acid (DHA), found in fish oil, and their dietary levels of vitamin C and selenium were tabulated. Higher levels of these antioxidants in their diet along with the omega-3 fatty acids helped to increase mobility.[184]

In a study of RA patients who took methotrexate, omega-3 fatty acids from fish oil (4,500 mg per day) improved their remission rates by more than twofold.[185] In guinea pigs prone to OA, a diet containing a high proportion of omega-3 relative to omega-6 fatty acids reduced the signs of OA.[186] In a study of people taking supplements, omega-3 fatty acids reduced markers of inflammation in the bloodstream.[187] A trial of a commercial product containing omega-3 fatty acids from fish oil, vitamin E, and an extract of nettles reduced joint pain and increased function in OA.[188] One reason for the efficacy of this combination is is that omega-3 fatty acids are susceptible to damage by oxidative stress because they are polyunsaturated. Fat-soluble antioxidants such as vitamin E are known to prevent degradation of PUFAs and thus to lessen the degree of oxidative stress in joints. Thus including vitamin E in this type of oil supplement is likely to prevent oxidation of the omega-3 fatty acids and further help to prevent OA. Indeed, natural vitamin E is purified from vegetable oils.[189]

Although it is not known exactly how omega-3 fatty acids help prevent pain and reduce OA and RA symptoms, long-chain omega-3 fatty acids such as EPA and DHA are anti-inflammatory. They are helpful in providing mobility for molecules in cell membranes, for example in chondrocytes in cartilage and osteocytes in bone. These omega-3 fatty acids are thought to inhibit inflammatory signals to the immune system, and this can prevent generation of free radicals. In this role, omega-3 fatty acids balance the inflammatory influence of omega-6 fatty acids on cytokines.[190] Omega-3 fatty acids tend to antagonize the level of arachidonic acid that would otherwise initiate inflammation.[191] Omega-3 fatty acids also have a variety of effects on modulating the expression of genes.[192] Essential PUFAs increase calcium absorption by enhancing the action of vitamin D, and they lessen the amount of calcium excreted in the urine. The result is that more calcium is available for deposit in bones, which can enhance the synthesis of collagen in bones and joints.[193]

Interestingly, omega-3 fatty acids may be useful in reducing the niacin flush.[194] Although many people find the warm niacin flush unpleasant, I (WTP) personally find it quite pleasant and enjoy the flush from 1,000 mg of niacin on a daily basis. The flush response occurs due to massive production of the prostaglandin signaling molecules PGE2 and PGD2. Omega-6 fatty acids are known to up-regulate inflammatory signaling pathways. Omega-3 fatty acids are precursors to anti-inflammatory prostaglandin signaling pathways, so the balance of omega-3 to omega-6 fatty acids influences how inflammatory the signal from these essential nutrients will be.

N-Acetyl-Cysteine and Alpha-Lipoic Acid

Glutathione is the most important antioxidant inside cells, and in arthritis patients it is depleted. It is not an essential nutrient because cells can synthesize it with their biochemical pathways. Glutathione can be obtained from the diet, but it is not well absorbed by the gut. When depleted it is helpful to take a precursor molecule for glutathione, N-acetyl-cysteine (NAC), which is well-absorbed in the gut, to allow more glutathione to be made. NAC is helpful in a variety of conditions where oxidative stress occurs.[195] When cartilage is exposed even briefly to blood, for example, after damage to the joint, it causes oxidative stress and long-lasting damage to the cartilage. This type of oxidative-stress related damage caused by blood is lessened by NAC.[196] In another study, NAC lowered the level of inflammatory markers present in the blood of mice with arthritis.[197] In a laboratory study of cartilage survival, NAC prevented chondrocyte death and cartilage degeneration.[198] This was due to the ability of NAC to raise glutathione levels. In a study of damage to cartilage tissue, a heavy weight load on cartilage caused chondrocytes to die, but this was prevented with antioxidants such as vitamin E and NAC.[199] In another study, NAC was shown to ameliorate lupus erythematosus.[200]

Taking supplements of NAC can prevent oxidative damage from a persistent chemical in the environment, PCBs, that can otherwise kill chondrocytes.[201] Many other artificial chemicals and drugs generate oxidative stress that can cause arthritis, and higher levels of antioxidants can help. NAC also helps to prevent DNA mutations in the synovial membrane.[202] Interestingly, NAC along with a compound of vanadium suppressed inflammation and ameliorated arthritis in mice.[203] Since antioxidants are synergistic, it is helpful to take several of them together, such as vitamins C and E, and NAC. Alpha-lipoic acid is another important related antioxidant that has been shown to ameliorate arthritis.[204]

Molecular Precursors to Articular Cartilage

Recovery of joints can be enhanced with other nutrients besides vitamins. Biomolecules such as collagen and aggrecan that make up the extracellular matrix of cartilage are synthesized from smaller building blocks such as single amino acids or small peptide chains (molecules made up of several amino acids). If these building blocks are provided in adequate amounts they can stimulate regrowth of articular cartilage and other tissues of joints.

Each protein in the body, such as collagen, contains a specific ratio of the twenty amino acids, and thus its synthesis will require amino acids in this proportion. If one or more amino acids become depleted within a cell that is synthesizing the protein molecule, the synthesis slows. Thus it is thought that for the highest efficiency of synthesis, the proper proportion of all the amino acids is necessary. This raises the question of whether, for example, eating eggs, which provide one of the most complete sources of protein, will give the best balance of amino acids needed to recover from OA. Although eggs don't contain much collagen, the proteins in the egg white and yolk do contain all the essential amino acids necessary to generate any protein in the body, including collagen and the other molecules necessary for joints. The same is true of any excellent diet that includes adequate protein and other essential nutrients. For example, a diet of sprouts, dark green leafy vegetables, and raw vegetable juices that contain protein, carbohydrates, and where necessary, supplements of other essential nutrients (vitamins B_{12} and D) is enough to provide excellent health. This raises the question of whether it is possible to improve upon such a diet that includes a balanced amino acid content.

In the stomach, protein in food is digested by enzymes and very strong acids that hydrolyze it (break it apart) into individual amino acids or small "peptide" molecules consisting of several amino acids. These molecules are transported into the bloodstream. In some cases, it is thought that larger building blocks digested from food can enhance recovery from OA, as some of them can also be transported into the bloodstream. Precisely how such larger molecules affect the synthesis of cartilage or an improvement of joint function is unknown. To help in remodeling cartilage, they must be transported by the bloodstream to the synovial membrane, which likely secretes them and other essential nutrients such as amino acids and vitamins into the joint's synovial fluid. Normally, new proteins are synthesized from individual amino acids. But the larger peptide molecules may also be involved in this process. For example, after eating gelatin (hydrolyzed collagen from cartilage), the amount of peptide building blocks for collagen increases in the bloodstream. These are thought to be helpful for stimulating the regeneration of collagen in joints and throughout the body.[205] Some recent evidence suggests that the building block molecules for articular cartilage in food or supplements that are at least partly hydrolyzed will reduce joint pain and increase mobility, and support regeneration of cartilage.[206]

Glucosamine and Chondroitin

Glucosamine sulfate and chondroitin sulfate are biomolecules normally present in the extracellular matrix of articular cartilage in joints. They are often described as "nutraceuticals" or "biologicals" because they not essential nutrients, but are nutritional supplements that provide some specific benefit for relieving symptoms of arthritis.[207] Glucosamine sulfate is a precursor for several glycosaminoglycans (GAGs) that are in cartilage. Thus supplements of glucosamine sulfate are thought to be helpful in regrowing cartilage.[208] Glucosamine is thought to be a signal to the synovial membrane and chondrocytes in cartilage to express enzymes that generate hyaluronic acid, which helps to lubricate the joint. Glucosamine is also thought to be a signal to generate more osteoblasts that increase bone mass.[209]

Chondroitin helps to add fluid to joints and also helps the joint to build cartilage.[210] In a study of Navy Special Forces personnel with knee OA, supplements of of glucosamine, chondroitin, and manganese ascorbate relieved OA symptoms reported by a physical examination and by a reduction in subjective OA pain.[211] In a study of people taking supplements, glucosamine and chondroitin reduced markers of inflammation in the bloodstream.[212] In a study of rabbits with OA, glucosamine and chondroitin were more effective when supplemented with fursultiamine, a derivative of thiamine.[213] Although not all studies have shown a the utility of glucosamine and chondroitin on OA, supplements of either or both of these natural biomolecules have helped some people recover significant joint function.[214]

The body can, of course, synthesize these precursor molecules from other molecules in the normal diet. However, it is thought that providing additional amounts of these precursors in the diet allows the osteocytes to synthesize new cartilage at a faster rate. Thus, it makes sense that supplements containing these precursor molecules will give joints a boost in regenerating their cartilage. Although orthopedic specialists may caution about the efficacy of this type of treatment, some continue to recommend it, advising that it is inexpensive and, at worst, will not hurt. Many will often candidly admit that some studies of glucosamine and chondroitin have shown benefit.

Hydrolyzed and Undenatured Collagen

As explained above, the right molecular precursors for molecules such as collagen can boost the efficiency of its synthesis. For this reason it was hypothesized that providing predigested cartilage would help joints to regenerate damaged articular cartilage. A recent RCT tested the effect of supplements containing hydrolyzed collagen, chondroitin sulfate, and a few other biomolecules on joints with OA.[215] Each individual in a group of eighty participants was given either capsules containing a total of 2,000 mg of these biomolecules or a placebo for seventy days. The amount of pain, stiffness and disability were tabulated at the beginning, halfway point (thirty-five days), and end of the study. The participants who received the hydrolyzed collagen and other biomolecules reported a significant decrease in pain and stiffness. The authors of the study suggest that these very positive results may originate in providing the right molecular precursors for articular cartilage. Another possibility is that the hydrolyzed collagen contains polypeptides (short-chain proteins consisting of only a few amino acids) present in collagen, such as proline-hydroxyproline, that can specifically stimulate the production of collagen and other constituent molecules of articular cartilage. The mechanism for such an effect is not currently known.

Vitamin C is necessary for synthesis of hydroxyproline,[216] implying that a deficiency in vitamin C might be ameliorated by supplements of hydroxyproline. Although these results are promising, this RCT did not test some obvious control cases; for example, to compare the results of providing a high-quality protein such as meat or eggs with the results of providing the hydrolyzed collagen and other molecules. However, it suggests that when present in sufficient levels, some predigested components of collagen taken along with vitamin C can help to prevent OA. In another study, collagen hydrolysates taken orally were well absorbed and one component was detected in the bloodstream as a small peptide (proline-hydroxyproline). This small peptide increased the amount of hyaluronic acid produced by synovial cells, suggesting a very promising treatment to reduce pain and improve function in OA.[217] Another likely possibility is that cartilage regeneration takes place at night when the joint has little weight loading, so that providing the precursor molecules along with a dinner that provides excellent nutrition might be helpful.

Several studies have shown the efficacy of supplements of undenatured (undigested and uncooked) collagen type II for reducing pain and symptoms of OA. This is the type of collagen in articular cartilage.[218] During normal digestion large proteins such as collage are thought to be broken down into smaller molecules. This raises the question of the mechanism for such a beneficial effect. One hypothesis about the mechanism is that when the collagen is being digested, immune cells in the lining of the gut are sensitized to the collagen and send cytokine signals that prevent an inflammatory immune response to collagen in the joint.[219] In one study, a supplement of undenatured collagen was compared to a supplement of glucosamine and chondroitin for efficacy in OA. The undenatured collagen was found to be more effective.[220] The mechanism for undenatured collagen is evidently different than for glucosamine and chondroitin, and also for hydrolyzed collagen. Supplements containing a mixture of these compounds are more effective than just one of them.[221]

ASU, SAM

Another food supplement, avocado and soybean unsaponifiables (ASU), has also shown promise in improving pain and function in OA.[222] This is the sterol-rich fraction of avocado and soybean oils that don't form soap when treated with lye. ASU is widely available as a supplement. It has anti-inflammatory properties with specific effects on chondrocytes, and can tip the balance towards regeneration of cartilage.[223] Several RCTs have shown significant benefit of ASU.[224] A sulfur-containing compound, S-adenosyl-methionine (SAM), has been tested on OA patients and found to be as effective as NSAIDs with fewer side effects.[225]

Injections into Synovial Fluid

As explained above, the synovial fluid is critically important for joint health because it carries the nutrients to cartilage and carries away the waste products. A common form of treatment is to inject a biochemical naturally present in synovial fluid that may be deficient in arthritis. For example, injection of hyaluronic acid (HA), one of the important viscous (thickening and slippery) components of the synovial fluid, has been shown to be beneficial in slowing progression of OA. In a normal joint, HA is synthesized by the synovial membrane and the surface layer of articular cartilage. It prevents inflammation and damage to the articular cartilage, but tends to get degraded in advanced OA into smaller molecules that aren't as viscous.[226] HA tends to reduce friction, which would otherwise cause cell death (apoptosis) in the chondrocytes within the articular cartilage.[227] In many studies of early arthritis, injections of long-chain or high-molecular-weight HA into the synovial fluid have had some success in improving function and recovery.[228] This treatment, when given early enough in OA, has even been shown to slow or stop its progression.[229] Of course, even mild joint pain indicates substantial progression of OA, so once pain is present, HA injections may be less effective. Thus, treating OA in the early stages before the pain gets severe is more likely to help. Also the presence of growth factors can be important. In many studies, growth factors or platelet-rich plasma containing them injected into the synovial fluid of early OA patients reduced pain and improved function.[230] One caveat for injections into synovial fluid is they can cause bacterial infections if not performed properly. A bacterial infection in the joint from whatever source is dangerous, because the body's immune system can't function well there. A joint infection can cause serious illness or death.[231] And as explained above, an infection in a joint can also cause arthritis.

Zinc, Copper, Selenium and Other Micronutrients

The micronutrients zinc and copper are both necessary as cofactors for enzymes. They are related because zinc inhibits the absorption of copper and also some of the effects of too much copper.[232] Zinc is an essential nutrient often deficient but helpful in OA and RA. It is an important antioxidant and enzyme cofactor for many functions throughout the body.[233] When the levels of harmful heavy metals in the body are high, the levels of the trace element zinc are lower.[234] This is especially true in RA, because toxic heavy metals such as arsenic, cadmium, and lead tend to be higher in RA patients than in the general population. This is thought to be associated to some extent with environmental triggers for RA, such as smoking or exposure to heavy metal dust. But it may also be associated with higher levels of oxidative stress in RA patients. Zinc levels tend to be lower in RA patients, but this is thought to be due to the oxidative damage from the disease process rather than a dietary deficiency.[235] In addition to oxidative stress, heavy metals in the body tend to interfere with the cofactor role of zinc, so a deficiency of zinc accentuates the damage from heavy metals. Zinc lowers the level of these heavy metals in RA patients, preventing the damage.[236] Zinc is also required for bone growth, which is necessary for recovery from arthritis.

Copper and manganese are required cofactors for the synthesis of collagen and elastin matrix.[237] In one study, copper levels were higher in synovial fluid of OA and RA patients compared with healthy subjects.[238] This suggests that this essential micronutrient is regulated by cytokines controlled by the immune system.

Both manganese and selenium are required for the synthesis of glycosaminoglycans and proteoglycans which are essential components of articular cartilage.[239] Selenium is an essential nutrient with important antioxidant and cofactor roles in the body. Deficiencies are common, depending on the location and diet, especially those who have OA or RA.[240] Patients with OA or RA have lower selenium levels in their synovial fluid.[241] Levels of inflammatory cytokines in rats and mice with arthritis were reduced when they were given selenium-enriched yeast.[242] The antioxidant role of selenium is synergistic with other antioxidants such as beta-carotene and vitamin E. Selenium is a necessary component of the enzyme glutathione peroxidase (GSH-Px), which along with glutathione plays an important antioxidant role inside cells.[243] Selenium-binding proteins that are essential for life have high affinity for selenium and can function with a moderate selenium deficiency. However, nonessential selenium-binding proteins tend to stop functioning with a moderate deficiency. Although they are not required for life, they are thought to have important antioxidant or regulatory roles. Loss of function due to selenium deficiency in these nonessential selenoproteins is implicated in some forms of OA.[244] The same triage principle holds for many other essential nutrients. Adequate (high) doses of essential nutrients, not just minimum doses, are important for health, especially in preventing OA and RA.[245]

Boron is another micronutrient thought to be involved in

arthritis. Areas of the world in which boron is deficient in the soil have much higher incidence of OA.[246] Further, an RCT showed that boron supplements (6 mg per day) improved pain and function in OA.[247]

Iron

Iron is an essential nutrient for the body, so an adequate amount in the diet is important for health. It is utilized in molecules of hemoglobin and myoglobin, which carry oxygen throughout the body into the tissues. It is also a cofactor in some of the crucial metabolic pathways in most cells. The body typically contains a total of several grams of iron, which is very closely controlled by a system of proteins for storage and distribution.[248] Iron is essential for most forms of life, including animals, plants, and most disease-causing and beneficial bacteria (but see "Iron and Bacteria" below). Inside cells, it acts as a cofactor for many enzymes used in energy metabolism, so it is crucially important for chondrocytes in cartilage and osteocytes in bone. Most people in the United States get sufficient iron, but deficiencies are common. Some people get too much, and others get too little and have a deficiency.[249] Women can lose enough blood during their menstruation to cause iron anemia, which can cause a lack of energy or general tiredness. Once diagnosed, a deficiency of iron is easy to treat, for many types of food are good sources, and it is available in many inexpensive multivitamin supplements.

The problem with iron in the diet is to get the right amount, for both too much or too little can cause oxidative stress and disease.[250] At high levels, iron can act as a pro-oxidant, actually increasing the level of free radicals in the body. This can cause oxidative destruction of body tissues including the heart, liver, pancreas, and bones. Thus, limiting the intake of iron to moderate doses according to need is extremely important. Because free iron is toxic, any excess is deposited inside cells in a protein molecule called ferritin. When too much iron is ingested, even a small excess over many months, stores of ferritin tend to accumulate, because iron is not actively excreted from the body. This accumulation of iron can cause toxicity. Problems of too much iron tend to be progressive and get worse with age.[251] When too much iron is accumulated, it may reflect a serious condition called hemochromatosis. This disease is often caused by a genetic predisposition. Excess iron accumulation can also be caused by alcohol abuse, inflammation, or metabolic syndrome.[252]

The amount of iron in the body is regulated by absorption in the gut, because once absorbed, there is no known physiological mechanism for its excretion.[253] Many vegetables and legumes are good sources of iron. The absorption of iron from these sources is relatively low but is regulated during digestion.[254] It can be increased by vitamin C. However, iron absorption from animal sources like meat, called "heme-bound" iron sources, is unregulated and relatively complete. Therefore, a common cause of iron overload (and many other serious problems) is eating too much meat.

An overload of iron can cause bone and joint problems because an excess of iron tends to prevent bone remodeling.[255] Genetic hemochromatosis (GH), an iron overload disease due to a specific mutation, often causes arthritis in the hands or other joints, typically at an earlier age than OA.[256] Before the excess of iron is detected, this type of arthritis is commonly misdiagnosed as OA or RA, but the symptoms are different. GH arthritis patients typically do not have pain at night or much morning stiffness.[257] GH is often treated with phlebotomy (bloodletting), which removes iron contained in hemoglobin of red blood cells. But this treatment usually does not prevent the arthritis symptoms. An excess of iron prevents osteoblasts from being formed, and thus changes the balance from bone formation to bone resorption.[258]

Lactobacillus and Probiotics

The gut contains thousands of different strains of bacteria. Many of these bacteria are helpful to the body and play an important role in digestion and absorption of nutrients. They can also synthesize some of the essential nutrients, including vitamins.[259] Some bacteria, perhaps all, have a preferred food that promotes their growth. Lactobacilli thrive in the acid environment of the stomach. They generate energy for growth by converting lactose (milk sugar) to lactic acid. The acid prevents the growth of some types of pathological bacteria. Lactobacilli are used in the production of beer, wine, sauerkraut, pickles, cheese, and yogurt.

Some types of gut bacteria are known to have antioxidant and anti-inflammatory functions which are helpful in recovery from arthritis. Other types of bacteria found in foods and living in the gut make vitamin K_2, which is readily absorbed and is necessary to prevent OA.[260] In two recent studies, the diversity and specific types of gut bacteria were shown to be related to metabolic issues, for example obesity, insulin resistance, and inflammation.[261] Those with low diversity in their gut bacteria had more inflammation and a higher risk of gaining weight and becoming obese. Further, when attempting to reduce their weight by eating more healthy foods, those with low bacterial diversity did not improve their inflammatory markers as well as those who had higher bacterial diversity.[262]

Lactobacilli are important for preventing inflammation. In several studies, oral administration of lactobacilli downregulated the body's pro-inflammatory cytokines and upregulated anti-inflammatory cytokines, leading to significant improvement in symptoms of arthritis.[263] When combined with oral doses of collagen and glucosamine, the improvement from lactobacilli was even greater.[264] In another study, RA patients were given an uncooked vegan diet that was rich in lactobacilli. Their stools were compared with those from RA patients who continued with their regular omnivorous diet. After a month following these diets, those following the vegan diet had significantly different microbes in their stools, and their RA symptoms were significantly improved over those on the standard diet.[265] Oral doses of another lactic-acid-forming bacteria, *Bacillus coagulans,* were tested in RA patients and found to improve RA symptoms and reduce inflammatory markers in the blood.[266]

One mechanism for the anti-inflammatory role of helpful lactobacilli is thought to be interactions with cells of the immune system in the lining of the gut. This suggests that lactobacilli can inhibit the autoimmune response from circulating antibodies in RA.[267] Lactobacilli are also able to bind and remove toxic heavy metals such as arsenic, lead, cadmium, chromium, and mercury from the gut. This ability makes lactobacilli very useful for RA patients because these metals can trigger RA.[268]

Lactobacillus acidophilus, Lactobacillus casei, Bacillus coagulans, Bacillus subtilis, and other helpful bacterial cultures are widely available in health-food stores as "probiotics" and in yogurt that contains active cultures. They promote health for the gut and for the entire body. The anti-inflammatory role of lactobacilli can play a very important role in prevention and recovery from OA and RA.

IRON AND BACTERIA

Unbound ("free") iron in body tissues can be hazardous because it encourages bacterial growth. Without iron, most bacteria cannot flourish, so the body has evolved ways of preventing iron from being available to microbes. Although red blood cells contain iron, the blood plasma contains little free (unbound) iron. All body fluids, including blood and lymph, are purged of free iron by a special iron-binding molecule called transferrin.[269] This helps to prevent bacterial infections. The body's cells can obtain the iron they need from the transferrin molecules.

Interestingly, milk contains very little free (unbound) iron, which is an essential nutrient for almost all forms of life, including most forms of bacteria. Cow's milk contains very little iron, and human milk contains even less. Infants do not need additional iron in their diet until six months of age. The lack of iron in milk limits the growth of harmful bacteria, which gives infants an important protection against bacterial infection. Further, all body fluids, including blood, contain very little free iron, which starves any bacteria that might gain entry. However, beneficial lactobacilli, which grow on milk in the gut, are one of the few forms of life that don't require iron.[270] Instead of synthesizing new molecules for their metabolic pathways, which requires the iron-containing enzymes required by most life forms, lactobacilli utilize existing molecules provided by milk. As an alternative to enzymes requiring iron, lactobacilli utilize other enzymes that contain manganese.[271] Thus infants can benefit from bacteria in their gut without problems from bacteria that cause disease.

The only other known form of life that does not require iron is the *Borrelia burgdorferi* bacterium that causes Lyme disease.[272] This allows it to live comfortably in the body of animals and humans. Iron and copper are toxic to this bacterium, and it contains a protein analogous to the ferritin used by mammals to sequester these minerals.[273] Instead of iron for its enzymes, it utilizes manganese. And insidiously, it tends to infect joints and cause arthritis as well as severe disease in the brain. Evidently it is well-adapted to the mammalian body.

Cherries and Berries

Interestingly, cherries are anti-inflammatory and lower the level of uric acid in the bloodstream. These properties make cherries an excellent food for preventing and helping recovery from several forms of arthritis.[274] The anti-inflammatory properties of cherries and other dark berries are thought to derive from a family of biochemical molecules they contain called polyphenolic flavonoids. These compounds inhibit the synthesis of nitric oxide (NO) and several other inflammatory signals for the immune system.[275] Similar properties have been suggested for other berries and dark fruits and vegetables, such as blackberries, black currants, blueberries, purple potatoes, pomegranate juice, citrus, and green tea.[276] Resveratrol is an antioxidant with anti-inflammatory properties found in grapes, peanuts, and cranberries.[277] Blueberries contain a similar compound called pterostilbene.[278] Resveratrol has a variety of beneficial properties. It inhibits the synovial cells from proliferating as they do in RA, and inhibits inflammatory pathways in joints, allowing their cartilage to regrow.[279] Polyphenols derived from pomegranate juice and rind inhibit the enzymatic degradation of articular cartilage, allowing it to be regrown.[280]

Cherries appear to be unique in their ability to lower urate levels. A few hours after eating a large helping of cherries, the level of urate in the urine goes up, and the blood level goes down.[281] Therefore, they are effective in treating gout, which is due to elevated urate levels in the body. Cherries also contain vitamin C, but the same amount of vitamin C taken alone does not duplicate the effect of cherries on lowering urate levels. In one study, after eating a generous portion of cherries every day for four weeks, inflammatory markers such as C-reactive protein (CRP) went down, without changes in blood sugar, lipids, or insulin.[282] This effect of cherries and other dark berries is likely to be helpful in preventing inflammatory diseases such as cancer, heart disease, OA, RA, and gout.

Cherries also contain high levels of melatonin, which is a hormone also synthesized in the body that regulates the circadian (daily) rhythms of sleep and activity.[283] The role of melatonin in cherries is thought to be its strong antioxidant properties to protect the fruit.[284] In one study, cherry juice reduced the severity of episodes of insomnia in volunteers, allowing them to get more and better sleep.[285] Cherry juice has also been suggested for improving the quality of sleep due to its anti-inflammatory and pain-reducing qualities.[286] These properties may be particularly important for OA and RA patients, because lack of sleep induces further inflammation.[287]

There has been some concern raised about antioxidants lowering the natural level of oxidative stress from exercise. It is thought that some oxidative stress is necessary in order for athletic endurance training to recover from exercise damage and generate more muscle. However, neither high doses of vitamin C or E, nor cherries appear to prevent such necessary adaptive responses of the body.[288]

The phenolic compounds such flavonoids and anthocyanins in cherries and other berries are typically dark and absorb light, so they are thought to help the fruit prevent oxidative damage from light. Many of these phenolic compounds are bioavailable and help prevent oxidative stress and inflammation.[289] Most varieties of cherries contain many antioxidants and essential nutrients such as beta-carotene, lutein/zeaxanthin, and vitamins B and C, as well as essential minerals such as calcium and magnesium. However, sour cherries contain less sugar and more beta-carotene and phenolic compounds, so they may be more effective for preventing inflammation. Hot days during ripening increase the level of phenolic compounds.[290] In cool climates, growing cherries in greenhouses can enhance their nutrient content. Canning hardly affects the amount of the beneficial polyphenolic compounds if their total levels are measured in both fruit and syrup.

Bottles of tart cherry juice, taken for several days before a long strenuous race, lowered the level of pain and inflammation in runners after the race.[291] This suggests that cherry juice can help to prevent acute oxidative damage and pain that occurs in muscles and tendons around joints in OA and RA, with less side effects than prescription medications.[292] A ten-ounce bottle of cherry juice is equivalent to about fifty cherries, and provides a natural alternative to nonsteroidal anti-inflammatory drugs (NSAIDs).

Other helpful polyphenols and flavonoids include compounds in vegetables, fruits, nuts, teas, extract of pine bark, cocoa, and spices. Many of these have been shown to inhibit pro-inflammatory cytokines, which can improve symptoms of OA and RA.[293]

Sulfur and the Cruciferous Vegetables

The nutritional approach to preventing and reversing disease is exemplified in a story about recovery from multiple sclerosis (MS). Dr. Terry Wahls is a medical doctor who was diagnosed with MS in the prime of her life. She had been a nationally competitive Tae Kwon Do athlete and marathon runner prior to initial diagnosis, but after MS struck, she was unable to walk without two canes. She was stuck in a tilted wheel chair, about to lose her job at the hospital. Her doctors told her that she would never be able to recover the functions she had lost. From her knowledge as a practicing doctor, she tried the best conventional MS treatments. They didn't help much. Then she began doing her own research into the problem, leading her to utilize nutritional treatments. She began a strict diet centered on green vegetables and other healthy foods. The regimen worked. Within about a year, she was able to run again.[294]

In her book, Wahls focuses on foods containing sulfur, primarily for its effect on the nervous system. She particularly recommends kale, collards, asparagus, brussel sprouts, broccoli, and cauliflower. With our knowledge about the importance of sulfur for OA, it makes sense to also consider these vegetables for treating arthritis owing to their high sulfur content. The sulfur contained in these foods is necessary to create disulfide bonds within the cartilage proteins, which helps them to fold into their proper shapes. Cruciferous vegetables such as broccoli, Brussels sprouts, cabbage, collards, kale, mustard, and radishes contain sulforaphane, a small molecule containing sulfur that has potent anticancer activities. These vegetables have similar antiproliferative activities that may help to prevent inflammation in RA. A study of the effect of sulforphane on articular chondrocytes and synovial fibroblastlike cells found that it inhibited the cytokine-induced metalloproteinase degradation pathway for cartilage, preventing cartilage degradation.[295] A diet of those cruciferous vegetables is excellent medicine! Dr. Wahls found that going off the healthy diet allowed her symptoms of multiple sclerosis to return. I (WTP) know from my own personal experience that whenever I have a little alcohol, I can feel it in my hip. An example recipe designed to provide most of these nutrients is included in Chapter 7.

HERBS AND SPICES

Some herbs used for centuries in traditional medicine, such as boswellia, are therapeutic for the immune system, and have been reported to lessen symptoms of RA. The resin from the boswellia tree is a component of the ancient compound called frankincense. Boswellia is thought to downregulate the cytokines that cause inflammation in the joint, and also to inhibit oxygen free radicals that cause inflammation and tissue damage.[296]

Turmeric

Another ancient cure is turmeric. It is an important spice of the ginger family that has been used in India as an ingredient in curry. Turmeric has also been used for thousands of years as a preservative and for treating many diseases. The active ingredient in turmeric is now known to be curcumin. This biomolecule gives turmeric its characteristic gold color. Curcumin has antioxidant and anti-inflammatory properties, as well as antiviral and antibacterial properties.[297] It inhibits the inflammatory cytokine pathways, and this helps prevent diseases such as cancer, heart disease, and arthritis.[298] Thus curcumin tips the balance away from inflammation and towards regeneration in both OA and RA. It also slows the excess growth of fibroblasts in the synovial membrane, thereby removing a target of inflammation in RA.[299] In this anti-proliferation role, curcumin and the omega-3 fatty acid DHA are synergistic in their effects.[300]

Curcumin works in a "dose-dependent" manner, so that higher doses are more effective. However, caution for high doses is given for those on antiplatelet or anticoagulation therapy.[301] Some evidence suggests that other compounds in turmeric may inhibit the anti-inflammatory properties of curcumin, so pure curcumin extract may be more effective. A clinical RCT of curcumin is currently underway to determine its efficacy in RA.[302] A commercial prescription food product, Limbrel (flavocoxid), is a mixture of natural ingredients from plants, primarily flavonoids.[303] It is designed for people with OA to inhibit inflammation, and is thought to be effective. However, like many foods, in some cases it can cause hypersensitivity or temporary toxicity.[304]

Natural molecules such as curcumin and resveratrol are also known to modulate transcription factors that control the genetic expression of anti-inflammatory pathways.[305] A new field called "nutrigenomics" has recently been focused on such natural molecules that can modulate genetic expression of cellular molecules to cure diseases. These molecules are considered to function much like powerful drugs, except that they are natural and do not generate huge profits for the pharmaceutical industry.

Ginger

Other herbs and spices such as ginger, tamarind, willow bark, capsaicin gel, chrysanthemum, and some types of mushroom are widely used as anti-inflammatory supplements.[306] Ginger contains many helpful biochemical compounds, including a high level of antioxidants and some anti-inflammatory biomolecules such as gingerol.[307] In recent studies, ginger or a mixture of ginger and other natural compounds was as effective as a NSAID or a glucocorticoid steroidal drug in relieving inflammation and pain symptoms of OA.[308] Ginger is safer than NSAIDs and doesn't affect the stomach lining as much.[309] Crude extracts of ginger have performed better in preventing joint inflammation and destruction than purified gingerol extracts.[310] Powdered ginger taken over a long period (months to years) also appears to be effective for relieving symptoms of OA and RA.[311] The mechanism for ginger's action in preventing inflammation is thought to be inhibition of prostaglandins and other inflammatory signaling pathways.[312] Ginger is also effective in preventing allergies, cancer, and cardiovascular disease.[313] Similarly, tamarind has antioxidant and anti-inflammatory properties.[314]

Other Anti-Inflammatory Foods

Some types of chrysanthemum are anti-inflammatory, and similar to curcumin (described above) can suppress proliferation of synoviocytes.[315] These are the cells in the inner lining of the synovial membrane that produce hyaluronic acid and proliferate like fibroblasts in RA. Green tea contains polyphenols, which have antioxidant and anti-inflammatory properties that inhibit of inflammation of chondrocytes and degradation of cartilage, and promote regrowth.[316] Some types of mushroom also have antioxidant and anti-inflammatory properties and may be useful in preventing symptoms of OA and RA.[317] Eating high levels of cruciferous vegetables (collards, kale, cabbage, Brussels sprouts, broccoli, and such) reduced risk for RA, with broccoli giving the biggest reduction of 35 percent.[318] Bioflavonoids such as quercetin or hesperidin are anti-inflammatory and are considered excellent for helping to prevent arthritis. They are found in a variety of fruits and vegetables such as grapes, grapefruit, onions, apples, black tea, and also in leafy green vegetables and beans.[319] Apples contain many antioxidant phytochemicals and are considered second only to cranberries in their antioxidant content.[320] The red pigment of tomatoes is lycopene, which is a powerful antioxidant with anti-inflammatory properties.[321]

Many other herbs and spices from traditional medicine, as well as common fruits and vegetables, have antioxidant and anti-inflammatory properties, and may be useful for their beneficial effects on arthritis.[322] However, because they often contain many different types of biochemical compounds, their specific effects are difficult to study comprehensively, and are unfortunately often considered as untested drugs by mainstream medicine. Indeed, some herbal preparations have induced temporary liver damage.[323] Yet most traditional herbs and spices (the ones mentioned in this book) are very safe because they've been tried-and-true remedies for centuries. They are natural foods and should not be regulated as drugs.

Nutritional Treatments for Gout

Several nutritional treatments are effective in preventing and reversing gout. They work by lowering the blood level of urate.[324] Red meat and seafood are typical triggers for gout, because these foods generate urate when they are metabolized. Another trigger is excessive consumption of alcohol or fructose. When these are metabolized in the liver, they increase the degradation of ATP to AMP (adenosine monophosphate, a purine compound), which is a precursor of urate.[325] The risk of gout is lowered by consumption of coffee, dairy foods, and vitamin C.[326] Although there is some evidence that vitamin A increases urate levels, beta-carotene, a precursor of vitamin A, appears to lower urate.[327] Vitamin C is an anti-inflammatory nutrient, and increases the excretion of urate, lowering its blood level and thus the risk of gout.[328] For a similar reason, drinking plenty of water can also prevent gout.[329] As described above, cherries or cherry extract can also lower the level of chronic inflammation and the risk of gout.[330] Fresh sour cherries work best.[331] The mechanism is thought to be inhibition of urate production, thus lowering the urate level in the blood. When taken over a two-day period, cherries or cherry extract lowered the risk of gout by 35 to 45 percent.[332] Eating cherries regularly over a longer period, along with adequate doses of vitamin C (3,000–10,000 mg per day or more to bowel tolerance, taken in divided doses) and water will help to prevent gout.

Summary of Treatments for Arthritis

This chapter has presented the rationale for preventing arthritis with an excellent diet and when necessary, supplements of essential nutrients. Flare-ups of arthritis can be triggered by many factors, but deficiencies of essential nutrients are usually the underlying cause. Genetic background can be a big factor, but arthritis occurs later in life because of an accumulation of cellular damage due to poor nutrition. Without adequate levels of vitamins, minerals, and other essential nutrients, the articular cartilage of joints cannot regrow and maintain its integrity. Deficiencies of many essential nutrients are common, but when these deficiencies are corrected the articular cartilage can regrow over time. The extent of regrowth depends on the amount of accumulated damage and the ability of the body to provide nutrients to the joints. There is robust evidence that vitamins C, D, E, K, the B vitamins, especially niacin, as well as essential omega-3 fatty acids can all help to prevent and reverse arthritis. Many vegetables and herbs contain natural biochemicals that are not essential but can play a very important role in preventing inflammation and providing the right environment to allow joints to heal.

CHAPTER 6

Restoring Cartilage After Complete Loss

When a limb has been amputated, it will not regrow. Taking a drug or nutritional supplement will not help to restore the limb. An analogous state of affairs can occur with arthritis. A "cartilage amputee" has lost all of the articular cartilage in a joint. The difference is that we cannot see the obvious lack of cartilage or chondrocytes without the aid of X-rays. When the cartilage is completely absent, one bone rubs directly on the other. This causes tremendous pain. Inside the capsule of a joint damaged in this way, there are no blood vessels to deliver vitamins and other biomolecules, and no chondrocytes to respond to to them. In this chapter we describe this problem and how to correct it. We describe the different types of stem cell therapies, clinical results focused on arthritis, the costs, and how vitamins can promote successful stem cell therapy to stimulate recovery.

Many arthritis patients are only aware of the surgical joint replacement option for treating advanced osteoarthritis (OA). Hip replacement involves cutting off the femur (thigh bone) and replacing it with a metal and plastic prosthetic joint. At this point, any ability to regenerate the joint is lost, because the chondrocytes (cartilage cells) are not present to grow new cartilage. If the prosthetic joint gets loose, it is likely to remain that way because normal bone cells cannot fill in the gaps. The only option is another replacement. For some people joint replacement is the best option, and the pain relief can be immediate and complete. But before making any major decision such as this, you should consider the full range of options, including natural ones such as nutritional supplementation.

Stem Cell Therapy

For most people, surgery is not the only option. Remarkably, there is a simple solution to the problem of complete loss of cartilage, and it works amazingly well. OA is one of the diseases most responsive and perfectly suited for stem cell therapy. There are a variety of stem cell therapies, and they represent the biggest advance in modern medicine since the discovery of antibiotics and vitamins. Don't miss the boat! Stem cell therapies are very effective in curing osteoarthritis. Simply inject stem cells back into the space where cartilage should be, add essential nutrients, and a healthy joint may be restored. This technique is increasingly being used with tremendously positive results.

Although human limbs cannot be regrown, it is widely known that amphibians can regrow their limbs or tails. Moreover, mammals, even humans, have some limited regrowth capability.[1] If the tip of a child's finger is cut off, it can fully regrow under some conditions. The amount of regrowth depends on several factors, including the child's age and how much of the tip was cut off.[2] This regrowth is due to stem cells present in the tissues near the finger tip.

Stem cells are a special type of cell that retains the ability to generate new tissues. Stem cells are similar to embryonic cells that develop from the fertilized egg into precursors of all the types of tissue in the adult. However, over the last few decades, stem cells have been discovered in most tissues of adults. They are the repair cells of the body. After an injury, they can divide and then differentiate (change) into any other cell type to reestablish the correct tissue and blend in with existing cells. Stem cells can be harvested from bone marrow, blood, and fatty tissue. These cells can then be purified and utilized to regenerate other tissues. More discussion about stem cell therapy is provided later in this chapter.

Core Decompression

When severe arthritis strikes, the physical destruction of the bone underlying a joint causes the bone tissue to die because of the lack of oxygen and nutrients supplied by blood vessels. To help keep bone more healthy, it is helpful to promote growth of blood vessels. One surgical technique commonly used is called core decompression. Holes are typically drilled in the femur head of a hip arthritis patient to promote the growth of blood vessels along with the corresponding delivery of nutrients. This technique can prevent the collapse femur head—a common form of disease progression in OA. This core decompression procedure is often advised by doctors for treatment of avascular necrosis (tissue death due to lack of blood vessels) in the head of the thigh bone before it collapses due to weakness. Some doctors then inject stem cells directly into the holes drilled for core decompression. Clinical trials have shown that stem cells along with core decompression results in a significant drop in risk for bone head fractures.[3] Most impressively, the effects continued to be observed five years after treatment! In one study, most of the patients (72 percent) who were treated only with core decompression got fractures, whereas only 23 percent of patients also receiving stem cell therapy got fractures.[4] The group treated with stem cells had dramatic reductions in pain and huge increases in joint function.

Angiogenesis

The goal of core compression is to develop new blood vessels in the necrotic zone of the bone. The growth of blood vessels, called "angiogenesis," can be promoted by nutrients and can enhance the benefit of core decompression and stem cell therapies. When I (WTP) directed my own research laboratory at the University of Cincinnati I collaborated with a major pharmaceutical company that was trying to identify biomolecules that would help new arteries grow in patients with coronary artery disease. The new arteries could help to supply more blood where it is needed in the heart. I found that niacin could stimulate angiogenesis. Niacin is being promoted for recovery from stroke because of this angiogenic property.[5] Many studies have shown that the metabolic product of niacin, NAD, can protect cells from death by anoxia (lack of oxygen). One recent paper found that pre-administered intranasal NAD protected one cerebral hemisphere in mice after blockage of the cerebral arteries.[6] The other hemisphere had twice as much tissue death. This is particularly impressive because it clearly shows the power of an essential nutrient.

Other nutrients that promote angiogenesis include thiamine,[7] choline,[8] and vitamin C. High-dose ascorbate (vitamin C) is angiogenic and promotes healing of an Achilles wound in mice.[9] Ascorbate is also angiogenic when placed in a stent (inside a blood vessel) designed to release it slowly.[10] Vitamin K, perhaps the least understood vitamin, plays important roles in controlling angiogenesis as well.[11] Also, lipoic acid promotes angiogenesis.[12]

Vitamin C is also known to prevent angiogenesis in cancer therapies, but this happens only in an environment specific to tumors. In fact, experiments have been performed using tumor anti-angiogenic amounts of vitamin C in pigs, which focused on normal angiogenesis for pig kidneys using advanced *in vivo* imaging techniques. The study concluded that increases in angiogenesis were apparent in the normal kidney because its redox environment (amount of oxidative stress present) is so different from that of a tumor.[13]

In summary, to promote angiogenesis in the arthritic joint as well as your entire body, we recommend taking a "mega-multivitamin" tablet at least three times a day along with 1,500–3,000 milligrams (mg) of niacin, taken in divided doses, and one additional tablet of vitamin K. A typical mega-multivitamin tablet typically contains 50–100 mg of each of the following: vitamins B_1 (thiamine), B_2 (riboflavin), B_3 (niacin as nicotinamide), B_5 (pantothenate), B_6 (pyridoxine); and also 100 micrograms (mcg) of vitamin B_{12} (cobalamin), biotin, inositol, Para-aminobenzoic acid (PABA), and choline bitartrate; and 400 mcg of folate. All of these molecules are water soluble, so they are excreted fairly quickly through the urine. None of these essential vitamins have any serious risks associated with high doses, and they all have a vastly superior safety record compared to any standard pharmaceutical medicine. However, depending on your need for iron, you may want to take a multivitamin that doesn't contain iron. Rather than a mega-multivitamin you could pay for separate pills for each of these molecules, but that would be less convenient and cost more. So the mega-multivitamin tablet is an excellent bargain. The best form of vitamin K to get is K_2 as the MK-7 form. Just 100 mcg per day is adequate, and this can be obtained in some of the best-designed multisupplements or individual pills. We also advise lipoic acid at 500 mg per day.

CREATING SPACE IN THE JOINT

Injecting cells into the joint capsule doesn't work well when there is no space left between the bones. This is often the case in advanced OA. Along with core decompression described above, other strategies are commonly used for creating space in the joints. You may also want to try to increase the space with a technique you can do all on your own (while you save those funds for your stem cell therapy, possibly along with core decompression). One very effective technique is the inversion table; another is yoga.

The Inversion Table

Instead of gravity crushing down on your joints, you can make gravity work for you to pull on the joints to create space between them. Most of the weight of your body is in your torso and head.

By hanging upside down you effectively eliminate joint pressure and create suction, pulling apart the joint spaces in your hips, knees, ankles, and spine. Most tellingly, bats and sloths that hang upside down a lot are the only known mammals that do not get osteoarthritis. But the extinct ground dwelling sloth put weight on its joints, and did get osteoarthritis.

The space in between the joints can be increased and pain can be reduced by inversion table therapy.[14] The time it take inversion to lengthen the joint is typically three to five minutes or more, but it's important not to overdo the duration. It's better to do many short inversions rather than a few long ones. And there are several cautions: don't do inversions if you have bone weakness, fainting spells, retinal detachment, cerebral sclerosis, or a recent stroke. And get the advice of a physician before you do inversion therapy if you have glaucoma, hiatal hernia, high blood pressure, certain orthopedic supports, acutely swollen joints, motion sickness, recent back surgery, cardiovascular insufficiency of extremities, or artificial hip joints. You should stop immediately if you feel dizzy or as if you are going to pass out. Also, depending on your weight and strength, it may be preferable to not invert completely upside down, but instead to try an angle adjusted to comfort. It may be beneficial to take a dose of vitamins a few minutes to an hour before the inversion therapy to better deliver the nutrients to the joint while it is getting expanded. Similarly, it may be helpful to take a hot-as-you-can-tolerate Epsom salt bath to deliver magnesium and sulfur to the newly created space in the joint, along with the nutrients needed for making cartilage and controlling excessive ossification.

Yoga for Joints

A very effective way to increase space in a joint is to do inversion yoga, which can be very helpful in reducing pain. Yoga is thought to move and renew the body's pools of lymph fluid, which helps to recovery from injury such as arthritis. The lymph system is a circulatory system extending throughout the body, similar to but separate from the bloodstream. It contains lymphocytes (white blood cells) that are one of the body's immune system defenses. The lymphocytes come from other neighboring tissues and move into the lymph ducts, where they drain into veins and the regular blood circulatory system. However, the heart is not directly involved in the flow of lymph fluid. Instead, the fluid and the lymphocyte cells it contains are pushed along by the body's movements. The lymphocytes in lymph fluid play a central role in autoimmune diseases such as rheumatoid arthritis.

The use of yoga to treat arthritis has been shown to be effective in clinical trials.[15] Several studies on yoga for arthritis found significant improvements in pain without adverse effects. It's also reassuring to know that yoga has been promoted for millennia in eastern cultures for its benefits in joint health. One of the standard questions a doctor asks an arthritis patient is, "What is your range of motion?" Yoga is beneficial for decreasing joint stiffness and increasing the range of motion. Yoga is quite different from using an inversion table, but may be used in conjunction with one. The inversion table pulls along the length of your body and is basically a passive process. Inversion yoga can actively create new available space for cells to enter the joints. It gently stretches joints to increase the range of motion, and it massages tissues throughout the body, including the lymph system. An otherwise healthy person with advanced osteoarthritis or rheumatoid arthritis may do well with inversion table therapy once or twice a day for at least five minutes, along with some yoga focused on the arthritic joints.

The use of yoga to achieve improvements in range of motion, available circulation space, movement of lymph, and general circulation are widely accepted. If you are on a really low budget and you are resourceful with the library and Internet, it can be completely free! For starters, there are literally thousands of free videos online showing how to do yoga correctly.

STEM CELL THERAPY FOR ARTHRITIS

Stem cell therapy is amazingly simple and noninvasive. It consists of harvesting stem cells by liposuction or use of a drill or mallet to get into the bone marrow. The cells are first purified by separating them according to cell type, and are then re-injected into the site of injury. A local anesthetic is generally used to obtain the stem cells from bone marrow. The injection is frequently performed with guidance from either arthroscopy or ultrasound. Arthroscopy involves inserting a miniature camera along with its own light source into the body. It allows the doctor to see exactly what is he/she is doing on a magnified screen. After injection, the stem cells transform into cell types characteristic of the local tissue environment. For joints, this includes chondrocytes, osteoclasts, and/or osteoblasts that can effectively grow and remodel articular cartilage and bone.[16] Some doctors advise favoring the joint that received stem cell therapy by avoiding placing any weight on it to prevent the injected stem cells from being crushed. Inversion table therapy is helpful in expanding the joint space to allow the injected stem cells to flourish.

Stem cells are characterized by their ability to differentiate into many different types of tissue. This ability is called their "potency." Stem cell potencies range from totipotent (can change into any cell type), to pluripotent (can change into most cell types), multipotent (can change into several types), oligopotent (can change into a few types), or unipotent (can change into one type). Embryonic stem cells are more potent than adult stem cells. However, since embryonic stem cells are derived from the blastocyst (a clump of cells that eventually becomes the fetus) they are difficult to harvest and are highly controversial on an ethical level. By contrast, adult stem cells can be easily harvested, and they are of sufficient potency to produce the chondrocytes needed in the joints to recover from arthritis. These cells are also termed mesenchymal stem cells (MSCs) because they are derived from the mesenchyme, which is undifferentiated connective tissue. Adult

MSCs are readily available in several types of tissue in the body, so they are increasingly being used for treating osteoarthritis.

Although stem cell therapy can be performed with cells from a different donor, it is most commonly performed using the patient's own cells, which prevents any risk of tissue rejection. This is referred to as autologous stem cell therapy. The alternative use of a donor's cells is termed allogeneic stem cell therapy. The alternative stem cell therapy may have advantages because some studies suggest that the stem cells of patients with osteoarthritis may be less potent. However, it is currently thought that the use of donor cells is not required to get the benefit of stem cell therapy for arthritis. Autologous stem cell therapy is usually the best option. Risks of complications are minimal, merely the standard risks associated with injections.

Sources of Stem Cells

For treating osteoarthritis, the stem cells are harvested from the bone marrow or fat (adipose) tissue. Stem cells from these two sources have different properties, and which is best is currently under study. Adipose tissue-derived stem cells are easily obtained through liposuction. This technique is not painful, but may cause a little discomfort in some people. Those with more fat generally have greater yields of potent mesenchymal stem cells. Surprisingly, adipose tissue has approximately 500 times more stem cells than does bone marrow.[17] Further, adipose-derived stem cells also typically provide more of a physical tissuelike matrix than do bone marrow stem cells. Many doctors advise that this is beneficial because this matrix can hold the stem cells in the joint space longer. By contrast, harvesting stem cells from bone marrow can be quite painful and may not be as effective.

Clinical Use of Stem Cells

It's a tragedy that so few people with arthritis are being treated with stem cell therapy. It is so simple and powerful. However, since no drugs are involved, there is little incentive for corporations to develop patents that generate profits. Further, there is little financial motivation for stem cell therapy to be promoted or approved for coverage by insurance. Thus, insurance providers often categorize stem cell therapy for osteoarthritis as "experimental" and as of 2013 they do not cover it. The procedure typically costs between $2,500 and $20,000 depending on the doctor, so it pays to shop around and research the physician and the treatment. A higher doctor bill does not necessarily mean higher quality stem cell therapy. The reason is that many other billable items besides the procedure itself can be included in the total cost. We hope that stem cell therapy for the treatment of osteoarthritis will become recognized by the Affordable Care Act. Stem cell therapy has also been proven to work for many other conditions besides arthritis.

Stem cells are effective in treating arthritis, and the benefit continues over the long term! This is very significant and exciting because many widely prescribed drug treatments treat only the pain of OA but do not treat its underlying cause. The data for arthritis is overwhelmingly positive. A summary analysis of publications about MSC therapies for OA identified one clinical trial, four case reports, and three cohort studies. One case study involving four women with hip or knee OA ranging in age from their twenties to seventies resulted in clear regeneration of cartilage and bone after co-injection of adipose-derived MSCs with hyaluronic acid and platelet rich plasma.[18] One of these patients had received hyaluronic acid injections many times prior to MSC therapy, but they never helped with the pain. After MSC therapy her pain was dramatically reduced. Another clinical study on six patients with knee OA that received bone marrow stem cell therapy found that all six had increased cartilage at a one-year follow-up.[19] Many other active clinical studies have not reported their outcomes yet. However, there are a large number of successful stories that simply have not been published. To learn more, check out a list of medical doctors practicing stem cell therapy.[20]

Dr. Nathan Wei is distinguished within this group by personal experience. His son suffered from juvenile arthritis that transformed him from a healthy soccer player to an invalid. Dr. Wei is a rheumatologist who has treated over 7,000 patients, including over 100 with stem cell therapies. Based on his success rate, he is in the forefront of stem cell therapy for treating OA. Stem cell treatment is also tremendously exciting because few significant changes or advances have been made for the treatment of advanced osteoarthritis in the past fifty years! The standard approach to date has been management of pain followed by surgical joint replacement. Dr. Wei points out that stem cell therapies serve two purposes: (1) pain relief and (2) regeneration of cartilage.

Stem Cells and Vitamins

To be most effective, it's important that the injected stem cells get adequate nutrition. Several vitamins and nutrients are important for stem cells. Vitamin C is known to be an essential nutrient for two types of stem cells required for recovery from arthritis: chondrogenic (cartilage-producing) and osteogenic (bone-producing) cells.[21] Recently, scientists discovered how to convert adult cells that have differentiated into specific types of tissue back into stem cells. This process seemed impractical because of its low efficiency until it was discovered that vitamin C can increase the yield of adult stem cells by a hundredfold![22] Further, it was discovered that vitamin C not only increases the yield of surviving stem cells, but also preserves pluripotency (ability to differentiate into most cell types).[23] Moreover, this treatment enhances the quality of these stem cells, because they develop fewer mutations in their DNA. This means less cancer and better quality of all the tissues derived from these cells.[24] In fact, this effect of vitamin C may contribute to its remarkable ability to improve health and prevent or reverse disease. To understand why vitamins are so important for stem cell therapy, we must first learn about how stem cells function in the healthy body.

Stem cells have a remarkable ability to home in on the site of an injury.[25] For example, stem cells injected into the tail of a rat that has been injured elsewhere on its body will move to the site of injury. When, in a rat model of stroke, the cerebral artery is blocked off, the stem cells will move from the tail to the brain. When the heart has become damaged, stem cells will move from the site of injection to the heart. So stem cells can be considered the "first responders." Even more important, after the stem cells have moved to the site of injury, they send out signals to recruit endogenous (naturally occurring in the body) stem cells to come to the site of injury. Thus it is a good strategy to boost the numbers of your own endogenous stem cells.

It is important to understand that in advanced osteoarthritis, a big part of the problem is that little space exists between the bones where stem cells can go to regenerate the cartilage. As we've already mentioned above, you can try to increase this available space with core decompression, inversion therapy, and inversion-based yoga. However, these space-creating techniques are unnecessary in many cases, because the simple act of injecting the stem cells into the afflicted joint may be sufficient to promote repair and recovery from even quite advanced OA.

Two types of adult stem cells are normally working very hard to keep the body healthy. These are the hematopoietic stem cells (HSCs) and endothelial progenitor stem cells (EPCs). HSCs make all of the cells in blood. They develop within our bone marrow. The EPCs are responsible for making new blood vessels, repairing them as required to avoid blockages, and performing maintenance on them throughout the body. For example, it's important to have excellent circulation through capillaries, the microscopically fine blood vessels that infiltrate and supply most of the tissues and organs, to provide adequate nutrition to all the body's cells. Recall that articular cartilage has no blood vessels, but the nearby tissues, bone, the capsule, and tendons and ligaments all are well endowed.

The numbers of the HSC and EPC stem cells are easily measured in the laboratory by detecting marker molecules on their cell surfaces, such as CD34, CD133, and several others. Recent studies have shown that the number of stem cells is reduced with age, and in Alzheimer's disease and cardiovascular disease.[26] This raises the issue of how to boost stem cells. Wouldn't it be fantastic if there was a supplement that could boost your own stem cells or those that were injected with for your arthritis? Well, Dr. Neil Riordan has been working on that exact question.

VITAMINS FOR STEM CELLS: CRUCIAL AND SAFE

It is quite striking that medical research relies heavily on the use of vitamins and essential nutrients to grow and propagate stem cells. Cells won't survive and grow robustly in the laboratory unless they are given adequate doses of all the essential nutrients. This mechanism for enhancing growth of stem cells with vitamins is similar to what is going on inside the body when robust doses of vitamins and essential nutrients (as provided by orthomolecular medicine) are taken to enhance the number and quality of stem cells. In this context, it seems ironic that we often hear the medical community criticizing the use of vitamins to promote health in favor of patentable medicines. The criticism often appears to be about vitamin supplement safety. Not surprisingly, the use of vitamins and stem cells by the medical profession to treat arthritis has been disappointingly limited. Yet vitamins and food supplements as a whole are far safer (by a factor of 1,000,000 fold) than many standard prescription drugs.[27] And stem cell therapy that includes adequate doses of vitamin supplements is likely one of the most effective treatments for advanced arthritis.

Enhancing Stem Cell Numbers Using Orthomolecular Methods

Dr. Neil Riordan is the son of the orthomolecular practitioner Dr. Hugh Riordan. These pioneers have been continually thinking "outside of the box." They knew how to make things happen. Hugh was an original medical maverick, and a major force in the development of orthomolecular medicine. His laboratory hosted much of the legendary pioneering work performed by Dr. Pauling that involved the use of high doses of vitamin C for the treatment of otherwise hopeless terminally ill cancer patients.[28] Neil has carried on this work to perform ground-breaking stem cell research and is currently very active in running the Stem Cell Research Institute based in Panama. He has developed a formula to boost an individual's stem cells prior to administration of stem cell therapy.

Dr. Riordan's group recently successfully treated a psoriatic arthritis patient using stem cells. Psoriatic arthritis is likely one of the most overtly obvious diseases. The skin is covered in red plaques. The joints are swollen and painful. It is an autoimmune disease. This particular patient had lost most of her hair, as her immune system was even attacking her hair follicles. However, all of these symptoms went away after the patient received stem cells with vitamin supplements, and she appeared to be a totally new person! This result is consistent with other reports showing that stem cells are typically deficient in patients with psoriasis.[29] Overall, this suggests that stem cell therapy is likely to be beneficial for other types of disease, including OA and RA (rheumatoid arthritis).

One unique feature of Dr. Neil Riordan's stem cell treatments is that the number of the body's natural stem cells are increased before more are injected. The reason is that stem cells injected into a site of injury send signals to the naturally occurring stem cells, enhancing their activity and mobilization to the site. Dr. Riordan's research has shown that higher levels of the body's stem cells tend to multiply the benefit from treatments of injected stem cells. This has been confirmed by many other studies.

A Vitamin Cocktail for Stem Cells

Riordan's group searched for natural biomolecules that boost the numbers of stem cells in cell culture and came up with a proprietary blend of nutrients that is quite inexpensive compared with other types of treatments. The food supplement has been tested in clinical trials and was shown to be effective in boosting the numbers of stem cells.[30] This supplement is made up of 2,000 IU of vitamin D in combination with proprietary fermented food products, including green tea, astralagus, goji berry extracts, food-derived lactobacillus, and also ellagic acid and beta 1,3 glucan. Beta-glucans help to increase the numbers of hematopoietic (blood cell-forming) stem cells. Supplements of beta-glucans are inexpensive and widely available.[31] However, one thorough study comparing different preparations of these beta-glucan molecules found they have huge differences in biological activity.[32] The most active preparation in this study included a product named B1,3 glucan #300, which is available for purchase. Alternatively, beta 1,3 glucans can be obtained through the diet, including oats and mushrooms (shitake and maitake). Oats are widely consumed and are known to to lower cholesterol and other risk factors for disease. By contrast with these natural and safe options, other therapies, for example injection of G-CSF, a glycoprotein that stimulates the production of progenitors of white and red blood cells, is known to have several harmful side effects, such as an increased risk of bone marrow depletion, formation of blood cells outside of bone (extramedullary hematopoiesis), and blood clots.

Thiamine

Stem cell numbers can also be enhanced by thiamine (Vitamin B_1).[33] One particularly impressive study examined eighty-eight diabetics versus ninety-one controls (people without the disease) while measuring the level of many different nutrients and their stem cell numbers.[34] The level of thiamine correlated better with stem cell numbers than any other nutrient. However, supplements of thiamine have not been carefully studied for their therapeutic potential for stem cells. As one of the earliest discovered B vitamins, thiamine just doesn't draw much attention, which seems unfortunate. Thiamine is essential in the metabolism of carbohydrates to generate other molecules required for cell growth and maintenance. It is especially important for stem cell growth and tissue regeneration at large. With the recent upturn in resources dedicated to stem cell research, thiamine may be rediscovered as central to boosting endogenous stem cell production. Thiamine is safe to take for most people at doses up to 3,000 mg per day. A dose of 500 mg taken three times per day is likely to be helpful. Although there is no study showing that supplements of thiamine are effective for boosting stem cell numbers, it is likely to give a huge benefit, especially when taken with other B vitamins.

Niacin

Another vitamin that can help to boost stem cells is niacin (vitamin B_3). It helps to increase the population of endothelial progenitor cells, which are important in regrowing blood vessels and can promote recovery from ischemic strokes.[35] Niacin has been shown to increase EPC recovery function.[36] One of the author's (WTP) primary focus areas of research has involved using zebrafish to identify hematopoietic stem cells. Since this vertebrate animal model is transparent it is a good choice for the identifying small molecules that increase hematopoietic stem cells, which are easily visualized using live animals that have been genetically modified to produce fluorescent hematopoietic stem cells. With this approach it is possible to screen literally thousands of molecules. One molecule that turned out to be the most potent at promoting increases in hematopoietic stem cells was a version of the prostaglandin E2 (PGE2).[37] This molecule PGE2 is made in massive amounts in response to niacin, where it is in part responsible the niacin flush response. Several studies have shown that niacinamide boosts white blood cells to fight off infections as well.[38] And, as described in previous chapters, high doses of niacinamide have been clinically proven by Dr. William Kaufman to provide dramatic recovery from otherwise debilitating arthritis when administered at 2,000 to 4,000 mg per day in divided doses. Most tellingly, he observed that more frequent dosings were more effective than higher individual doses; in other words, for 4,000 mg per day it's better to take 250 mg sixteen times per day at regular intervals, than to take 1,000 mg four times per day. This divided dose protocol for niacin is helpful for all of the B vitamins.

Vitamin C Dosing for Stem Cell Growth

Based on the research described above showing that adequate doses of vitamin C can enhance the number of adult stem cells by a hundredfold in culture, along with Dr. Riordan's protocol in which the number of host specific or "endogenous" stem cells are boosted prior to stem cell therapy, we recommend high doses of vitamin C (1,000 mg every hour or two for four to eight hours or more, taken to bowel tolerance) taken before and right up to the stem cell therapy procedure. Because cell replication takes at least several hours, it may be helpful to take a robust vitamin C dose, for example, 3,000–5,000 mg, immediately prior to the stem cell therapy procedure.

In summary, stem cell therapy goes like this:

Step 1: Boost your endogenous stem cells with supplements prior to the stem cell procedure. If necessary, make sure that your joint has space by physical therapy such as yoga or inversion table.

Step 2: The doctor harvests your stem cells and injects them directly into the afflicted area. In the case of advanced OA, the circulation is usually very poor at this location, and the stem cell population there may be low.

Step 3: The stem cells begin to do the work for you at this point. They send out signals to the other stem cells your body has been making to come to the site of injury and get to work in repairing the injury. You support this repair with supplements of vitamins and other essential nutrients.

In the context of this very effective cell therapy, it's helpful to understand the importance of an excellent diet and adequate doses of vitamins and other essential nutrients. The next chapter reviews foods and essential nutrients for best health and fastest recovery.

CHAPTER 7

Prevent and Reverse Arthritis through Lifestyle and Food

This chapter summarizes how proper diet, including adequate doses of vitamins and other essential nutrients, can prevent or reverse the progression of arthritis. Most types of arthritis, including osteoarthritis (OA) and rheumatoid arthritis (RA), are chronic diseases that are considered to be age-related. But the evidence in the preceding chapters suggests that most arthritis and other chronic diseases appear age-related mainly because they originate in nutritional deficiencies that get worse with age. They can be treated by satisfying the nutritional deficiencies that have created them. An excellent diet is essential to maximize health and recovery from arthritis. For many who purchase inexpensive processed foods at their local supermarket, it may seem difficult to find good buys on nutritious food. In contrast, processed food is tasty and convenient. But an excellent and nutritious diet can be easy and inexpensive by following a few simple rules.

THE DECLINE IN NUTRIENTS

Compared to our forefathers a century ago, we are lucky to be able to purchase fresh produce throughout the year. Much of the vegetable produce sold in the United States is grown in the Central Valley of California, where the land is generously irrigated and cultivated year-round. The cultivation and harvest methods are heavily mechanized, and yields have improved steadily.

California grows most of the tomatoes used for canning and tomato paste for the United States, and more than a third of the world's supply.[1] During the winter season most of the produce sold throughout the country is grown in California, Florida, and other southern states, as well as Mexico and other more southern countries such as Chile. The nutrition we get from fresh produce is essential for our health.

Yet, the soil in many states across the country including California is being depleted of micronutrients by industrial agriculture.[2] And standard tilling practices cause erosion of topsoil at a rate (one millimeter per year) that exceeds the rate of natural erosion or topsoil creation by a factor of ten.[3] No-till methods of farming can reduce the rate of soil erosion, but industrial no-till methods rely on herbicides and pesticides with genetically-modified organisms (GMOs). This sacrifices the soil in a different way, by polluting the environment and killing off insects as well as organisms and microbes in soil, many of which are beneficial and help provide nutrients to plants. These losses in soil and its nutrients can directly affect the nutrient content of food. Some promoters of artificial fertilizer for industrial agriculture deny this, saying that plants can only grow to the extent that they get essential nutrients from the soil, and that robust growth implies sufficiency of soil nutrients.

However, before the advent of modern industrial scale farming, many crops contained higher levels of minerals than they do today.[4] This suggests several possibilities: a) some soils used for farming today have inherent deficiencies not made up for by modern methods; b) heavy cultivation of the soil has depleted it of some nutrients due to loss of topsoil; c) heavy cultivation depletes soil of some essential minerals because widely used artificial nitrogen- phosphorus-potassium (NPK) fertilizers do not contain or replenish them; d) heavy use of industrial fertilizers, herbicides, and pesticides damages the soil organisms that help to supply nutrients to plants; f) modern varieties of plants are selected for looks, fast growth, and yield, but not nutrient content; g) produce is trucked across country so it is not fresh when sold.[5] All of these mechanisms are likely causes for loss of nutrients. Some studies suggest that that the decline in nutrients is mainly due to the modern varieties of plants that are selected for higher yield, because the decline in nutrients came after the modern semidwarf high-yielding cultivars were introduced.[6] This suggests that a balance may exist between yield and nutrient content in typical modern crops such as wheat and corn. But the nutrients we get in our food are critical for preventing and recovering from arthritis.

ORGANIC FARMING GENERATES NEW TOPSOIL TO BALANCE LOSS

Topsoil is required for plants to obtain robust amounts of nutrients. It is eroded by rainfall and wind after tilling. It is washed into streams where it progresses through rivers to the ocean. The erosion of soil and loss of its nutrients is balanced in nature by new topsoil created by geological processes along with compost from plant matter and bacteria, molds, fungi, and critters such as worms.

In order to practice sustainable agriculture, it's important to tip the balance away from erosion and towards renewal of nutrient-filled topsoil. Just as it's important to shift the balance away from resorption and towards regrowth of articular cartilage and bone, it will be imperative to stop the erosion of soil and loss of nutrients. Organic farming uses natural compost without pesticides or herbicides to grow produce, utilizing a layer of mulch on top of the soil to preserve moisture and reduce soil runoff. Another similar method utilizes sustainable perennial polyculture, in which several species of perennial plants are grown together.[7] This is similar to the prairie ecosystem. The different types of plants support each other physically and ward off pests and diseases together. The complex ecosystem in a prairie can produce high yields of natural foods that have more nutrients in a sustainable manner, without loss of topsoil. The perennial polyculture system can be adapted to wet or dry climates.[8] A prairie requires neither fertilizers nor fossil fuels, and is nature's way to create a sustainable ecosystem. Expensive fertilizers are not necessary to produce nutritious fruits and vegetables sustainably, but organic compost is important. Perennial polyculture requires no tilling, and generates its own layer of compost to enhance the topsoil. Compost for organic farming can be created from manure from animals, biosolids from water treatment plants, autumn leaves, food scraps, chaff and straw, and other leftovers from plant harvest. The aim in organic farming is to retain the topsoil and increase its nutritive value, so that the soil becomes more alive, and the plants absorb more nutrients and produce healthier fruits and vegetables. If you eat more nutritious vegetables, your joints will have better support for regrowth.

ORGANIC FOODS AND THE SUSTAINABLE FOOD MOVEMENT

Over the past several decades, as awareness about the importance of eating healthy food has developed, a more general understanding has grown about the urgency of following sustainable practices. Our world is progressing towards several environmental disasters: global warming, pollution of air, water, and soil, and the loss of invaluable resources: fossil fuels, minerals, and topsoil, as well as the loss of wilderness and the threat of extinction of species. We must reconsider how to feed the people of the world.[9] Eating meat produced by industrial farming is unsustainable. It takes much more water and other resources such as grain and fossil fuels to produce meat than vegetables and grains, which produce the equivalent amount of protein. The grain fed to cattle in feedlots is wasteful, because the grain that feeds the cattle could feed many more humans than the meat that is ultimately produced.[10] This wasteful use of resources is a major factor in global warming.[11]

Moreover, along with these problems, our food sources are increasingly controlled by a handful of large corporations that are developing new varieties of seeds and plants. They argue that the only way to feed everyone in the world is to grow genetically modified (GM) food. To go in this direction, however, would mean that everyone would be dependent on seeds that carry potentially toxic genes and are produced and marketed by just a few corporations for huge profits. Farmers are being prevented from raising healthy crops because of this industrialization of food, which limits our choices for healthy food at the local market.[12] Many of the foods widely sold throughout the United States and the world are processed (as described in Chapter 2) to the point that they lack basic nutrients necessary for health.

With all these considerations, the local, sustainable, organic food movement is a crucial addition to food production. Purchasing organic produce has several advantages. The organic label means that the produce was grown using natural methods without synthetic chemicals: no artificial pesticides, herbicides, or fossil-fuel based fertilizers were used. Organic foods are grown with compost, often rich manure from animals combined with plant material.[13] This is sustainable because it does not require fossil fuels. The compost provides organic matter and soil nutrients, which helps microbes and worms in the soil make the nutrients more available to the plant crops.

Organic foods generally do have more nutrients and much lower levels of pesticides than produce grown by "conventional" methods, and they often taste better.[14] This is likely due to slower growth and higher levels of available minerals and beneficial organisms in the soil of organic farms. Further, produce grown locally is fresher and likely contains higher levels of vitamins. It is not trucked long distances, which minimizes the amount of fossil fuel required. Thus, nutritionally, purchasing fresh fruit and vegetables from the local organic food outlet has several advantages: depending on the particular crop, organic cultivation will produce higher levels of nutrients; it will be fresher, so more nutrients will be available: it will be more sustainable in a future without fossil fuels; and it will support local farms and communities. If you are wondering why this topic is important to arthritis patients, keep reading. Eating local produce, especially from your back yard or a neighborhood garden, is one of the best ways to get and remain healthy.

ARTHRITIS PREVENTION BASICS

Several basic principles from common sense are helpful, along with excellent nutrition, in providing health. In this section we explain how important it is to keep hydrated with pure water, keep warm, chew your food properly, and avoid harmful and toxic chemicals. You'll want to avoid sugar, food additives, and trans fats.

Keep Hydrated

For prevention and recovery from OA or RA, keeping hydrated is very important. Drinking plenty of water helps joints recover. An adequate water intake is important for preventing joint disease because it allows the body to rid itself of waste products that otherwise would contribute to inflammation and damage to cartilage. Further, the articular cartilage depends on an adequate amount of fluid in the synovial capsule. If you become dehydrated, the cartilage may also become dehydrated, which can cause its surface to become wrinkled or dented. This can cause damage from abrasion on its surface when you move the joint.

Consuming an inadequate amount of water is surprisingly common, especially in older adults. It happens in part because drinking water increases the need to urinate, which may be inconvenient for some. Everyone knows that on a hot day you will get thirsty, but this is also common on a cold winter day, when the humidity is low. Typically, the ability to sense thirst tends to decrease as we get older, so many older patients get dehydrated. When your mouth becomes dry, you should consider drinking a glass of water. This will help your joints to function more smoothly without pain.[15]

The water in many towns and cities contains chlorine and

other harmful chemicals at low levels.[16] If you live where the water supply is chlorinated or tastes bad, you can remove the chlorine and other harmful chemicals by installing a carbon water filter. You can install one in your kitchen sink connected to a cold water tap, or you can purchase a pitcher that contains a carbon water filter. You can also remove chlorine from water by adding a sprinkle of vitamin C powder. Either way, make sure you fill your water bottle regularly with clean water. Normal perspiration and breathing uses five to eight cups of water every day. In very hot weather with low or high humidity, perspiration can take several additional quarts.

The municipal water supply of many towns and cities also contains minerals such as sodium, calcium, and magnesium. If these minerals are present at high levels, they provide a supplement every time you drink the water. It's best if the level of magnesium is at least half the level of calcium.[17] Hard water contains calcium, which precipitates with ordinary soap, leaving a soap film. Calcium carbonate dissolved in water can cause buildup of scale in pipes and faucets. The calcium is not harmful for health, except when it is present at a high level more than twice the level of magnesium.[18] You can check with your local water utility company to find out its levels of sodium, calcium, and magnesium.

Some people prefer to drink bottled water. Often bottled water originates in a natural spring, but usually it is filtered for purification. It may contain helpful levels of minerals such as calcium and magnesium. These minerals make spring water taste better than ultrapure distilled water and, as described above, can help to supply your body's need for them. Although distilled or deionized water is pure and healthy, it lacks the helpful minerals contained in typical bottled spring water or municipal drinking water. Water from the faucet is less expensive than bottled spring water, so when passed through a carbon filter, it may be preferable.

Drinking coffee, tea, or other beverages containing caffeine can cause you to lose most of the water they contain by excretion. This is a common source of dehydration. Some fluids like milk or juice require additional water to digest. Therefore, these fluids will not give your body the full amount of water they contain. They should not be counted 100 percent in your five to eight cups per day. If you weigh 200 pounds or more, you should consider consuming eight to ten cups of water or more per day. This may seem like an excessive amount, but drinking this extra water will have the effect of flushing your bloodstream of wastes a little faster. This is important when you have inflammation and oxidative stress.

However, you need not obtain all this water from drinking water. Most vegetables and fruits contain approximately 80 to 90 percent water, and watermelon, peppers, and cucumbers contain 90 to 95 percent water. Vegetables also contain a healthy dose of with minerals and vitamins. The water in these vegetables can give you 50 percent or more of your water if you eat generous servings. They release their fructose content and other nutrients slowly so they don't overwhelm your body like sodas or fruit juices. That is why whole raw fruits and vegetables are healthier than a commercial soda or fruit drink. For example, a quarter of a cucumber, a carrot, a stalk of celery, and half of a pepper before dinner will give you one or two cups of water (depending on the serving size) along with the generous dose of nutrients they contain. If you have difficulty with the fiber content of raw vegetables, start with a small portion and gradually build up to a larger portion.

Further, on a hot day, sweat takes electrolytes (potassium and sodium) from the body,[19] which should be replenished with vegetables, fruits, and salt. Most fruits and vegetables contain relatively high levels of potassium. Along with taking plenty of water, it helps to take a pinch of sea salt with each glass, especially on hot days, because the body excretes salt and needs it to be resupplied. Sea salt contains many essential trace elements that the body needs. It is good for the brain, muscles, joints, and digestion. You should consult your medical professional about the right doses of water and salt. However, drinking vegetable juice or eating lots of vegetables is an excellent way to get electrolytes.

It's best to avoid drinking water or other fluids during a meal and just after. Fluid will dilute the acid and digestive enzymes in the stomach, which will slow digestion. Although water is absorbed fairly quickly by the stomach, the time that food stays in the stomach for digestion is limited to an hour or so. When food moves out of the stomach, the acid is neutralized and absorbed in the duodenum (first section of the small intestine). After the acid is absorbed, breakdown of large food molecules is terminated, so any slowing of digestion in the stomach will prevent optimal absorption of nutrients in the rest of the gut. The best time to drink water or other fluids is a few minutes before meals or two hours after meals.[20]

A good water bottle is helpful for keeping hydrated throughout a hot summer day. You can purchase an excellent water bottle at many camping supply vendors. The best ones are unbreakable, light, and do not contain the type of plastic that leaches chemicals into water. Look on the bottom of the bottle to see what kind of material it contains. Avoid plastic types with the numbers 3 (polyvinyl chloride), 6 (polystyrene), and 7 (other), for these may contain harmful volatile chemicals that can contaminate your water, especially if it gets hot. Good choices are 2 (HDPE), 4 (LDPE), and 5 (polypropylene), or a stainless steel bottle. Even if you don't finish drinking all of the water in the bottle, empty it every day or so and refill it to lessen bacterial growth. This is especially important when you've filtered the water through a carbon filter, for this removes chlorine that normally prevents bacterial growth in the water system's pipes. You can clean a water bottle by adding a half teaspoon of laundry detergent, filling it one-third full with hot water, and shaking hard, then rinsing out all the detergent several times with hot water.

If you keep your water bottle full of clean water and look forward to drinking it instead of coffee, sodas, or sugary juices, you will stay in better health, especially in your joints.

WATER, CALCIUM, AND MAGNESIUM: KIDNEY STONES

One reason to drink plenty of water is to prevent formation of kidney stones, which are much more likely when you get dehydrated. Kidney stones are not uncommon, with a rate of 9 percent per year.[21] They are very painful, but most kidney stones can be prevented by following simple rules. There are many types of kidney stones, but the most common type is formed from calcium oxalate, a compound in vegetables but also made by the body.[22] The reason why some people tend to get kidney stones while others don't is not well understood. Some rare genetic conditions cause high levels of calcium in the urine and tend to increase the risk of kidney stones. Calcium binds to oxalic acid and together they precipitate in the urine to cause crystals that form the stones. Some vegetables such as spinach, rhubarb, beets, and sorrel have high levels of oxalate. The leaves have higher levels of oxalate than the stems. But many of these vegetables also contain calcium, which binds to the oxalate in the gut, preventing both the calcium and the oxalate from being absorbed. Thus eating foods that contain calcium is one way to lower the risk of kidney stones. Other foods such as chocolate, soybeans, legumes, nuts, berries, kiwi fruit, potatoes, wheat germ, and drinks such as coffee, black tea, and beer contain relatively high levels of oxalate, so they may contribute to oxalate levels in urine.[23] However, unless the diet includes a large amount of foods containing oxalate, the level of oxalate in the urine is usually not closely related to the amount of oxalate in the diet. Thus, for most people, moderate amounts of oxalate are not a big risk factor for kidney stones.[24] Some bacteria in the gut can metabolize oxalate, which prevents it from being absorbed. For this reason oral antibiotics, which kill gut bacteria, may be a risk factor for an increase in absorption of oxalate from food.[25] Oxalate is also formed in the body and in most people is eliminated safely in urine.

To prevent kidney stones, drink plenty of water because it lowers the level of calcium and/or oxalate in the urine. Citrate can dissolve calcium oxalate crystals, and lemonade, (which contains citric acid) and/or magnesium is recommended to prevent this common type of kidney stone.[26] Magnesium citrate has been shown to help prevent kidney stones.[27] Small daily doses of magnesium citrate (100–300 mg of elemental magnesium) are helpful. The reason is that magnesium competes with calcium for binding to oxalate in the urine. Compared to calcium oxalate, magnesium oxalate is much more soluble in water. Therefore, magnesium in the urine prevents calcium oxalate from forming stones. An adequate amount of magnesium in the diet or magnesium supplements, along with adequate intake of water, will prevent most kidney stones.[28] And plenty of water with magnesium helps to prevent arthritis.

Keep Warm

For best joint health, it's important to stay warm. Many people are deficient in iodine, which is required by the thyroid gland. This gland controls the overall level of energy metabolism in the body which can regulate body temperature when you're sleeping. If you have morning stiffness, this may be due to the cooler temperatures at night. It can be caused by an inactive thyroid, so iodine supplements can help.[29] Cold extremities (hands and feet) can be due to an abnormal reaction to cold, in which blood flow is restricted more than normal. This can be treated using magnesium to help relax the blood vessels.[30]

Of course, in the summer, it's also important not to get too hot. Overheating can cause nutrient deficiencies such as loss of sodium, potassium, calcium, magnesium, and iron.[31] These must be made up for in the diet. And on a hot day you can lose so much water that it can directly affect your joints.

Keep Chewing

It's important to chew your food thoroughly.[32] The reason is that small food particles can be digested more readily than large ones. This is because the acid and enzymes in the stomach can only digest the molecules on the surface of a food particle. Food that has been chewed into smaller food particles has more surface area than the same food chewed only into larger particles. This may seem a trivial point, so it is easy to neglect. However, it is of major importance in the context of age-related disease such as arthritis. We can only absorb nutrients from food that gets digested. For example, nuts and other fibrous foods such as raw carrots can provide excellent nutrition, but only when they're chewed to a fine consistency without large particles. Food in the stomach only gets an hour or so to digest, and during this time even the strong enzymes and acid in the stomach can't digest large particles. Another example is pasta or rice, which is often only partially cooked (*al dente*) and must be chewed thoroughly to be digested. Chewing stimulates the production of saliva that contains enzymes to start the digestion of starch and other biochemicals that protect the gut.[33] When chewing starchy foods such as pasta, bread, and rice, it's important not to drink water or other liquid, because it will dilute the enzymes from saliva in the stomach. Fresh fruit and vegetables also require thorough chewing. An alternative way to be sure you are getting the full benefit of the fruits and vegetables you eat is juicing (see below).

Avoid Smoke, Alcohol, and Coffee

When considering which foods will give the most nutrients, it's also important to consider which foods and chemicals to avoid. First on the list is smoking. Smoke from any source, including cigarettes, pipes, and cigars, contains thousands of chemicals that damage the body and prevent good health.[34] Smoking directly causes inflammation and oxidative stress throughout the body. It is a major risk factor for all the age-related progressive diseases such as heart disease, cancer, and OA and RA.[35] You should avoid smoking, breathing any type of smoke, and air polluted by chemicals or automobile or diesel exhaust, for it causes oxidative stress. This contributes directly to tissue damage that causes arthritis. Stopping smoking is associated with improved health and a lower risk of all types of arthritis. And for best health and to avoid generating inflammation and oxidative stress (as described in Chapter 3), it's imperative to reduce exposure to air polluted with harmful chemicals such as phthalates (found in cars during a hot day), fire retardants, and other chemicals that harm the body.[36] Electronic cigarettes may have fewer toxic chemicals, but the drug—nicotine—they provide is addictive and harmful. Nicotine and caffeine are created by plants to deter insects.

Similarly, alcohol is damaging to many parts of the body, including the liver, brain, and joints. A recent study of RA patients showed that those who had fifteen servings of alcoholic beverages or more per month had a faster rate of progression of joint damage.[37] Several studies have shown that alcohol consumption raises the risk of gout.[38] Although some studies have shown that RA patients drink moderate amounts of alcohol, possibly suggesting a protective effect, they only reported a correlation and could not establish a causative mechanism. In fact, this type of correlation may indicate that heavy alcohol consumption is perceived as risky to patients with severe RA.[39] It's also important to note that the recent book, *The Vitamin Cure for Alcoholism,* advises that alcoholics tend to be deficient in nutrients, especially vitamin B_3 or niacin.[40] Once these deficiencies are corrected, often with supplements of multivitamins and niacin, the need and urge for alcohol consumption vanishes and the addict can recover. High-dose niacin is also known to provide relief from the symptoms of OA.

In a diet without adequate calcium and magnesium, coffee and tea cause the body to take these essential minerals from the bones and excrete them in the urine.[41] To maximize your recovery from arthritis, avoid black tea and coffee, either regular or decaffeinated. Although you may rely on these drug-containing beverages or even feel addicted to them, you won't feel the need to consume them after a few months. For a quick pick-up, substitute unfiltered fruit or vegetable juice diluted 50 percent in water, or a green smoothie (see below). Then continue to drink plenty of water. Your entire body, and especially your bones and joints, will thank you!

Sugar

Another risk for arthritis is the consumption of refined sugar. In commonly available forms such as sugary desserts and sodas, sugar overwhelms the body with empty calories and causes inflammation. Sucrose (cane sugar) contains equal amounts of glucose (blood sugar) and fructose (fruit sugar). Glucose is utilized by tissues throughout the body for energy, but fructose must be metabolized into glucose by the liver before it can be utilized.[42] A temporary excess of glucose is stored by the liver as glycogen, a molecule similar to starch. However, many sodas and fruit juices contain large amounts of fructose. The result of drinking a large glass of fruit juice or soda is an enormous dose of fructose that temporarily overwhelms the liver. The liver cannot metabolize the fructose quickly, but it is readily converted into fat within the liver and throughout the body.[43] This is a leading cause of nonalcoholic fatty liver disease, which is linked to metabolic syndrome.[44]

There is an evolutionary rationale behind our tendency to convert fructose into fat. Plants have evolved to make their fruits attractive to animals by incorporating large amounts of fructose. Animals have evolved to eat the fruits and spread the seeds, which gives the plants an advantage in procreation. Because many fruits ripen at the end of the growing season, their ready availability would normally cause an excess of fructose. This could be converted to glucose and stored as glycogen in the liver. But the storage capacity of glycogen is limited. After the growing season ended, food may have been scarce. Thus, there may have been an evolutionary advantage for our distant ancestors to convert abundant fructose directly into fat rather than converting it to glucose and storing it as glycogen.[45]

The overall problem with sugar in the modern diet is that it's often present in large quantities in processed food. An eight-ounce glass of orange juice contains 15–20 grams (that's 15,000–20,000 milligrams!) of fructose.[46] A large glass of apple, grape, or orange juice, or a soda, can easily overwhelm the liver. Sucrose is nearly as bad as pure fructose, because when it is consumed in excess it is also converted into fat. A tablespoon of jelly contains 10 grams of sugar, as does a glazed donut. A cup of sugared commercial breakfast cereal contains 10–15 grams of sugar.[47] The total amount of refined sugar in the processed foods consumed in a typical modern diet often adds up to 200 grams or more per day. At 4 calories per gram, that equals 800 calories just from refined sugar. And that is not counting the long-chain carbohydrates in starchy foods.

The taste of sugar is a clue to the brain that a fruit or vegetable is ripe and ready for eating, for sugar is a ready source of energy. Sugars are addictive and toxic, almost like alcohol, and their overconsumption directly contributes to metabolic syndrome, which is closely related to inflammation.[48] Fructose tastes sweeter than sucrose. However, because it must be converted to glucose before it can be utilized for energy, it does not satisfy hunger as readily as glucose. Both of these factors encourage its consumption. Sugars added to foods such as frozen dinners, juice drinks, and sodas have been refined, so they have lost the other nutrients that existed in the original plants that created them. Along with the inflammation caused by overconsumption, this causes diseases such as heart disease, cancer, diabetes, and arthritis.[49]

The main source of fructose in a typical healthy diet is fruits and vegetables. Yet, when an apple is consumed, its fructose is released more slowly and in a lower amount than it is from an eight-ounce glass of apple juice. Filtered apple juice is almost pure fructose (along with some electrolytes and water). But an apple also contains more essential nutrients and a healthy dose of fiber. Many of these nutrients are in the apple skin, which requires chewing and digestion.[50] This does not overwhelm the liver, which can readily metabolize its sugar content more gradually into glucose because it is digested more slowly. Juices such as fresh cider and orange juice are not as refined, and therefore contain many other essential vitamins and nutrients.[51] However a large glass of any of these sweet juices may easily overwhelm the liver because of their high sugar content.

To avoid the consumption of large amounts of refined sugars, it is best to abstain from foods and drinks with a lot of added sugar, such as commercial sugared cereals, cookies, cakes and pastries, sugar donuts, jellies, juices, punches, and sodas. Many of these foods contain large amounts of high fructose corn syrup, which is unhealthy.[52] Although consuming jelly spread on a piece of bread, or a sugar donut, or a large glass of 100 percent whole juice such as orange juice or cider may not seem toxic on the first dose, its effect is more insidious because in the long run consuming these foods will tend to cause inflammation and disease.

Although starch is made by plants from sugar and releases glucose when digested, it is not as toxic as fructose or sucrose because it is digested more slowly in the gut. However, some foods that contain starch tend to cause high blood sugar and should be avoided to prevent inflammation.[53] The measure of the tendency to cause a rise in blood sugar after a meal is the "glycemic index." Foods with a high glycemic index include refined sugar, white rice, taro, waffles with syrup, white bagels, and commercial refined breakfast cereals. These foods release sugar quickly when digested and should be avoided. Take only moderate portions of potatoes, and focus on vegetables with color. To lose weight and optimally improve symptoms of OA, replace high-glycemic-index foods with raw vegetables such as tomatoes, sprouts, carrots, red peppers, dark green leafy vegetables, along with a generous portion of essential fatty acids from fish oil, flax meal, or walnuts.[54]

Food Additives and Artificial Sweeteners

Modern processed food often contains many food additives, and a variety of sugar substitutes and other artificial food additives are widely available. Some food additives are preservatives to prevent spoilage, others are dyes to give the food color, and others are added for flavor, pourability, or texture. Artificial dyes made from petroleum are widely considered to be harmful.[55] Some artificial dyes and pigments contained in pills such as ordinary one-a-day multivitamins, for example, FD&C Blue 2 Aluminum Lake, contain aluminum or titanium in a form (nanoparticles) that could cause harm.[56] Many of these additives are included in small amounts in processed food. In large amounts, some of them may be harmful. Some meats such as ham, salami, and commonly available hot dogs are often preserved with nitrate or nitrite, which can be toxic in large doses.[57] Nitrite can combine with amino acids in the diet to generate nitrosamines, which are known carcinogens. Preservatives and dyes are usually added in small amounts but may irritate or cause food sensitivity, allergies, or worse in some people. Although foods without preservatives may spoil sooner, modern refrigerators kept at 40 degrees Fahrenheit can keep foods without preservatives fresh for up to a week, and freezers can keep foods fresh for months. Double-acting baking powder contains aluminum, which is thought to be toxic and should be avoided. Single-acting baking powder is safer. Antacids containing aluminum are thought to contribute to osteoporosis and also should be avoided. Butylated hydroxytoluene and butylated hydroxyanisole are artificial antioxidants sometimes added to food to prevent spoilage. They are thought to be safe in small quantities but some studies have linked them to cancer. Another additive, sulfur dioxide, is added to dried fruit (apricots, peaches, apples, golden raisins) to preserve color and flavor. It is thought to be safe in small quantities but it is an irritant for some people. When there is an alternative, food additives should be avoided. For example, hot dogs and sausages are available without preservatives. Although you may read that "there is no evidence that they are harmful," this usually means that the proper studies of these potentially harmful additives on humans have not been done.

Artificial sweeteners are often considered safe when taken in small doses, but they may cause toxicity if used over long periods and should be avoided.[58] Xylitol, a 5-carbon sugarlike alcohol, is toxic to dogs.[59] Several sugar substitutes have been shown to cause cancer in animals. Diet sodas contain artificial sweeteners and should be avoided. The effect of these substances on the body has not been carefully studied, and there is some evidence that they disturb the body's metabolic pathways.[60] Artificial sweeteners tend to confuse the sugar sensing system in the body and may cause some individuals to overeat.[61] It is thought that artificial sweeteners may cause metabolic imbalances such as inducing increases in hormone and insulin levels, and may induce cognitive deficits.[62] There is little reason in an excellent diet for using artificial sweeteners. Drinking diet sodas regularly may be harmful. An excellent alternative is to drink water instead. And, of course, juicing is also excellent!

Empty Calories in Processed Foods

Let's face it, processed foods are convenient! They are designed to taste good and to have a long shelf life. But a disadvantage of processed foods is that they are made from components that have been refined, so they don't contain their original complement of essential nutrients.[63] These nutrients are required for health and to prevent diseases such as heart disease and arthritis. As described in Chapter 2, most wheat products today are made from "enriched flour," which, as we've seen in the previous chapters, lacks some of the vitamins and essential minerals in the whole grain. The bran and germ is removed from the wheat, leaving the white endosperm. This is then ground into white flour. In past centuries, the resulting long shelf-life made white flour highly prized, but it lacked essential nutrients. To prevent acute vitamin deficiency diseases, some vitamins and minerals (vitamins B_1, B_2, B_3, folate, iron) are now added back into the flour. Unfortunately, this "enriched flour," while it looks and tastes good, still cannot support life. It is missing several of the essential nutrients found in whole grains, vitamins B_5, B_6, B_7, and E, and also magnesium and other minerals. These essential nutrients are mostly contained in the bran and germ components that were removed in the refining process. A slice of whole wheat bread contains approximately 25 milligrams (mg) of magnesium, but a slice of white bread contains only 7 mg, a loss of 72 percent.[64] A cup of whole-grain cornmeal has 155 mg of magnesium, a cup of degermed cornmeal has 48 mg, and a cup of white corn grits contains only 12 mg, a loss of 92 percent![65]

The same problem haunts other refined foods, such as refined sugars and oils. Raw unrefined sugar is full of calories and contains some essential nutrients. When most of the sugar has been removed, the molasses that remains contains a robust dose of many nutrients such as calcium, magnesium, potassium, and iron. But refined sugar has none of these, and is harmful for several reasons, as described above. Similarly, many good oils are inexpensive and widely available, such as peanut, palm, coconut, canola, soy, corn, and olive. Some of these have a large saturated component and are suitable for cooking because of their high smoke-point temperature and relative freedom from rancidity. Others, with a larger mono- or polyunsaturated component are widely used as an ingredient in prepared food and salad dressings. While many of these oils have important health benefits, they all have the disadvantage that they provide a robust amount of calories without the essential nutrients contained in the food from which the oil was extracted.

For example, olive oil is rightly promoted as an oil with many health benefits. It contains a modest amount of vitamins E and K, along with a large amount of monounsaturated oil. It is widely used as a salad oil. However, it also has 100 calories per tablespoon. The olives that were crushed to extract the oil also contained those calories, but they also contained many other nutrients such as protein, vitamin A, calcium, magnesium, and iron. Moreover, the salad eaten with the dressing that contains the tablespoon of oil may only contain 10 or 20 calories[66] compared to the oil's 100 calories!

The calories in refined foods such as white flour or olive oil are not necessarily unhealthy, because some carbohydrates and oils in the diet are essential. Olive oil is for good reason associated with health in the Mediterranean diet. The problem is that the calories in refined flour and oil will replace calories from other foods in the diet. If those other foods are (or would be) unrefined whole grains and vegetables that contain healthy oils along with other essential nutrients, the net result of eating the refined foods instead of other more healthy foods is a lower dose of nutrients. Thus, the essential nutrients missing in processed foods cause deficiencies and damage to body tissues that can add up over decades, causing illnesses such as heart disease, cancer, and arthritis.

A recent sale at the local supermarket exemplifies the problem. The market offered a special sale with low prices on large packages of cane sugar, long-grain white rice, and vegetable oil when purchased together. All of these items are refined. They lack essential nutrients that would help to prevent arthritis. The special sale depended on industrial production and refining of these so-called staples, which allows inexpensive distribution and sale. But a special sale of such refined products sold in bulk at a very inexpensive price may not be such a good deal. Although they have a longer shelf life, they are a source of nutritional deficiencies that can cause age-related disease such as arthritis.

To prevent long-term nutrient deficiencies, it is best to avoid sources of refined calories. For example, avoid foods made from enriched white flour such as white or "wheat" bread, bagels, cookies, crackers, cereals, cake, pastries, and pasta. Whole grain versions of these foods that contain moderate amounts of brown sugar instead of refined sugar are excellent alternatives. Also avoid refined grains such as white rice and corn grits, and commercial cereals made from refined grains. Substitute brown rice and whole grain corn products. Wheat germ is an excellent addition to breakfast and baking. Avoid the use of large amounts of vegetable oil for salads and cooking. Remember that oils have lots of calories, along with some essential fatty acids, but have lost most of their other nutrients. Salad dressing is OK if it is used very sparingly, especially if made with fresh virgin olive oil.

Hydrogenated Fats

Another food category to avoid is partially hydrogenated fats. These fats have a higher melting point than the oils they are derived from, and are solid at room temperature.[67] This makes them ideal to prevent oil separation in many processed foods. Margarine, made artificially by hydrogenating (adding hydrogen to) vegetable oil in an industrial process, contains a high proportion of trans fats. Although partially hydrogenated fats are less prone to rancidity than natural fats and have other good qualities, they are toxic because they contain unnatural molecules, called trans fats that, when incorporated into cells, confuse the natural functions of fatty acids in the cell membrane.[68] They raise cholesterol levels, accumulate in the body, and cannot be metabolized to provide energy like natural cis fats. The terms "trans" and "cis" are taken from Latin and refer to the orientation of side-groups, or side-chains, on the carbon backbone of molecules. Trans means "on the opposite side" and cis means "on the same side."

Saturated fatty acids (such as palmitic acid found in palm oil) have a straight side-chain that allows them to pack closely together, causing them to have a high melting point. These fatty acid molecules are an essential component of cell membranes throughout the body. Excess carbohydrates are converted by the liver to palmitic acid, which can then be stored as fat in the body or metabolized further to other fat molecules. They can be converted by the body back to blood sugar if no other source of sugar is available.[69]

Polyunsaturated cis fatty acids (PUFAs) have a bent side chain that prevents close packing, which causes them to have a lower melting point.[70] This property is responsible for the fluidity of vegetable oils. This fluidity is an important and essential property for the lipid bilayer of cell membranes, which require their fatty acids to be fluid to allow diffusion of proteins within the membrane. The body cannot make omega-3 or omega-6 PUFAs but must get them from the diet. PUFAs that have a low smoke-point temperature should not be used for cooking because when heated they go rancid very quickly. PUFAs such as peanut oil with higher smoke point temperatures are better for cooking because they don't go rancid as quickly.

Trans fatty acids are also unsaturated, but they have a relatively straight side-chain, which gives them a higher melting point.[71] Trans fats are resistant to breakdown by bacteria, so they provide a longer shelf-life when incorporated into foods. The liver cannot easily metabolize them, however, so they tend to build up in the liver and cause accumulation of fat.[72] This contributes to metabolic syndrome, which causes inflammation throughout the body.[73] It is best to avoid foods such as margarine, crackers, and biscuits that contain partially hydrogenated fats.

Good alternatives to partially hydrogenated fats are moderate quantities of saturated fats such as palm oil, coconut oil, and grass-fed butter. These naturally saturated fats are widely used for cooking because they don't go rancid as quickly as PUFAs. However, it is important to note that much of the world supply of palm oil is produced in huge, unsustainable monoculture plantations that have displaced the natural ecosystem of the jungle in tropical climates. You may want to limit your use to palm oil that is grown more sustainably.

For many decades, partially hydrogenated fats were added to peanut butter and other products containing vegetable oil to prevent the oil from separating. With the recent revelations about the toxicity of trans fats, many brands of peanut butter have replaced the partially hydrogenated fats with saturated fats (palm oil or fully hydrogenated vegetable oils) that are not as toxic. Of course, natural peanut butter made from 100 percent peanuts is likely more healthy, because it contains no added fats. To prevent the oils in natural peanut butter from separating, you can stir in the oil and then either store it in the refrigerator, heating in the microwave for ten seconds to allow spreading, or keep the jar turned upside down when the top is on. And it is likely that organic natural peanut butter is healthier! For those who cannot eat peanuts because of an allergy, other nut butters such as almond butter are excellent alternatives. And you may find that with an excellent diet, along with supplements of vitamin C and E, your allergies disappear.[74] Vitamin C is an excellent antihistamine and, along with magnesium, can prevent allergic reactions, for example, asthma.[75]

Avoid Too Much Meat

Although protein is one of the main nutrients essential for health, it is often consumed in excess. Red meat, duck, and turkey can provide protein along many other essential nutrients. However, when meat is consumed exclusively, it must be metabolized to provide blood sugar for tissues. This process is inefficient, and some of the metabolic products cause toxicity in the liver. It also causes calcium to be taken from bones and excreted, which can be prevented by eating foods such as leafy green vegetables and beans, or taking additional magnesium.[76] Further, a diet high in fish and animal products tends to result in a greater intake of persistent toxic chemicals and heavy metals than a mostly vegetarian diet. The reason for this is that these compounds get concentrated through the food chain.[77]

The Inuit, who traditionally ate large amounts of raw meat, stayed remarkably healthy.[78] Their diet provided adequate vitamin A and D from the meat and fat of fish and marine mammals. Cooking at high temperature destroys vitamin C, but they obtained vitamin C from eating raw meat, which contains just enough to prevent scurvy.[79] They avoided the problem of eating too much protein by consuming generous amounts of fat along with the meat. More than half of the calories in their diet originated from marine animal fat that contains mostly PUFAs, including a high level of omega-3 fatty acids.

However, most meat sold today contains high levels of saturated fat as well as hormones and antibiotics, which should be avoided. Organic grass-fed beef grown by a local farmer is generally best, and should be consumed in moderation. The grass diet provides higher levels of omega-3 fatty acids, vitamin K, and other essential nutrients.

Although many plant foods such as beans, legumes, and wheat germ contain high levels of protein, they do not cause the problem of protein toxicity because they also contain sugars that can be converted more directly to blood sugar. And a purely vegetarian diet is healthy as long as you make sure you get adequate doses of vitamins.

WHAT TO EAT

Many popular books provide a rationale for one diet or another to stay healthy and prevent and reverse arthritis.[80] In this book we have attempted to provide the scientific basis for the nutritional approach. We focus on encouraging the growth and regeneration of lost cartilage typified by the most common form of arthritis, OA. However, following an excellent nutritionally oriented diet is equally important for regrowing cartilage in other forms of arthritis, such as RA. For the best health and recovery from arthritis, it's important to eat a variety of fresh vegetables and fruits that contain robust amounts of the essential nutrients. This will prevent the deficiencies of these essential nutrients that over decades can cause progressive age-related diseases such as heart disease, cancer, diabetes, and arthritis. A diet of vegetables and fruits has successfully reversed heart disease[81] and can also reverse diabetes.[82] Those who stay on such a diet live longer and remain in better health throughout their life.[83]

An excellent diet that provides all the essential nutrients consists of generous servings of dark-green leafy vegetables, a variety of cooked colored vegetables such as broccoli, Brussels sprouts, green beans, summer and winter squash, sweet potatoes, items made from whole grains such as whole wheat bread, whole wheat pasta, brown rice, bulgur, millet, oats, quinoa, beans and lentils, and seeds and nuts, along with yogurt and small amounts of meat. It should also include fresh raw vegetables such as carrots, tomatoes, celery, lettuce, peppers, fresh sprouts, and a variety of fruits such as apples, oranges, pears, plums, peaches, and berries. Cooking increases the levels of some nutrients because it releases polyphenols and antioxidants from the fibrous matrix in raw vegetables, making them more available to human digestion.[84] However, it can decrease the levels of some other nutrients such as vitamins B_1 and C. Many cultural dietary traditions exist, and most of these are compatible with this basic plan. Green smoothies are excellent nutrition. They make it easier to consume a large portion of raw green leafy vegetables.[85]

Eating a big salad without dressing before lunch and dinner can help to provide excellent nutrition and fill the stomach before the main course. Some people find this method helpful to limit the calories they consume. Juicing can simplify getting large amounts of nutrients from raw vegetables. Juice from fresh vegetables such as carrots, peppers, and radishes, without their fiber, helps many people maximize their nutrition.[86] Some specific foods are known to be helpful in preventing inflammation (for instance, dark-green leafy vegetables, cherries, and ginger), so they should be included in an excellent diet for preventing arthritis. You should plan your meals to include generous servings of leafy green vegetables such as collards, kale, spinach, other colored vegetables, nuts and seeds, fruits, and modest amounts of meat. Dulse and other sea vegetables are especially healthful because they contain robust levels of essential trace minerals.

For those who have arthritis that flares up now and then, such as with an autoimmune disease like RA, consider going onto an "elimination-challenge" diet as described in Chapter 3. You first eliminate a food group such as corn or dairy from your diet for two weeks to see if this improves your symptoms. Then restart that food and try eliminating another food group. When one or more food groups are found by this method, then challenge yourself by eating the foods in that group, one at a time, to see whether it worsens your symptoms. This procedure, of course, should be done in the context of an excellent diet, where you are always getting adequate nutrition. You should also check possible sources of oxidative stress in your environment, such as contaminants in the air you breathe in your house or car as described in Chapter 3. You may benefit by discussing your plan with your medical doctor.

A feature of many nutritional strategies focused on treating inflammatory diseases like arthritis is to limit the diet using a technique such as the Gerson diet, which includes regular juicing. The Gerson diet protocols are quite strict: completely vegetarian, no dairy, no sugar, no legumes, no nuts, all organic, deionized water only, with occasional coffee enemas, depending the severity of the disease. We note that the Gerson technique has been primarily used to treat cancer patients, but it works remarkably well for arthritis too.[87] Gerson therapy can help combat the excessive growth and proliferation of tissues that occur in both cancer and autoinflammatory diseases like RA. Although we do not emphasize the importance of such a strict diet, we do recognize its efficacy, and it may be worth trying if you find other approaches don't work well for you.

Juicing and Green Smoothies

An excellent way to get a robust amount of nutrients is to drink vegetable juice, prepared either commercially or at home with a juicer. Low-sodium vegetable juice is great for quenching thirst on a hot day. It can help to make up the loss of electrolytes such as potassium and magnesium that are lost through sweating. Vegetable juice is preferable to fruit juice because it contains less sugar along with high levels of nutrients. On a hot summer day, an excellent beverage is made by diluting low-sodium vegetable juice with water (one-half cup juice to one cup water). And when you're stressed out, as a supercharger or quick pickup, stir in one-half teaspoon (2,000–4,000 mg) of powdered vitamin C. You will hardly notice the acidity of the vitamin C because it's buffered by the vegetable juice.

Juicing vegetables at home is an excellent way to get high levels of nutrients that can prevent and reverse OA.[88] Although we advise eating whole vegetables, the advantage of juicing is that it encourages consumption of more vegetables than many individuals would normally eat. The juice contains most of the nutrients in the original vegetables, without the fiber content. Although juicing does lose some of the nutrients in the skin and fibers of the vegetable, it can be the path to health if you find eating lots of vegetables difficult. You can drink the juice without chewing, so you can get more nutrients from the juice than you might if you chewed the vegetables. There are many different brands of juicers. You can start with an inexpensive one and graduate to a more expensive and powerful one when you feel you are getting good results. A juicer cuts up the vegetables very finely, which allows the juice to be separated from the fiber. The fiber contains nutrients and a small amount of the juice, and can be included in baking recipes. You can start with raw vegetables such as carrots, radishes, squash, tomatoes, green beans, and pea pods, and then add seeds and nuts, and fruits such as apples, pears, and peaches.

Home-made green smoothies are another great way to get excellent nutrition.[89] You can make them with an ordinary kitchen blender. To a cup of water, blend in several big collards or kale leaves, along with other vegetables such as peppers and tomatoes. You can substitute any dark green leafy vegetable such as spinach, dandelions, Swiss chard, or mustard or beet greens. If the "green" taste is too strong, you can add fruit such as apples, peaches, grapes, berries, or fruit juices. The advantage of green smoothies over juicing is that the entire vegetable is pureed, so you get all the nutrition and fiber. Amazingly, a green smoothie that contains several big leaves of collards or kale is a complete meal! It contains protein, carbohydrates, oils, fiber, and essential nutrients such as vitamins and minerals in nearly optimal proportions. The actual amount of protein and omega-3 and omega-6 fatty acids in collard greens is relatively small. Yet the proportion of omega-3 to omega-6 is outstanding. If you eat only green smoothies containing collards, you can get all the nutrients, including protein, that you need. Green smoothies can be difficult for beginners to digest because they have a lot of nutrients and fiber, but if you persist and consume green smoothies every day, your digestion will likely improve. The extra nutrients you'll get will make the gut more efficient at the digestion process.[90] Green smoothies and fresh raw vegetable juices will give you a great mix of nutrients that is highly effective for preventing and reversing arthritis.[91]

Raw Vegetables and Sprouts

Salad and raw vegetables are an important part of an excellent diet. They provide essential vitamins and minerals, a good mix of omega-3 and omega-6 fatty acids, and fiber. Dark greens such as spinach, collards, kale, Brussels sprouts, Swiss chard, dark lettuce, dandelion leaves, and beet, mustard, and turnip greens are excellent. They contain high levels of vitamins and minerals along with protein and a good proportion of omega-3 oils. Finger food such as raw carrots, radishes, celery, cherry and grape tomatoes, red and green peppers, and cucumbers all contain many essential nutrients and a healthy dose of fiber. Few foods can compare with sweet tender pea pods or tomatoes picked from the vine. A good way to combine these raw vegetables in a meal with more caloric cooked dishes is to eat a large plate of raw vegetables and/or salad (without dressing) as the first course of the meal. When you get to the second course of cooked food you will not feel the need to overeat, because you're already partly satisfied from the raw vegetables. To get the full benefit of raw vegetables, it's important to avoid excess salad oil, and chew them thoroughly.

Sprouts are an excellent way to get complete nutrition. You

can buy them at many supermarkets and health food stores. But you can also grow your own from seeds very inexpensively. Many different types of seeds are available for sprouting, including alfalfa, wheat, clover, cabbage, lentils, mung beans, radish seeds, soy beans and fenugreek.[92] To grow your own sprouts, pour the seeds two or three layers thick into a container and add water. Over the next twelve to twenty-four hours the seeds will absorb water and grow in size severalfold. Over the next days, while the seeds are sprouting, rinse them by adding water (pure, without chlorine), swirl them very gently (to avoid breaking the emerging sprouts), and drain the container carefully. This minimizes the growth of bacteria. Rinse the seeds twice every eight to twelve hours. Gradually the seeds will send out sprouts (which are their new roots), and then leaves. The initial sprouting may take only two days in the heat of summer, or four to six days in cooler weather. Once the seeds have sprouted they are ready for eating. You can store them in the refrigerator for a few days, rinsing them again every day, while you eat them. If you want to get even more nutrition place the sprouts in sunlight, which will prompt them to make green leaves.[93] Avoid eating the greens of sprouted buckwheat because they contain a toxic substance.[94] The groats (seeds) themselves, either unsprouted or sprouted, are okay to eat and they are quite nutritious.

Backyard Gardens

A backyard garden can help keep you healthy. Fresh produce is easy to grow and is inexpensive, even for an apartment dweller in a city. You only need some soil, a few seeds, and four to six hours of summer sunlight. Collards, kale, green beans, peas, summer and winter squash, tomatoes, carrots, and peppers are very easy to grow. It's very satisfying to fresh-pick some greens, beans, and tomatoes out of the back yard and eat them for lunch or dinner. You can make a green smoothie quickly and easily, starting by picking several leaves from your backyard garden, blending them with other vegetables, drinking the smoothie, and cleaning the blender. This entire process takes less than five minutes. Many excellent books explain how to grow the most produce from the smallest space.[95] If you have only a few square feet, you can put your plants in pots or other containers. A few seeds or plants purchased at the local garden center will give produce for several months. You only need to take care of them a few minutes per day.

In my (RGS) back yard I have a small twelve-by-twelve-foot plot with several rows of tomatoes, green beans, peas, collards, kale, broccoli, and carrots. It takes me a weekend in the spring to prepare the soil by adding several bags of manure and pulverized dolomite that I purchase at a local garden center. I plant small seedlings I've either grown or purchased. At the edges of the garden plot, adjacent to a small lawn, I also plant two mounds of summer squash and two of winter butternut squash. When the squash seedlings sprout, I remove all but two from each mound. They spread out over the lawn and in ten weeks produce ten summer squash and ten to twelve winter squash (if the squirrels don't get them!). I eat out of this small plot for the whole summer, trading the extra produce with my neighbors. In the winter, I rely on the local market and purchase the same types of produce relatively inexpensively. The winter squash keep for several months, contain more essential nutrients than potatoes, and are excellent when cut in chunks and steamed for ten minutes. I also eat sprouts year-round, usually alfalfa or mung bean sprouts. They're excellent nutrition and taste good.

Buy Local, Farmers Markets, CSAs, and Neighborhood Gardens

If you don't have the time or resources to maintain a small garden, you can likely find neighbors who will share or trade their produce. The local food movement has blossomed in the last two decades, and includes traditional farmers markets, community-supported agriculture farms (CSAs), backyard gardens, small-scale permaculture, mini farming, and urban community farming.

Many books are available that cover a wide range of topics on the local food movement.[96] Often there is a farmers market or CSA outlet nearby where you can purchase fresh greens and other vegetables.

A farmers market can offer fresh produce at low cost. The farms are within easy driving distance of the urban market where the farmers sell you their fresh produce. You buy from the very farmers who grow the produce. Organic farms close to a town or city can get good prices on their produce without the delay and cost of long transportation routes. This means fresher, healthier produce and more sustainable production and sales. You can find farmers markets online, where there are lists of farms and locations of the urban farmers markets.[97]

In many regions throughout the United States there is a CSA nearby that you can join to get fresh produce throughout the growing season.[98] A CSA is a farm that is supported by its customers, who pay in advance for a season's worth of fresh produce. This may be the least expensive way to get fresh produce without growing it yourself. The CSA concept connects you with your local farmer and the land, and benefits both farmer and consumer by encouraging community.[99]

In many markets, local produce is available even during the colder months. Tomatoes, peppers, and other fresh vegetables are widely grown in heated greenhouses. They are grown in Mexico and in Southwest states such as Arizona, but also in Maine and Canada. Using the hydroponic growing method, the roots of tomato plants are fed a solution of minerals in artificial soil (rock wool) that provides their nutritional needs. Light for their growth comes from the sun or artificial lights run on hydroelectric power. Vine-ripened tomatoes are picked every day and trucked to be sold at a premium price. Unfortunately, the environmental cost for these vegetables is high because the greenhouses are heated with fossil fuels.[100] Solar-heated greenhouses are possible in some regions but require a large investment. With even a larger capital investment a seasonal heat storage can provide nearly free heating during the winter, even in the northern states and Canada.[101]

Cooperative food markets are widely established in many cities throughout the country. You can join the co-op to get inexpensive prices on fresh organically-grown produce and most types of dry goods you would find in an ordinary food market. Some co-ops require members to volunteer several hours per month or per year, but many are large enough to support full-time employees who do the work.[102]

A NEIGHBORHOOD GARDEN

In many cities, you can join a neighborhood garden to grow vegetables in a small plot. Compost and water are made available, so you only need to plant seedlings. A local cooperative neighborhood garden was started recently in Philadelphia, Pennsylvania. An unused lot was available, but it had no electricity or running water, and the soil was of unknown quality. A local gardening group had the soil tested by a local environmental laboratory, which found it to be acceptable for gardening. A well was drilled and gave water at 120 feet. A well pump was purchased that could run from battery power. The water was tested and found safe for irrigation. The gardeners purchased a shed with funding from a local foundation, and a solar panel was placed on the roof of the shed. The solar panel charges a 24-volt battery, which powers the well pump. However, the well pump is limited to two gallons per minute. This rate is not high enough for several gardeners to simultaneously water their plots, so the gardeners installed a system of fifty-five-gallon drums to hold enough water for a few hours of watering. The water storage drums sit on a platform six feet above the ground, giving enough pressure for gardeners to water through a hose. Gardeners pay a small yearly fee for a garden plot that covers the purchase of compost, fencing, and other necessities such as garden tools.

Several of the gardeners have arthritis, but they note that gardening keeps them active, and the greens and other fresh produce they grow benefit their joints. Favorites are kale and collard greens, which grow well throughout the spring, summer, and fall. These vegetables are among the best for preventing and reversing arthritis. After a few years, the garden has established a vibrant community that supports newcomers with advice and help in gardening.

Joining a neighborhood garden of this type is an excellent choice for urban dwellers who don't have sunlight in their backyards. Gardening will give you exercise, vitamin D from the sunlight, excellent nutrition, and social relationships with like-minded people who want to improve their diets and health. And this type of moderate activity helps prevent arthritis.

The Best Food Buys for Nutrition

Healthy foods can also be inexpensive at an ordinary supermarket. Greens such as collards, kale, cabbage, Swiss chard, and beet and mustard greens are among the best buys, for they provide excellent nutrition at very low cost. In many markets they are available throughout the year. Collards and kale have the highest content of vitamin K_1 of the most common vegetables.[103] They contain high levels of vitamin A, lutein/zeaxanthin, vitamins C and E, calcium, magnesium, iron, and many other nutrients. Although their levels of polyunsaturated fat is low, it has a higher proportion of omega-3 to omega-6 fatty acids than most other foods. Other cruciferous vegetables such as broccoli, bok choy, Brussels sprouts, cabbage, cauliflower, cress, and turnip are also very good. In some markets, broccoli, Brussels sprouts, and cabbage can be purchased during sales in the fall months at reduced prices. (Note: Individuals who are susceptible to goiter should steam cruciferous vegetables for thirty minutes or more.) Other inexpensive raw vegetables that contain high levels of nutrients include carrots, peppers, tomatoes, pea pods, dark lettuce, and sprouted seeds. A good rule is to fill up on raw vegetables: eat one or more carrots, a few slices of a pepper, and other inexpensive raw vegetables such as radishes, a stalk of celery, cherry or grape tomatoes, and a few slices of cucumbers every day. Sprouts contain lots of nutrients, and are easy to grow. All of these vegetables are inexpensive and available year-round. Other vegetables excellent for cooking include corn, peas, green beans, carrots, winter squash, and potatoes (sweet and regular). Frozen vegetables such as peas, green beans, carrots, and broccoli contain more nutrients than canned, are often fresher than fresh produce, and can be purchased inexpensively on sale. Canned beans on sale are often good buys and are convenient. You can elaborate on choices at your local market.

Some fruits are also excellent buys, especially when grown locally. Apples, pears, and peaches are excellent buys in season. They are chock full of antioxidants and essential nutrients.[104] Locally-grown apples can be purchased in many locales throughout the winter. A favorite is the traditional Winesap, which does not keep as well as other varieties but is excellent for eating and cooking. I (RGS) pick several bushels at a local orchard at a low price and store them at 40 degrees Fahrenheit for up to five months. I prefer to eat them raw throughout the fall and winter months for their fiber and many nutrients such as antioxidants.

Berries such as blueberries, blackberries, currants, raspberries, and strawberries are excellent buys during the summer months. Many of their nutrients are retained in preserves or when kept frozen over many months. However, commercially-grown berries such as strawberries are widely treated during growth with pesticides that are difficult to wash off. Organically-grown berries don't contain pesticides. Also, local organically-grown fruit is usually better because it is fresher, more nutritious, and sustainable. Several types of fruit are grown in remote states or countries and must be trucked or airlifted long distances for sale. Bananas are grown in Central America, and while they are inexpensive and contain vitamins and essential minerals, they are less sustainable for people in North America than other fruits grown locally because of the required transportation from tropical regions. Bananas are promoted as an excellent source of potassium, but do not have much higher levels of potassium than most other fruits and vegetables. Indeed, greens, potatoes, and beans contain higher levels of potassium.[105] Oranges and orange juice are promoted for their content of vitamin C, but only contain 100 mg of vitamin C per eight ounce cup. Yet oranges also have high levels of potassium, bioflavonoids, and other healthful nutrients. As explained in Chapter 5, cherries and cherry juice are excellent buys because even though they are expensive, they are anti-inflammatory and lower the level of urate in the body, which can prevent gout.

Getting fresh fruit inexpensively during the winter can be a challenge, but it's not always necessary. Dried fruit is an excellent source of nutrients, but it's best to avoid the varieties that contain preservatives such as sulfur dioxide. Brown raisins are an excellent buy, because they are inexpensive and contain many of the essential nutrients in the grapes they come from, with exceptions being vitamin C and a few other nutrients that get oxidized in the drying process. This is not necessarily a big problem because these essential nutrients can be supplied by other sources in the diet or supplements.

Other excellent buys are dry foods such as beans, chickpeas, lentils, peas, brown rice, and oats. These contain high levels of many nutrients such as protein, B vitamins, and magnesium, and also are very inexpensive. Oats contain the most protein of the common cereal grains (16 percent), and rolled oats provide excellent nutrition and fiber without the need for cooking. They can be purchased inexpensively in bulk at organic food stores, or in clearance sales at regular supermarkets. Whole grains (wheat, barley, rye, oats, whole-grain bulgur, and others), are a good buy because they are inexpensive and contain more nutrients than their refined counterparts. Other more expensive items, such as buckwheat (also called kasha, high in magnesium and B vitamins), quinoa (high quality protein and minerals), and nuts are excellent buys because of their very high levels of nutrients. Millet contains robust levels of magnesium, copper, and manganese. Most ground and tree nuts, including peanuts, almonds, cashews, and pistachios, are are very good buys, though their protein is not complete.[106] But eating a variety of vegetables over several days will provide an adequate supply of complete protein.

Most nuts and seeds (including buckwheat, chickpeas, millet, quinoa, and peanuts, almonds, and Brazil nuts) have a large component of omega-6 fatty acids and only a small amount of omega-3 fatty acids. This imbalance is considered to increase inflammation. However, walnuts have high levels of alpha-linolenic acid (the essential omega-3 fatty acid), and so are very good buys even though they cost significantly more. Brazil nuts are very nutritious, but have an exceptionally high content of selenium (540 micrograms (mcg) in one ounce, or six to eight nuts), so high that eating more than a few per day can cause selenium toxicity. Although selenium is an important antioxidant and essential nutrient (50–200 mcg per day), a mild overdose can cause cracked nails and broken hair. It may be best to limit your consumption of Brazil nuts to prevent toxicity, especially when you take a daily multivitamin tablet that contains more than 50 mcg of selenium. Brazil nuts are often found in packages of mixed nuts.

Flax seeds are an excellent buy because they are relatively inexpensive and are one of the best sources of alpha-linolenic acid. This essential omega-3 fatty acid taken from flax seed will go rancid when exposed to air or bright light at room temperature. However, the seed coat protects the alpha-linolenic acid from oxidation, so whole flax seed does not need refrigeration. The practical problem is that the seeds are small and difficult to chew, and will often pass undigested through the gut. Flax oil can be purchased in opaque bottles and stored in the refrigerator. However, the oil is relatively expensive and contains fewer nutrients than whole flax seed. A good alternative is flax meal, which is relatively inexpensive, but it is often purchased several months after milling so it may not be as wholesome as fresh-ground flax meal. You can grind your own flax meal inexpensively from flax seed. Two tablespoons of flax seed make about three tablespoons of flax meal. Flax seed mills are inexpensive and available online. An inexpensive coffee mill can also be used to make flax meal. For some mills, it is helpful to pass the meal through the mill a second time to grind it more finely. A friend eschews flax seed meal and simply chews the flax seed thoroughly.

Wheat Germ and Yeast

Wheat germ, brewer's yeast, and nutritional yeast are in a special category, for although they cost more than dry beans and whole grains, their levels of essential nutrients are higher. They are excellent buys. Wheat germ contains high levels of protein (as much as meat), B vitamins, vitamin E, and magnesium. Although it originates from the refining process and is thus not "whole-grain," it is an excellent food supplement because it contains the nutrients that were removed from white flour in the refining process. It is often sold in vacuum-packed glass jars or in plastic packaging with an inert gas to prevent rancidity. After opening, wheat germ must be refrigerated like meat and fish to prevent rancidity and spoiling. It is excellent for boosting nutrients in breakfast cereal and baking. One concern is that wheat germ contains phytate, a compound that can bind to minerals and prevent them from being absorbed in the gut. However, this is not a problem for most people who are eating an excellent diet that provides an adequate level of minerals.

Brewer's yeast and nutritional yeast have excellent levels of protein, B vitamins, magnesium and selenium. In addition, nutritional yeast is fortified with enough vitamin B_{12} to make it a good source for vegetarians. Brewer's and nutritional yeast can be safely stored at room temperature. They are excellent for boosting nutrients when added to a variety of foods and sauces. Brewer's yeast has a strong nutty flavor and makes a terrific dip for raw vegetables. Nutritional yeast, with a cheeselike taste, is good for sauces, soups, and stews.

Rice bran is similar to wheat germ because it contains high levels of nutrients and also is promoted as being a healthy food additive. But many rice brans contain unhealthy levels of heavy metals such as arsenic, cadmium, and lead. The amount of these heavy metals in rice bran depends on their level in the soil where the rice was grown. However, the bran concentrates arsenic at a level tenfold higher than whole grain brown rice.[107] Thus, depending on the brand and origin, rice bran may be unhealthy and should be avoided.

Dairy

Just plain milk is a great buy, either in jugs or as dry powder. It contains an excellent combination of protein, vitamins, and minerals. Nonfat dry milk can be added to many other foods such as sauces, soups, stews, and cereal. Whole milk is excellent nutrition, but it contains twice the calories of nonfat milk. Some people cannot tolerate milk because of lactose intolerance but find they can tolerate yogurt, which contains all of the nutrients in milk as well as beneficial probiotic *lactobacilli* cultures. It is more expensive than milk but the probiotic cultures may be worth the extra expense. Hard cheeses with lowfat content, such as Parmesan, mozarella, Swiss, and feta, are excellent. They contain most of the nutrients of milk as well as beneficial bacterial cultures that provide vitamin K_2. Although they are expensive, their high level of nutrition may be worth the added expense. We recommend dairy products such as milk, yogurt, and cheese in moderation along with a diet that includes plenty of vegetables.

Soy Products

Some soy products such as soy milk, tofu, and fermented soy foods are also great buys. The best soy foods are traditionally fermented organic soy foods such as soy sauce, tempeh, miso, and natto. These have high high levels of protein and other essential nutrients, especially B vitamins, except vitamin B_{12}. Natto has high levels of vitamin K. Soy sauce and miso may have high levels of sodium, but this is not usually a problem because they are used in small quantities for flavoring. However, most soy products produced in the United States that are not grown organically are made from genetically modified (GM) soy plants which are potentially harmful. Avoid soy protein powder that may contain GMO soy products.

Meat, Fish, and Eggs

Although many meats and seafoods have excellent levels of essential nutrients, they are generally more expensive and less sustainable than vegetables, fruits, and grains that supply the equivalent amounts.[108] Exceptions are liver, which has outstanding amounts of most essential nutrients; and oysters and clams, which have the highest levels of vitamin B_{12} of any food, and very high levels of other essential nutrients such as zinc, iron, copper, and selenium.[109] Although these foods cost a little more, they are exceptionally nutritious. Sardines, herring, and other small fish are a good source of the omega-3 fatty acids EPA and DHA. They are safer than tuna and other large fish, which contain higher levels of mercury and other heavy metals. When purchased on sale, canned sardines and herring are excellent buys because they also contain high levels of protein and other essential nutrients. Duck and dark chicken and turkey meat are excellent sources of protein and B vitamins as well as other nutrients. Eggs are one of the best values because they contain all the essential nutrients and are relatively inexpensive. They contain high levels of omega-3 oils when they are produced by range-fed chickens. Although eggs contain saturated fat and cholesterol they do not increase risk of disease when consumed in moderation as part of an excellent diet along with appropriate doses of vitamin supplements and other essential nutrients such as omega-3 fatty acids.[110]

RATIONALE FOR VITAMIN AND MINERAL SUPPLEMENTS

If we all could eat an excellent diet and lead an active lifestyle, the risk of progressive age-related disease would be low, and supplements might not be necessary. However, in the modern world, processed food is inexpensive and ubiquitous. Processing removes many of the essential nutrients. People who eat processed food over decades tend to build up deficits that cause diseases such as arthritis. Most people in today's modern society have one or more of these nutritional deficiencies. They are caused by lifestyle, a poor diet that lacks enough fresh vegetables and fruits, and eating processed foods that lack nutrients. Deficits of vitamins such as vitamins C, E, and B_{12} and minerals such as magnesium, zinc, copper, and selenium are common. All of these nutrients are essential for preventing arthritis. Nutrient supplements, such as vitamin and mineral tablets and essential polyunsaturated fatty acids can provide the essential nutrients and make the difference between disease and health.

Supplements can provide additional nutrition that is crucial when the diet contains insufficient levels of the essential nutrients. For example, I (RGS) enjoy several items on the "avoid list" above. I enjoy a peanut butter and jam sandwich for lunch. I enjoy yogurt with a spoonful of brown sugar or sweet preserves stirred in. At a party, I'll enjoy crackers, a small serving of pasta, cookies, or cake made with refined white sugar and enriched white flour. At a lab party we'll often eat a a tasty and nutritious oriental takeout meal, which comes with white rice. I'll take a few spoonfuls. And when dining out I enjoy a small amount of dressing on the salad. Each of these items sets up a deficit. Jams and preserves such as strawberry, blackberry, elderberry, or black currant are favorites of mine. They are very tasty and have a generous portion of antioxidants and other helpful biomolecules. But they often contain 75 percent or more refined sugar, which lacks essential nutrients such as magnesium that would be provided by its original unrefined source. Most crackers, pasta, cake, and other items made from refined grains lack some of the essential nutrients that were in the whole grains before refining. This is true even of items made from enriched flour. The oil in the salad dressing contains several times more calories than the salad and lacks several important nutrients. I've learned to eat salads with minimal or no dressing. But after occasionally eating these refined foods, I take supplements that provide the missing nutrients to make up the deficit. For example, a multivitamin tablet and a magnesium tablet are helpful to make up for the B and E vitamins and magnesium that are missing in white rice and enriched flour.

Getting the Right Doses

Adequate doses of supplements are crucial. Many studies testing the efficacy of nutrient supplements have not determined or utilized a large enough dose, predictably giving disappointing results.[111] The recommended daily allowance (RDA), for vitamins and minerals is only a bare minimum, and most people should take higher doses. The RDA doesn't address the actual levels of vitamins and minerals required to prevent disease. The reason is that an extra amount of essential nutrients, above and beyond the bare minimum, helps the body's metabolic reactions proceed more fully.[112] This is especially true for the body's maintenance functions that regenerate tissues such as cartilage in joints.[113] High levels of nutrients allow the body to tip the balance from cartilage resorption to regeneration.

A further complexity, described in Chapter 2, is that individuals vary in the amount of essential nutrients they require for optimal health.[114] Individuals have different stresses in their daily lives, and they have genetic differences in their metabolic pathways. Also, their diet varies day by day, providing different amounts of nutrients. So their biochemical needs differ.[115] Further, nutrients are absorbed differently by each individual, depending on many factors such as age, microbiota in the gut, and apparently mundane details such as how much water is consumed with food during meals. The amount of fat in the body affects the blood levels of the fat-soluble vitamins such as vitamin A, D, E, and omega-3 and omega-6 fatty acids. Heavier individuals need more of these essential nutrients. As we age, we need to eat more nutrients because the gut absorbs less of them. Ironically, this age-related effect is due in part to nutrient deficiencies.

For most individuals in today's modern society, it is helpful to take supplements containing much higher doses of vitamins and minerals than the RDA. Most of the vitamins and minerals, except vitamin A, iron, copper, and selenium, are very safe when taken at these much higher doses. One way to get essential nutrients is with a nutrient-dense, low-calorie, high fiber supplement bar. A study of this type of supplement was found to lower inflammation due to nutrient deficiencies.[116]

Vitamin A

Vitamin A is important for the whole body, including the joints. It is fat soluble, so the level in the body rises and falls slowly. It is considered a hormone because it is required only in very small amounts and has many effects on receptors throughout the body. Many people are deficient in vitamin A, but it's usually easy to correct. Eating a robust amount of carrots and dark green leafy vegetables will give an adequate dose. Other excellent sources are liver, cod liver oil, eggs, and whole milk products. Vitamin A comes in two forms, retinol, which is found in meat and liver, and beta-carotene, found in plants such as carrots and greens.

One concern about vitamin A is potential toxicity. High doses of the animal form, retinol (or retinyl), can cause the liver to become enlarged or hair to fall out. Liver contains robust amount of vitamin A, and can be toxic if a large enough quantity is eaten. In fact, eating a portion of a liver of a polar bear or seal can cause illness and death.[117] So it's important not to get too much of the animal form of vitamin A. However, even though taking an extra large dose of vitamin A in supplement form (20,000–50,000 international units (IU) per day) may give toxic symptoms, it will not likely kill anyone. Vitamin supplements are safe when taken in appropriate doses.[118]

Another concern is that in some studies, it has been reported that beta-carotene slightly increases the risk of lung cancer in smokers. The risk appears to be limited to smokers, because when beta-carotene is given to nonsmokers, it does not increase the risk. The effect is thought to be due to the high level of oxidative stress in smokers' lungs. In this environment, vitamin A is thought to be converted into a biochemical that damages DNA and initiates cancer. This chemical also prevents carotenoids from being converted into the active vitamin A hormone. Moreover, when smokers take beta-carotene along with vitamin C and E, it does not cause an increase in risk.[119] The reason for this is likely that vitamin C and E together can prevent the oxidative stress in smokers' lungs. Carrots, which contain a healthy dose of beta-carotene as well as many other essential nutrients, are not implicated in the risk. In one study, beta carotene lowered blood urate, and was suggested as an excellent treatment for gout.[120]

A common dose of vitamin A is 5,000–10,000 IU per day (25–50 IU per pound per day), which is thought to be safe for most people.[121] However, people who have special circumstances such as kidney disease or women who are pregnant are at higher risk for toxicity from vitamin A. A four-ounce portion of liver can contain 100,000 IU, so it's important to keep track of your total intake from animal sources and from any supplements you may take. Because vitamin A is fat soluble and its level rises slowly in the body with moderate doses, you must take it for several months to get the full benefit. Drinking alcohol can increase your requirement, so it's best to avoid alcohol, drinking it rarely and only in moderation. The plant form of vitamin A, beta-carotene, is not toxic, and the body will automatically convert as much beta-carotene as it needs into vitamin A.[122] Beta carotene obtained from eating carrots and other vegetables is about 10 percent as effective as vitamin A. Many multivitamin supplements contain both a moderate dose of retinol and also some beta-carotene. This limits the dose of the animal form and allows the body to make additional vitamin A from the plant form. But you can get your required vitamin A very easily, simply by eating carrots. It's safe to eat as many carrots as you want. A large carrot contains the beta-carotene equivalent of 3,000 IU of vitamin A, without any potential toxicity. Other excellent sources include dark-green leafy vegetables, winter squash (any kind), and sweet potatoes.[123] A good plan is to take a modest amount of vitamin A in supplement form (5,000 IU) along with an excellent diet that includes lots of green, yellow, and orange vegetables. If you eat too much beta-carotene, your skin may turn light orange, but this is not harmful and will disappear once you reduce your intake.

Vitamin Bs

These vitamins are essential for health because they are required cofactors for the body's metabolic pathways, and thus are important for maintenance of joints. They have been shown to have specific benefits for preventing and reversing arthritis. B vitamins are normally taken together because the body's biochemical pathways work best when they are provided together. Many one-a-day multivitamin tablets include relatively low amounts of the B_1-B_6 vitamins (1–10 mg), but it's usually best to take mega-multivitamin tablets that contain higher doses (50–100 mg per day). As explained in Chapter 5, deficiencies of these vitamins can cause a variety of symptoms throughout the body, and are responsible for age-related diseases such as heart disease, cancer, and arthritis. Because they're all water soluble, a dose is typically excreted within a few days. Therefore, it is best to take a supplement for these vitamins every day. If you do, you may notice an orange-yellow color in urine, which is caused by vitamin B_2 (riboflavin). Although some serious conditions can be signaled by colored urine, the yellow color from taking vitamin B_2 in a multivitamin tablet is harmless. Remember that taking amounts of the B vitamins in excess of the minimum requirement is helpful to allow the body to optimally perform maintenance functions such as regrowth of collagen in articular cartilage.

Niacin

Particularly important for arthritis is niacin (vitamin B_3), which, as explained in the previous chapters, can prevent the pain and stiffness of OA when taken in adequate doses (50–2,000 mg per day or more in divided doses). Kaufman discovered this inexpensive and very effective treatment seventy years ago[124] and it is still valid today.[125] At high doses, niacin helps metabolic pathways proceed at optimal rates. This is particularly essential for maintenance functions such as rebuilding articular cartilage. Kaufman found that high dose treatment of niacin in divided doses reliably reduced pain from arthritis. Niacin has many benefits, including lowering your cholesterol and blood pressure and helping to prevent anxiety, depression, and alcoholism.[126] Further, if taken regularly, niacin (as well as vitamin C) can protect against anaphylactic shock in those prone to this allergic reaction.[127]

NIACIN FLUSH AND SAFETY

The correct dose of niacin to take is dependent on your body's needs. You can determine the right dose by starting with a small dose and gradually increasing it. If you take a large dose, you may notice an itchy reddish rash on your skin, known as a "niacin flush." If taken on an empty stomach, niacin will cause a flush within about thirty minutes, and if taken with a meal, the flush may be delayed by an hour or more.[128] The flush is not harmful, and depending on the dose will usually disappear within thirty to sixty minutes. It indicates that the niacin is functioning correctly to lower cholesterol.[129] The flush gives a warm sensation on the skin, which is welcome to many people because it feels good and means the niacin is working to lower cholesterol. However for some people the niacin flush is uncomfortable. You can avoid getting a flush by taking small doses at first and gradually building up to a larger dose (see the main text). The body takes several weeks to adapt to higher levels of niacin. This is due to slow upregulation of the biochemical pathways that utilize niacin in the liver and throughout the body. After several weeks, a higher dose can be given without causing the niacin flush. Or you can take niacinamide, which does not cause a flush but also doesn't lower cholesterol.

In some individuals, niacin can slightly increase blood sugar, but this is not usually a problem. Vitamin C helps to prevent cytotoxicity and other complications from high blood sugar in diabetics.[130] Further, high dose niacin can often cause a remission (cause lower blood sugar) in diabetics, and is helpful in preventing and recovering from heart disease.[131] Niacin can also temporarily increase the level of liver enzymes found on a blood test, causing an alarm about potential toxicity for those who are misinformed about its effects. However, an increase in liver enzymes is a side effect of niacin's beneficial effect on metabolic function in the liver.[132] Niacin is used by the body to make NAD (nicotinamide adenine dinucleotide), which is a cofactor for many liver enzymes. Many liver enzymes require NAD for their activity. Because taking niacin increases the level of NAD, it also elevates the activities of those liver enzymes. This is not a measure of the liver responding to toxicity. Instead it is merely a measure of enzyme activities available with the high level of NAD cofactor to deal with normal body metabolites and toxins. You can prevent any confusion about liver enzymes by stopping the niacin dose several days before a blood test.

At doses up to about 1,000 mg per day, niacin can temporarily increase blood pressure. This effect is related to the niacin flush, and can largely be prevented by taking niacin along with vitamins C, D, E, and magnesium, which work together to allow arteries to relax and reduce high blood pressure. Very high doses of niacin (more than 3,000 mg at one time) can sometimes cause blood pressure to temporarily drop quickly. Much higher doses of niacin (more than 10,000 mg at one time) have led to persistent decreases in blood pressure that lasted for over twenty-four hours. Another complication with very high doses (more than 3,000 mg per day) is that niacin can cause problems in the eye, including cystoid macular edema. This is condition is rare, and only 1 percent of individuals who take the very high dose report this symptom. In this condition, niacin causes fluid to build up within the retina, but this goes away in a few weeks when the dose of niacin is lowered below a certain threshold; for example, 1,000 mg per day. This is not due to leakage from blood vessels in the eye that typically occurs with diabetes, because it is reversible.[133] If you notice any problems with your vision when reading (which uses your macula), you should consult your ophthalmologist, who may recommend reducing your dose of niacin.

Overall, niacin and niacinamide are very safe, and are highly recommended for preventing pain and stiffness in arthritis. Niacin has been widely studied and shown to be safe in thousands of studies over many years.[134] A daily amount of 1,000–2,000 mg per day, taken in smaller divided doses (250 mg four to eight times per day). is safe and can greatly reduce or stop pain and stiffness from OA. Consult your doctor before taking high-dose niacin (more than 1,000 mg per day).

Niacin comes in several forms, including standard "fast-release" niacin, and niacinamide. Both of these help to prevent pain and stiffness of arthritis. They both increase cellular NAD, an essential metabolic molecule for all life. Only niacin raises HDL (high density lipoprotein) more than any statin drug, while simultaneously lowering LDL (low-density lipoprotein) and total cholesterol.[135] However, in many cell types, niacin also elevates NAD more than niacinamide, making niacin superior to niacinamide for helping to prevent disease.[136]

Finding the right dose for niacin is similar to finding the right dose of vitamin C. The idea is to take small doses at first, then gradually increase the dose day by day. A good way to accomplish this is to purchase a bottle of 100 mg tablets of niacin. Break a tablet into four pieces so that you can take 25 mg at first. Take one 25 mg dose for the first few days, then gradually build up to take two, three and four of these 25 mg doses taken several hours apart each day, so in a few days you're taking a total of 100 mg. After several weeks, you can build up to larger amounts, always taken in divided doses throughout the day. This is more effective than taking one large daily dose. The optimal dose may vary from one week to the next, depending on the foods consumed and the level of stress.

The alternate form of niacin, called niacinamide, is also inexpensive and effective at preventing pain and stiffness from OA. Kaufman used this form to successfully treat arthritis in his patients because it does not cause the niacin flush.[137] Niacinamide helps to prevent a wide variety of diseases, including cancer, neurodegenerative diseases, and obesity. You may find it helpful to compare the effects of niacin and niacinamide on improving arthritis symptoms. As with niacin, it is helpful to start with small doses of niacinamide and gradually build up to 1,000–4,000 mg per day. Dr. Kaufman found the best results with frequent low doses of niacinamide (250 mg sixteen times throughout the day), rather than single daily high doses (4,000 mg). Several other forms of niacin, often termed "slow-release," "extended-release," or "no-flush" niacin, are promoted to prevent or reduce the occurrence of the niacin flush. However, they are not reliably more effective than plain niacin. Some have been reported to cause liver damage at high doses, and they cost more.[138] Therefore, it's best to stick with niacin for all of its benefits, or niacinamide to avoid getting a flush. Before starting high-dose niacin, niacinamide, or other niacin compounds, get the advice of your medical doctor.

Vitamin B_{12} and Folate

Vitamin B_{12} and folate are water-soluble B vitamins necessary for the metabolic pathways of every cell in the body. They are essential cofactors in the synthesis of DNA and for the production of energy. Vitamin B_{12} is necessary to regenerate folate, so a vitamin B_{12} deficiency can mask a folate deficiency. They work together and so should be taken together. As described in Chapter 5, arthritis patients often have a deficiency of these essential nutrients. They are necessary for bone growth, and adequate amounts are necessary for preventing and reversing OA and RA.

The body only needs a tiny amount of vitamin B_{12} (cyanocobalamin or methylcobalamin), about 1 mcg per day, but the mechanism that the body uses to absorb it is one of the most complex, and many things can go wrong.[139] That is why it's best to take a much higher dose. A special protein-binding factor from saliva binds to vitamin B_{12} to prevent it from being degraded by the stomach acid. When the B_{12}-binding factor is carried into the small intestine, the binding factor gets degraded by enzymes released by the gut, releasing the B_{12}. Then an "intrinsic factor" (IF) released by the gut binds B_{12}, and forms a IF-B_{12} complex. This is recognized by cells in the small intestine and is then absorbed into the bloodstream. The B_{12} is then transferred to another protein, a transporter that allows it to be carried into cells where it is finally utilized in metabolic reactions. This complex transport system can fail at any point, either by a genetic mutation in the various binding proteins, an insufficiency of the stomach or intestinal enzymes, or an immune reaction to the binding factor or intrinsic factor. In normal individuals, only a small fraction of ingested vitamin B_{12} is absorbed. In many cases a dietary insufficiency or problem with digestion or the absorption mechanism prevents absorption of enough B_{12}, which can cause a deficiency.

Many people are deficient in vitamin B_{12} without realizing it, because a deficiency can cause several seemingly unrelated problems.[140] A mild deficiency of vitamin B_{12} can cause numbness or tingling in the extremities, tremors, balance problems, fatigue, depression, and memory loss. A severe deficiency can cause pernicious anemia, cognitive impairment, loss of brain function, and brain damage. Vitamin B_{12} is stored in the liver, which can hold enough for several years, so an insufficiency in the intake or absorption of vitamin B_{12} may go unnoticed. A vitamin B_{12} deficiency is easy to misdiagnose.[141] Many older individuals have a B_{12} deficiency because they lack good digestion or absorption. This is a common cause of "age-related" dementia. In fact, this problem may be a simple deficiency and, if so, can usually be easily corrected. An inexpensive blood test is available if you suspect a vitamin B_{12} deficiency.

Vitamin B_{12} is not made by plants or animals, but only by bacteria. Although bacteria in the gut can make it, this happens beyond the point in the intestines where B_{12} is absorbed. Therefore it must be absorbed from foods. Good sources are meat, fish, poultry, dairy products, eggs, and nutritional yeast (not brewer's yeast). The best sources are clams (raw, cooked, or canned), liver, liverwurst, sardines, and salmon.[142] A deficiency of vitamin B_{12} is common among vegetarians, but several vegetarian sources are available, such as fermented soy foods like miso and tempeh, and some seaweeds.[143] Interestingly, if you grow your own vegetables, you can get some vitamin B_{12} simply by not washing them, for some bacteria in the soil that gets splashed onto vegetables make their own. We do not recommend eating dirt, but unwashed vegetables will provide some since vitamin B_{12} is preserved to an extent during cooking of short duration, such as steaming.

Most multivitamin tablets contain an adequate dose of vitamin B_{12}. The best form of vitamin B_{12} for oral supplements is considered to be methylcobalamin. But individuals who lack even one of the absorption mechanisms cannot absorb B_{12} from a multivitamin tablet. An alternative is a "sublingual" tablet that you place under the tongue. The tablet is dissolved in the saliva and can be directly absorbed through the skin under the tongue. Although the recommended daily amount is 2.5 mcg per day, like other B vitamins it is safe to take in much higher amounts (100–1,000 mcg per day). Although the gut typically cannot absorb all of the higher dose, having an excess amount available may increase the absorption, especially in those who are deficient. If you suspect that you are deficient in vitamin B_{12}, you may benefit by consulting your medical doctor.

Folate

Folate (folic acid) is a water-soluble B vitamin essential for growing and dividing cells to synthesize DNA, so like vitamin B_{12} it is used throughout the body. Direct sunlight overhead (11:00 A.M. to 3:00 P.M.) can degrade folate in the bloodstream under the skin, which is thought to be a major reason why skin color has evolved to be dark in equatorial climates.[144] Other common reasons for a deficiency of folate are heavy consumption of alcohol and use of contraceptive pills.[145] Folate is made by plants (folate comes from the Latin word *folium* for leaf), and dark green leafy vegetables are excellent sources. All animals need folate, and it is passed up the food chain. Good sources include liver, beans, dark-green leafy vegetables, asparagus, and nutritional yeast.[146] Folate in vitamin supplements is better absorbed than from food. The recommended daily amount is 400 mcg per day, or 600 mcg for pregnant women, but higher doses up to 1–5 mg are thought to be safe.

However, there is one concern about high doses of folate. For many decades, babies were born with neural tube defects. It was found that this was due in part to a folate deficiency. In 1998, folate was included in the fortification of enriched flour, which immediately reduced the rate of these neural tube defects.[147] Many studies have shown that adequate levels of essential nutrients including folate during fetal development improves the survival of children and lowers the risk for cancer and heart disease later in life. However, cancer cells are continually growing, so once cancer gets started it requires folate. Therefore, folate is suspected to increase cancer risk, and a chemotherapeutic target of cancer drugs is the folate pathway. Some studies of folate have found it increases the risk of low birth weight and of chronic diseases such as cancer later in life. In adults, one study suggested that folate supplementation increased the risk of lung cancer in smokers. These studies are controversial and were likely faulty, because the cancers may have started before the supplements were given.[148]

In contrast, folate also helps to prevent cancer, because a deficiency of folate can cause defects in DNA similar to those caused by radiation. Therefore an adequate level of folate is helpful in prevention of cancer. A recent study verified that folate reduces the risk for lung cancer.[149] Another concern is prostate cancer. Some studies have found that folate supplements increase the risk of prostate cancer, especially in those who may already have this disease, but many studies have shown the opposite, that folate and other nutrients reduce the risk of prostate cancer.[150] Many nutritionists believe that very high levels of folate greater than 1,000 mcg per day (that's 1 mg) do not provide much benefit. However, it's important to get an adequate amount of folate, either though supplements or diet. The simplest and perhaps best way to get folate is a well-balanced diet that includes lots of leafy green vegetables!

Vitamin C

Although many antioxidants are important for the body, vitamin C (ascorbate) has a special status because it is the most important water-soluble antioxidant in the bloodstream.[151] It is involved in preventing arthritis for several reasons.[152] As an antioxidant, it helps to prevent oxidative stress that damages tissues of the joint. It is also essential in the synthesis of collagen, the most common protein in the body and a major constituent of articular cartilage of joints. Further, vitamin C is essential for the immune system, and it helps to prevent inflammation.[153]

Vitamin C is essential for the entire body. It strengthens arteries and increases their elasticity through its function in collagen synthesis. This helps to lower blood pressure, and lowers the risk of heart disease and stroke.[154] A slight deficiency of vitamin C can cause these age-related diseases because the damage to collagen in arteries builds up over decades.[155] As described in Chapter 2, vitamin C is only necessary for higher primates, guinea pigs, and a few other animals. All other species can make their own ascorbate, so for them it isn't a vitamin. Primates have a special recycling mechanism to regenerate vitamin C once it has been oxidized in performing its antioxidant function.[156] But higher levels of vitamin C than the 100 mg

RDA are helpful to prevent age-related diseases such as heart disease and arthritis.

A typical diet that includes lots of raw vegetables may supply 100–500 mg per day of vitamin C. But we typically need much more, depending on our daily stresses; for example, 3,000–10,000 mg per day, depending on body weight. These higher doses are equivalent to the amount of vitamin C that apes get from their diet, and also to the dose of vitamin C in guinea pig chow (25–50 mg per kilogram (kg) per day). Thus, to get an adequate amount of vitamin C, it is helpful to take supplements, as it can play an important role in preventing and reversing arthritis. Vitamin C is degraded in water by high temperatures, so high temperatures during cooking can lower the amount found in food. Interestingly, boiled or baked potatoes and many other cooked staple foods still have enough vitamin C (20 mg per cup) to prevent scurvy.[157] Many poor people have relied on this inexpensive source of vitamin C. This is one reason why the Irish potato famine of the 1840s caused an outbreak of scurvy.[158]

Although concerns have often been suggested about supplements of vitamin C, megadoses are nontoxic and safe.[159] It is a small molecule and therefore does not generate an immune reaction or allergy. Vitamin C is an antihistamine and can stop an allergic reaction.[160] Like other water-soluble vitamins, it is excreted in urine, so its half-life (the time it takes to decrease by 50 percent) in the body is short, about four to eight hours.[161] For this reason, it is helpful to take vitamin C in divided doses throughout the day rather than all at once. This keeps the blood level high throughout the day.[162]

Both blood sugar and vitamin C are transported into cells by glucose transporters. This causes high levels of sugar to compete with vitamin C for entry into cells. Therefore, vitamin C is most effective when taken without food containing sugar. It's also a reason why diabetics, who have high blood sugar, often get symptoms caused by a deficiency of vitamin C such as damage to arteries or cartilage. Smoking causes lower levels of vitamin C and E in the blood because the toxins in the smoke increase oxidative stress.[163] A similar effect is caused by bacterial or viral infections. The oxidized vitamin C can be recycled in red blood cells or it can be replaced by a fresh source of vitamin C in the diet. Because vitamin C is so important for preventing and reversing arthritis, it's important to take higher doses when stressed by infections or chemical or environmental toxins.

Concerns about Vitamin C

There are several concerns about supplements of vitamin C. One common myth, often repeated by medical professionals, is that vitamin C can increase the risk of kidney stones. The myth was started because vitamin C tends to raise the level of oxalate in the urine. Oxalate can precipitate to make kidney stones in the presence of a high level of calcium. But for several reasons, vitamin C doesn't cause this problem. There is no evidence in the literature that vitamin C taken by people with normal kidney function actually causes kidney stones.[164] In fact, vitamin C is a diuretic, and tends to increase the volume of urine, which prevents formation of any type of kidney stone.[165] Vitamin C actually prevents formation of calcium oxalate stones by binding to calcium in the urine.[166] Many foods, such as coffee and tea, spinach, rhubarb, chocolate, and beets contain oxalate at much higher levels than those caused by vitamin C. To prevent oxalate stones, it is now recommended to take moderate amounts of calcium and magnesium supplements along with vitamin C and other antioxidants. Dietary calcium binds oxalate in the gut, which prevents oxalate from being absorbed.[167] Adequate magnesium prevents calcium from binding to oxalate in the urine, which prevents calcium oxalate stones.[168] In some people, vitamin C can increase the amount of urate in urine, which is a benefit in preventing gout. However, urate can also cause kidney stones. Both of these types of stones can be prevented by adequate intake of magnesium and water.[169] Further, a recent study tested the effect of a diet high in fruits and vegetables, nuts, legumes, and whole grains, and low in sodium, sugar, and red and processed meats. Participants on this diet showed a reduced risk of kidney stones. Ironically, the diet increased the participants' level of potassium, calcium, magnesium, oxalate, and vitamin C.[170]

In summary, to prevent kidney stones, drink plenty of water along with supplements of vitamin C (3,000–10,000 mg per day), calcium (200–600 mg per day), and magnesium (200–600 mg per day for a 1:1 ratio with calcium), avoid drinking large amounts of coffee and tea, and avoid foods containing high levels of oxalate. The high intake of water, vegetables, fruits, and vitamin C is important to prevent arthritis, especially on a hot summer day. You and your doctor may benefit by discussing this topic.

Another concern about vitamin C is its acidity. It is a weak acid, a little stronger than vinegar but weaker than lemon juice. First, you should not chew tablets of vitamin C because it can stick to teeth and the acid can etch them. This can be a problem with chewable vitamin C tablets, which contain sugar. Sweet-tasting chewable vitamin C tablets can be used to entice children to get their vitamin C, but these should be buffered with either sodium, calcium, or magnesium-ascorbate. However, if you take vitamin C tablets without chewing them, they will not harm your teeth. When taken at high doses, such as 10,000–20,000 mg or more per day or more in divided doses, for example, to prevent joint damage or a viral infection, vitamin C tablets can cause an upset stomach. But it's important to understand that the acid in even such a large dose is much weaker than the normal hydrochloric acid in the stomach. In some cases, vitamin C tablets don't dissolve well in the stomach, and this may cause the upset. To prevent this, you can purchase buffered ascorbate powder (sodium, calcium, or magnesium ascorbate) which is not acid and won't upset your stomach.

Another myth, spread innocently by many people—including my college organic chemistry teacher—is that the acidity of vitamin C can upset the body's acid balance (pH), which might cause other health problems. However, this usually isn't a problem, because the body closely regulates its acidity, given a healthy diet that includes robust amounts of fruits and vegetables. The autonomic nervous system sets the amount of acidity in the body over a short timescale (minutes to hours) by controlling the rate of breathing. Faster breathing removes more carbon dioxide, which reduces the acidity of the blood. Slower breathing increases the acidity. And over a longer time period, the kidneys control acidity by excreting urine with either acid or alkaline components.[171] My college chemistry teacher apparently had not studied physiology and didn't understand how the body regulates acidity! After vitamin C has done its antioxidant job, neutralizing oxidative stress in the blood and tissues, some of its oxidized form (dehydroascorbate, DHAA) is recycled in red blood cells and the remainder is excreted in the urine. Because vitamin C is a weak acid, taking even large doses is relatively easy for the body to counteract with its respiration and excretion mechanisms.

Regulation of Iron Uptake

Another concern about vitamin C is that it increases the uptake of nonheme iron by the gut. For those who have iron overload, or hemochromatosis, this can be a problem. As explained above, the body does not excrete much iron in the urine, so iron must be regulated in absorption.[172] But heme-bound iron, found in red meat, is almost fully absorbed, and this absorption path cannot be regulated.[173] On the other hand, absorption of nonheme iron, found in vegetables and in supplements, is closely regulated by the body according to its level and need for iron.[174] Because vitamin C increases this absorption of nonheme iron, it is often blamed for the excess of iron in hemochromatosis. To limit iron intake, a good plan is to eat red meat in moderation and continue taking vitamin C. You can control the amount of iron you get by eating higher or lower amounts of iron-containing foods, and when necessary by taking a multivitamin that contains iron.

Rare Genetic Concerns

A final caution is that some individuals with impaired kidney function or some rare genetic mutations should not take supplements of vitamin C.[175] Those with glucose-6-phosphate dehydrogenase (G6PD) deficiency should avoid very high doses (greater than 6,000 mg per day) of vitamin C supplements, for this condition can cause hemolytic anemia.[176] However, lower doses pose little risk for those who have G6PD without symptoms.[177] Further, vitamin E tends to prevent the hemolytic anemia from occurring.[178] You should consult with your doctor to determine that you have normal kidney function, and do not have any of these genetic conditions before taking high-dose vitamin C.

Finding the Right Dose of Vitamin C: Bowel Tolerance

Throughout this book, we have inserted the recommended doses of vitamin C, which differ depending on the situation. Each individual is different and has different needs for vitamin C and other vitamins.[179] Therefore it is necessary to find the appropriate dose of vitamin C for each relevant condition. Vitamin C is transported from the gut by a special transporter protein. This uptake mechanism is slowed when the level of vitamin C in the bloodstream increases, which limits the amount of vitamin C that can be absorbed from one dose.[180] When a large dose of vitamin C is taken, for example, 2,000 mg at one time, some will be absorbed into the bloodstream and the rest will stay in the gut. The larger the dose, the smaller the absorbed fraction. However, a larger dose will invariably give a larger total amount absorbed.[181] The vitamin C that remains in the gut encourages bacterial growth, and this attracts water into the gut, causing gas and a laxative effect. The highest amount of vitamin C that can be taken without causing the laxative effect is a limit called the "bowel tolerance."

The bowel tolerance limit is not hard and fast. For example, the level of vitamin C in the bloodstream drops when the body encounters oxidative stress, such as damage to tendons and muscles during exercise, breathing smoke or other environmental toxins, or during a bacterial or viral infection. It also drops in response to sources of inflammation such as heart disease or arthritis. This is a normal function of vitamin C, for it will sacrifice itself (chemically speaking) to neutralize a free radical, getting oxidized in the process. But when this happens, the body requires more vitamin C. It can recycle some by transporting the oxidized vitamin C into red blood cells, where it is converted back into vitamin C. But with low blood levels of vitamin C, the gut will also actively transport a larger fraction of ingested vitamin C into the bloodstream.[182] This implies that the requirement for vitamin C, and the dose required to prevent a deficiency, varies according to the degree of oxidative stress in the body.[183] With a cold or flu, or when breathing vehicle exhaust or smoke,[184] oxidative stress jumps up, and the bowel tolerance for vitamin C jumps up accordingly. To find this higher limit, when you know you've been exposed to stress or an infection, it's necessary to be proactive and take an additional amount of vitamin C. You may be surprised at how your need for vitamin C varies from one day or week to the next.

The idea that the need for vitamin C varies over time and between individuals may explain the negative results and confusion implicit in many health studies testing the effect of vitamin C. Many studies have determined the effect of relatively low doses of vitamin C, for example, 500 mg per day. Although this is fivefold larger than the RDA, it will not reach the bowel tolerance for most people. Further, the increase in the level of vitamin C from a single dose will fade within a few hours. Someone under little oxidative stress may have a low requirement for vitamin C (1,000–3,000 mg per day) because the level in the body from an excellent diet including fruits and vegetables may be adequate. But with an increase in oxidative stress the same person may readily oxidize some or even most of the vitamin C present in the body. Under this condition, much more vitamin C is transported from the gut into the bloodstream, and a higher dose of vitamin C can be taken with benefit. Many studies have not taken this mechanism into account and have given hardly enough vitamin C to make any difference. Yet, when adequate doses are given, the results can be dramatic.

PERSONAL CASE HISTORY OF VITAMIN C

An acquaintance who had rather severe back pain, upon hearing advice about the importance of vitamin C for arthritis, took 10,000–20,000 mg per day in divided doses for several weeks. At first he got diarrhea because he had taken too much at once without an understanding of the advice about determining the proper dose by checking for bowel tolerance. But after decreasing the divided doses to just below bowel tolerance, he found after several days that his back pain was greatly reduced. He was amazed and thankful. He then went on to modify his diet to get larger amounts of the other essential nutrients, and was on the path to recovery.

I (RGS) have found when gardening that I sometimes develop joint or tendon problems due to the unusual stress of holding a long heavy gardening implement in my hand. When I was younger (in my thirties), I once found that after an hour using lopper shears, my wrists hurt so much that I had to stop. Favoring my wrists, I hoped they would recover. They did, but it took four to six weeks before the pain went away. A similar problem occurred on day hikes when my sister was showing me the Cascade mountains of Oregon. Just a short one-hour hike caused such pain in my hips that it forced an embarrassing retreat from the mountain. It took my hips several months to recover. At that time, I was taking only 500–1,000 mg of vitamin C per day. This helped but was not enough.

More recently, I've found that, although my wrists hurt a little after too much manual work, when I take adequate doses of vitamin C they recover quickly, usually overnight. With adequate vitamin C, I can now go on strenuous all-day hikes without any problem. And on a day when I notice a scratchy throat or a slight headache, I take 1,000 mg every half hour for four to eight hours to prevent a viral infection. The mega doses of vitamin C to bowel tolerance, along with adequate levels of the other essential nutrients in an excellent diet have made the difference. I take a half-teaspoon (3,000–4,000 mg) of vitamin C powder in a four-ounce of orange juice at breakfast, along with a multivitamin tablet and other supplements. At midmorning after riding to work on my bike, I'll take another 1,000 mg capsule of vitamin C. At lunch I take another 1,000 mg of vitamin C, and again during the afternoon. If it's been a very stressful day, I take another half-teaspoon of vitamin C powder in vegetable juice before dinner. Then, before going to bed, I take my last divided dose of magnesium (200 mg), niacin (200–500 mg), and vitamin C (4,000 mg). When these doses cause a laxative effect or gas, which they sometimes do when I'm not so stressed, I'll reduce the dose over the next several days by 30 to 50 percent. An excellent diet of vegetables and supplements has given me better health, which allows faster recovery from injury. And most important, it has given me the confidence about my abilities to do more than I thought was possible!

Doses: Importance of Finding Bowel Tolerance

When you have an infection or other oxidative stress, including OA or RA, it's important to determine your bowel tolerance with small doses taken frequently, gradually building up to a higher daily dose. The reason is that the bowel tolerance for vitamin C is higher when totaled over a twenty-four-hour period with smaller more frequent doses. The smaller doses are better absorbed by the gut, resulting in a higher total amount absorbed. Typical doses for average individuals are 500–2,000 mg taken four to six times per day, for example, before breakfast, lunch, and dinner, and before going to bed at night. This helps to prevent many age-related diseases such as heart disease, cancer, diabetes, and arthritis. Typical doses for an acute infection of a cold or flu virus are 1,000 mg taken every ten to twenty minutes for several hours, until bowel tolerance is reached. Then continue with smaller doses to find a lower bowel tolerance, 1,000 mg taken every hour or two. Continue this lower dose for several days until the infection is gone.[185] For sufferers of OA and RA, typical doses to reach bowel tolerance may be in the range of 1,000 mg per hour during an episode of pain, or 1,000 mg every three to six hours under nonstressful conditions. With experience, it's possible to feel the amount of stress and predict the bowel tolerance and dose of vitamin C that the body needs.

The importance of the vitamin C transporter for the body was highlighted by a recent study of mutations in the gene that codes for the transporter protein. This mutation was associated with a three- to fivefold higher risk for heart disease.[186] The hypothesis implied by this study is that when vitamin C cannot be transported from the gut into blood and tissues, the resulting lack of vitamin C causes heart disease. Although the study did not test the association of the defective transporter gene with arthritis, given the close association of arthritis and heart disease, the risk is likely to be similar for arthritis.

Oxidative stress and inflammation are known to occur in OA and RA, so it's important to find your bowel tolerance for vitamin C under the conditions of stress you are exposed to from one day to the next. The dose is important for arthritis because vitamin C has several functions, all relevant to OA and RA. When oxidative stress causes vitamin C levels to drop, it becomes less available for its other essential functions such as synthesis of collagen and strengthening the immune system. Because vitamin C is synergistic with other antioxidants, if you keep your level of vitamin C and other antioxidants high with adequate doses, more vitamin C will be available to help regrowth of cartilage.

Forms of Vitamin C

Vitamin C (ascorbic acid) is available in several forms. Ascorbic acid is the least expensive and is exactly the same molecule as vitamin C in food.[187] Tablets of vitamin C containing 500 or 1,000 mg compressed into a solid are convenient and widely available. Chewable buffered vitamin C tablets that contain sugar are helpful to convince children to take their dose. Capsules containing vitamin C powder encapsulated by a thin gelatin shell are also widely available. Vitamin C is also available unencapsulated in crystalline powder form. Timed-release tablets of vitamin C contain an additional ingredient, a long-chain carbohydrate to delay digestion, which is useful to allow the vitamin C to be absorbed slowly over several hours. Although this form of vitamin C costs more than standard tablets, it can provide a continuous dose during sleep and can help to avoid taking pills throughout the day. Which form is best for you depends on your preference.

For those who prefer or need a nonacid form, vitamin C is also available in buffered form as sodium ascorbate, or in several other forms such as calcium or magnesium ascorbate. These forms are nonacid but also contain sodium, calcium, or magnesium. They are a little more expensive than plain ascorbic acid, but may be worth the extra expense. Powdered sodium, calcium, or magnesium ascorbate are helpful because they can be readily dissolved in juice or water. In this form, they don't need to be further dissolved in the stomach, so they may have greater absorption in the gut. If you take magnesium ascorbate, you get the bonus of extra magnesium along with your vitamin C. Sodium ascorbate is recommended for those who have difficulty with the acidity of ascorbic acid because it is less expensive than calcium or magnesium ascorbate. The extra sodium does not cause high blood pressure, because it is not associated with chloride as in salt.[188] Ascorbyl palmitate is a fat-soluble form of vitamin C. It is more expensive than regular vitamin C but has been shown to help prevent oxidative stress in fatty tissues and cell membranes.[189]

The form of vitamin C you take can help you get the best absorption into the body. Often, large tablets of vitamin C do not dissolve completely in the stomach. This may prevent their contents from being fully absorbed in the gut. Vitamin C in thin flexible gelatin capsules will dissolve faster in the stomach and may be better absorbed than some types of hard tablet, because inside the gelatin shell the vitamin C is in powder form. The gelatin will swell and open up so the vitamin C inside can get digested more readily than it would with a tablet. When the vitamin C dissolves within the limited time that food stays in the stomach (about an hour), it can be better absorbed in the remainder of the gut. An excellent alternative is to purchase vitamin C in powder form and stir it into low-sodium vegetable juice. This buffers the sour vitamin C acid so it's barely detectable, and it makes a great boost after a stressful day. The powder form (small crystals of vitamin C) costs about the same as tablets, and is more readily absorbed. If you take a huge dose (for instance, 10,000 mg at one time) that gives you too much vitamin C you may exceed your bowel tolerance and notice a laxative effect along with gas, and with huge doses a slight acidity in the stools. However even such large doses are nontoxic and won't damage the body.[190] And if you have difficulty with the acidic form, try sodium or magnesium ascorbate powder.

You can get an idea about easily a vitamin tablet dissolves by placing one in a glass of warm water and stirring it occasionally while observing it for thirty minutes. If it disintegrates and starts to dissolve by then, it probably will be dissolved in your stomach. However, many pills are compressed so tightly that they don't readily dissolve. You can get them to dissolve better by breaking them into several pieces, for example with your incisors (without chewing) or a knife, and swallowing the pieces with a glass of water. If you chew a vitamin C tablet that contains the acid form (ascorbic acid), it may get stuck in your teeth and this can etch them if the ascorbic acid stays there for more than a few minutes. This is especially a concern with chewable tablets. To prevent etching from chewable tablets, purchase only those that contain fully-buffered vitamin C.

Liposomal Vitamin C

Recently a new form of vitamin C has become available, in which the vitamin C is packaged inside tiny phospholipid nanospheres called liposomes, which comprise a membrane formed from fatty acids. This is analogous to how a cell protects its contents with a cell membrane made from fatty acids. The liposomes protect the vitamin C from oxidation and are absorbed by the gut more efficiently than vitamin C in solution. This liposomal form of vitamin C is five- to tenfold more powerful than plain vitamin C at raising the levels of vitamin C in the blood. This means that a 1,000 mg packet of liposomal vitamin C gives the same blood level as 5,000–10,000 mg of vitamin C in tablets or capsules. It is also more expensive, but because of its efficacy, it may be a good buy. Along with the vitamin C, the phospholipids are healthy because they are utilized throughout the body in cell membranes. To take the liposomal vitamin C packets, cut them open, squeeze the contents out into a glass of water or vegetable juice, and stir vigorously until it is thoroughly mixed. Because each packet is equivalent to 5,000 mg of vitamin C but doesn't give a laxative effect, you can take a much higher dose if required, for example, one 1,000 mg packet every one to three hours.

Alternatively, you can make your own homemade liposomal vitamin C. All you need is an ultrasonic jewelry cleaner, which can be purchased for less than fifty dollars, a blender, vitamin C powder, and a good source of lecithin. A typical recipe involves three cups of cold water, one cup of liquid lecithin, and one tablespoon of vitamin C powder. Blend this mixture, then pour it into the ultrasonic cleaner and turn it on for ten minutes. The ultrasound causes the lecithin to form liposomes that absorb and encapsulate the vitamin C. Stir this mixture to improve the encapsulation of the dissolved vitamin C. Repeat this step to the desired texture. This solution can be stored in the refrigerator and used for about a week. Lecithin has many health benefits. Since this liposomal form of vitamin C is five to ten times more effective than oral vitamin C, the price of the ultrasonic cleaner and lecithin will pay for itself in a short time compared to just taking oral vitamin C tablets.

Intravenous Vitamin C

To achieve the highest blood level of vitamin C, an intravenous (IV) preparation is best. It is safe and can directly raise blood levels without any of the limitations of absorption with oral administration.[191] We recommend this treatment because several recent studies have shown that it is particularly effective at reducing pain and inflammation in RA. In one case, a patient with severe pain from RA was given an IV of 15,000 mg of vitamin C in a 500 milliliter (ml) sterile phosphate buffer solution at 6 ml per minute, followed by glutathione (600 mg, 200 mg per ml). The pain stopped for six hours, and when it recurred it was less severe.[192] Subsequent flare-ups were attenuated (eased) with intramuscular (IM) injections of glutathione. Another study showed that markers of inflammation dropped dramatically in eleven RA patients when they were given IVs of 7,500–25,000 mg of vitamin C.[193] Participants were screened for glucose-6-phosphate dehydrogenase (G6PD) deficiency, and any with this deficiency were not given the IV. The authors found the results very hopeful and suggested further studies. They suggested that the increase in vitamin C levels downregulated the production of pro-inflammatory cytokines. This finding is exciting because the improvement in pain and the drop in inflammation that occurred during the IV sessions was immediate. If you want to pursue this treatment, you must have it supervised by a medical doctor who understands the rationale for the treatment, how to perform it, and its possible complications.

Vitamin D

For many decades, vitamin D (cholecalciferol, vitamin D_3) was thought to be involved mainly in the regulation of calcium for bone health. It is effective for this purpose at a relatively low level in the bloodstream (20–30 nanogram (ng) per ml, equivalent to 50–75 nmol/L). This is one reason that vitamin D is thought to be important in preventing and reversing arthritis. However, over the last two decades research has shown that vitamin D at a higher level (40–60 ng/ml) is required for many other functions in the body, including the proper function of the immune system.[194] Thus, vitamin D helps in several ways to prevent OA and RA. Many researchers working on vitamin D suggest intakes in the range of 3,000–10,000 IU per day, depending on the individual, to reach blood serum levels of 40–60 ng/ml. Blood levels of vitamin D are not always directly proportionate to intake, so to achieve a twofold higher blood level may take more than a twofold increase in dose.[195]

In the summer, you can readily get vitamin D from exposure to direct sunlight between the hours of 11:00 A.M. and 2:00 P.M. With arms, legs, and face exposed, individuals with light skin can get a dose equivalent to 10,000 IU in about fifteen to thirty minutes (about one quarter of the exposure time it takes to produce a slight sunburn twenty-four hours later).[196] Those with dark skin may require one or two hours or more for the same dose of 10,000 IU depending on the skin color. Note that these exposure times are approximate, and only for summer midday sunlight when the sun is 45 degrees or more above the horizon. Below this angle, the sunlight can give a tan, but it doesn't give much vitamin D. This sounds hard to believe and contrary to common sense, but when the sun is below 45 degrees above the horizon, the amount of UVB (that generates vitamin D in the skin) is less than 5 percent of the amount generated when the sun is directly overhead. This means that most people in the United States and southern Europe get little vitamin D from the sun in the winter months, and people in Canada and northern Europe get little in summer and almost none in winter. The amount of vitamin D made in the skin by UVB is also dependent on the altitude (the higher the altitude, the more UVB), cloud cover, use of sunblock, and age.[197] Further, window glass removes the UVB rays, even in conditions where sunbathing in a window gives a tan.

It's easy to get adequate vitamin D levels from UVB rays of sunlight in the summer, or from supplements in the winter. An adequate dose of vitamin D for most people is 25–50 IU per pound per day, which for most adults is in the range of 3,000–10,000 IU per day. In many people this dose will produce the optimal level of 40–60 ng/ml. Note, however: if you take a twofold higher dose, your blood level may not rise twofold. The highest advisable level is 70–80 ng/ml, but no ill effects are observed until much higher levels are reached.[198] Vitamin D made by sunlight in the skin never causes an overdose even with long daily exposure, because the skin stops making it when the level rises. It is known that vitamin D prevents skin cancer, so the vitamin D you get from exposure to thirty minutes of sunlight will tend to lower rather than raise your risk of cancer.[199] It is also thought that vitamin D obtained from the sun stays in the body longer than vitamin D from supplements.[200]

To determine what dose you need, you can get a standard blood test for vitamin D. The blood test typically measures the level of 25-hydroxyvitamin D_3 (abbreviated 25(OH)D, also called calcifediol or calcidiol), which is a precursor for the active form of vitamin D used in the body. Because vitamin D is a fat-soluble vitamin, its level rises and falls slowly, with half-life of several weeks to months. After a summer full of exposure to sunlight, the level will be high. During the fall and winter months in regions far from the equator such as North America, Europe, or southern Africa and Australia, little vitamin D is obtained from the sun, so the level will fall without supplements. By early spring, the vitamin D level will be very low. Therefore winter supplements of vitamin D are necessary for most people in these regions. If a blood test shows you have a level on the low side (less than 40 ng/ml), you should take supplements at an increased dose for at least two months before getting tested again. This is the time it takes for the level to rise to a plateau level in the body.

The Institute of Medicine recommended a daily dose of 600 IU per day of vitamin D for most adults, with an upper recommended dose of 4,000 IU.[201] This recommendation was based on bone health, but excluded the beneficial effects of vitamin D in preventing cancer, heart disease, and in supporting the immune system. Therefore this recommendation is widely believed to be too low for most people.[202]

Other sources of vitamin D include cod liver oil, milk, and wild oily fish such as salmon and sardines. Cod liver oil is not recommended for vitamin D because to get enough, the higher level of vitamin A in the oil would cause toxicity.[203] Milk typically is enriched to contain only 100 IU per cup, so you'd need to drink two gallons to get 3,000 IU. Salmon and sardines typically contain 250–500 IU per three-and-a-half-ounce serving.[204] These amounts are too low to be relied upon to give an adequate dose. An excellent buy are gelcaps containing 2,000 or 5,000 IU. To achieve an adequate blood level during the winter months, you should take one or two of these daily, depending on your body weight and need.

Vitamin E

Vitamin E is the main fat-soluble antioxidant in the body. One function of vitamin E is to neutralize free radicals that otherwise would oxidize the fatty acids and proteins in cell membranes. It has been widely used for six decades to prevent heart disease, cancer, and inflammation. Doses in the range of 400–1600 IU per day are very safe and have a long record of efficacy.[205] One of the roles of vitamin E in preventing arthritis is thought to be through its anti-inflammatory function. Another of its roles is slowing blood clotting, which is helpful in maintaining good circulation.[206] As explained in Chapter 2, vitamin E comes in eight different forms, alpha-, beta-, gamma-, and delta-tocopherol, and alpha-, beta-, gamma-, and delta-tocotrienol. Although they all have antioxidant activity, they perform different functions in the body.[207] They come in natural forms, derived from natural oils, or artificial forms, synthesized from fossil fuels. The d-alpha-tocopherol form (the natural form of alpha-tocopherol, also called RRR-alpha-tocopherol) has been considered to have the most biological activity because it is actively taken up by the body. Gamma-tocopherol is an important form of vitamin E for arthritis, because it facilitates bone growth.[208] However, the tocotrienols are more potent antioxidants.[209] They are more expensive than tocopherols, but because of their high potency, they may be worth the extra expense.

The different forms of vitamin E may seem confusing. Many studies of its efficacy have used an artificial, less effective form of vitamin E, which confounded their results. A widely sold artificial form of vitamin E, dl-alpha-tocopherol (also known as *all-rac*-alpha-tocopherol) has only half the biological activity of the natural form. Further, high doses of d-alpha-tocopherol are known to deplete the body of the other forms of vitamin E, including gamma-tocopherol.[210] Since the gamma-tocopherol form is thought to help bone regrowth, a mixture of the different forms is considered the best for arthritis. Some studies have used the esterified form of vitamin E, alpha-tocopherol-acetate. This form must be cleaved by enzymes in the stomach to be active, so it is dependent upon the level of enzymes, and therefore often has reduced biological activity. Many studies performed with low doses of the artificial form of vitamin E predictably showed little effect. Vitamin E should be taken as "mixed tocopherols and tocotrienols," the natural mixture of all of its forms.

Another concern about vitamin E is exemplified by a recent study that concluded vitamin E increased the risk of prostate cancer. Participants in the study were given a dose of 400 IU per day.[211] The form of vitamin E utilized in this study was dl-alpha-tocopheryl acetate (the artificial esterified form of vitamin E with low biological activity). This dose is equivalent to less than 200 IU per day of d-alpha-tocopherol, which is known to be moderate.[212] Because the dose of vitamin E was moderate, it could not be expected to have much effect. Indeed, the risk of prostate cancer was apparently increased by only about 0.1 percent per year. Further, the study showed that there was no significant increase in risk for prostate cancer for patients taking both vitamin E and selenium. Overall, the study's methods and results make its conclusions highly questionable. The form and dose of vitamins and antioxidant supplements are likely to be important for preventing cancer.[213] Other studies showing increases in mortality risk from vitamin E are also suspect because they were performed on people who were heavy smokers or drinkers, and/ or already very sick with cardiovascular disease or diabetes.[214]

In normal people, many studies have shown that oxidative stress and the resulting inflammation are leading causes for most cancers, including prostate cancer, and that antioxidants lower the risk.[215] Other recent studies have shown that vitamin E given with other antioxidants lowers the risk of prostate cancer.[216] Thus, the concerns about vitamin E increasing risk of stroke or prostate cancer appear mainly to be the result of special cases; for instance, with the very sick, those with rare mutations, or in studies where vitamin E is given in inappropriate doses without other synergistic essential nutrients. In fact, many studies have shown that vitamin E is safe and very effective at reducing the risk of many serious diseases, including liver disease, ALS, lung cancer, and heart disease.[217]

Vitamin E is an essential component of an excellent diet that includes vitamin supplements. It is synergistic with vitamin C and other antioxidants in preventing oxidative stress. Vitamin E works best in combination with other nutrients and antioxidants, such as vitamin C, zinc, selenium, coenzyme Q10 (coQ10), alpha-lipoic acid, and glutathione. The best form of vitamin E to take is a natural mixture of tocopherols and tocotrienols that contains a robust amount of gamma-tocopherol. It's important to start with a moderate dose, for example, 400 IU per day of mixed tocopherols and tocotrienols.[218] After several weeks to a month, individuals sixty-five or older should gradually increase to 800–1,600 IU per day. In some cases it may be helpful to take higher doses, up to 3,200 IU per day. Those with cardiovascular conditions should consult with their doctor before taking vitamin E at high doses.

VITAMINS C AND E PREVENT RISK OF STROKE

Along with its important antioxidant and anti-inflammatory benefits, vitamin E also slows the rate of blood clotting. This is good for circulation, but it can increase the risk of hemorrhagic stroke (bleeding) in patients whose blood vessels are weak or damaged by inflammation.[219] However, when the starting dose is moderate and then increased gradually over a period of several weeks to months, vitamin E strengthens blood vessels.[220] Moreover, vitamin C strengthens blood vessels and lowers high blood pressure, preventing strokes.[221] Therefore, vitamin E is most effective when taken with adequate doses of vitamin C.

Patients taking anticoagulant drugs such as warfarin are often advised not to take supplements of vitamin E because of its anticoagulant effect. Doctors may advise that vitamin E interferes with the drug's action. However, instead of eliminating supplements of vitamin E, it may be better to reduce the dose of the anticoagulant drug instead, for the drug is likely to cause serious side effects, including an increased risk of hemorrhagic stroke. The same is true for aspirin, which is widely prescribed to slow clotting but has several serious and potentially dangerous side effects. An excellent plan is to start with a moderate dose of natural (mixed tocopherols) vitamin E (200–400 IU per day), along with vitamin C (3,000–10,000 mg per day to bowel tolerance), and over several weeks gradually ramp up the dose to high levels (800–1600 IU per day or more). This lengthens the clotting time, improving cardiovascular function throughout the body. And it has fewer side effects than aspirin.

On the other hand, because vitamin E slows blood clotting, it also lowers the risk for ischemic stroke (a blood clot blocking an artery).[222] The number of ischemic strokes is about five times greater than the number of hemorrhagic strokes in the general population.[223] This implies that vitamin E taken alone reduces the overall rate of strokes. Further, in combination with vitamin C and/or other antioxidants, vitamin E is even more powerful. Vitamin C reduces the rate of hemorrhagic strokes because it strengthens arteries and prevents bleeding and inflammation.[224] In critically ill patients, vitamin C and vitamin E taken together reduce the risk of multiple organ failure and the length of stay in intensive care.[225] And, as described above, vitamin C can regenerate vitamin E, and together their effects are synergistic. Vitamin C taken along with vitamin E, coQ10, and selenium increases elasticity of arteries and lowers blood pressure.[226] Thus, when taken together, antioxidants such as vitamin C, E, and selenium reduce risk for both hemorrhagic and ischemic strokes, and for progressive age-related conditions such as heart disease and arthritis. Further, these essential nutrients will help to prevent and enhance recovery from arthritis. Individuals who are deficient in any of these essential nutrients are at higher risk for many serious diseases. Studies that do not test these essential nutrients together at adequate doses will likely not observe these synergistic positive benefits.

Vitamin K

Vitamin K is a fat-soluble vitamin necessary for bone and joint health. There are two forms of vitamin K, one available from eating plants (K_1), and another available in animal products (K_2). Both are thought to be helpful in preventing OA, but K_2 has received much recent attention because a deficiency is found in OA, and it is important in controlling calcification of arteries.[227] Relatively high levels of vitamin K_1 are found in dark green leafy vegetables such as kale, collards, spinach, Brussels sprouts, parsley, lettuce, and mustard, beet, turnip, and dandelion greens. These provide about 1,000 mcg of vitamin K_1 per cup when cooked with butter. It is also found in canola and soybean oil, sprouts, asparagus, broccoli, peas, peanut butter, beans, onions, celery, and a wide variety of fruits and berries.[228] Because vitamin K is fat soluble, its absorption is enhanced by dietary fats.[229]

Vitamin K_2 has several subtypes, MK-4 to MK-10. The relative efficacy of the different subtypes is unknown, but they are typically found in different levels in organs throughout the body. Vitamin K_2 taken as a supplement can increase the level of vitamin K in the body higher than provided by food, and this is likely to be useful in improving bone health.[230] It has been estimated that approximately 1,000 mg of vitamin K is typically needed to fully perform its function (to carboxylate osteocalcin) throughout the body. This may indicate a subclinical deficiency in most people[231] and would likely require supplementation.[232] However, it is thought that complete carboxylation of osteocalcin is not achievable, and may not even be optimal, because undercarboxlylated osteocalcin is thought to be a signal in the glucose metabolism.[233]

The lifetime of vitamin K in the body is relatively short for a fat-soluble vitamin. The half-life of vitamin K_1 and the MK-4 subtype of K_2 have been estimated to be four hours, compared to several days for MK-7.[234] The reason for this difference is thought to be due to their molecular geometry. Both K_1 and MK-4 have a relatively short side-chain, making them more water soluble (hydrophilic), whereas MK-7 has a longer side-chain, making it less water soluble and more fat soluble (lipophilic). In practice, this means that the level of MK-7 will rise over several days to a higher level than the same dose of K_1. Evidently the consequence of this is that vitamin K_2 is available longer in the body and therefore can be absorbed better into tissues outside the liver.[235] So, to achieve roughly similar concentrations in the body, the recommended dosage of MK-4 is 15 mg taken three times per day, while the recommended dose of MK-7 is just 100 mcg per day.

One concern with vitamin K is its interaction with vitamin E, which slows blood coagulation.[236] High levels of vitamin E can counteract vitamin K and slow blood clotting, which can induce bleeding in some people, especially those deficient in vitamin C. Although this is not relevant for most people, it can be prevented by supplements of vitamins C and K, along with an excellent diet with plenty of leafy green vegetables.

A related concern is the interaction of vitamin K with anticoagulant drugs such as warfarin, which block the action of vitamin K and thus prevent blood clotting. This type of anticoagulant is widely prescribed for those with cardiovascular disease to prevent blood clots that could cause ischemic stroke. But this treatment has some very severe potential side effects, such as hemorrhagic stroke.[237] Those who are taking warfarin are often advised by their doctor to eat a diet low in vitamin K, for example, no leafy green vegetables. This diet will prevent high levels of vitamin K from lessening the effect of the anticoagulant drug. One problem with this advice is that vitamin K is necessary for joint health and to prevent arteries from getting calcified. The use of anticoagulant drugs tends to cause calcification of arteries and loss of bone density, which increases the risk of OA.[238] It may be better and safer instead to take vitamin K along with vitamin C, vitamin E, and other antioxidants, which together reduce the risk of stroke, and to get on an excellent diet, as explained above. This is a much safer way to lower your risk for cardiovascular disease.[239] You may benefit by discussing this with your doctor.

The action of vitamin K is dependent on sufficient levels of vitamin D, calcium, and magnesium.

A dose of 5,000–10,000 IU per day of vitamin D taken with 45 mg of vitamin K_2, along with adequate calcium and magnesium, either in the diet or as supplements, should be sufficient.

The best sources of vitamin K_2 are fermented food products, such as hard cheeses, sauerkraut, and the Japanese food called natto, which contains high levels of MK-7. Three ounces of natto contains about 1 mg of vitamin K_2. Natto is made by fermenting soybeans with *bacillus subtilis,* a common bacteria sometimes used as a probiotic.[240] Natto is quite an acquired taste. If the taste is too strong, it can be blended with other foods. Goose pâté contains high levels of MK-4. Other foods containing K_2 are liver, hard cheeses, egg yolks, butter from range-fed cattle, and most meats.

Supplements of vitamin K are widely available. MK-4 is available as 1–15 mg pills from several vendors. MK-7 is also available as 100 mcg pills. Although this is a much smaller amount than available in tablets of MK-4, the MK-7 form has a longer lifetime in the body, so only a lower dose is needed. Therefore, we recommend this MK-7 form of vitamin K_2. The MK-7 form is also synthesized by bacteria in the gut, and probiotics can help provide sufficient K_2. For many people, this bacterial source of K_2 is the most important. However an excellent diet that supplies K_1 may allow the body to convert some of it to K_2.

Vitamin K_1 and K_2 are safe to take in large amounts, because no toxicity has been observed with very high doses and consequently no upper limit has been set. However, synthetic forms of K_2, including menadione, can be toxic in large amounts.[241] As explained above, one concern is that K_1 interacts with anticlotting drugs. However, vitamin K_2 does not interact much with these drugs, so it is relatively safe. If you are taking anticoagulants, you should consult with a doctor before taking vitamin K.

Omega-6, Omega-3 Oils

It's important to consume a healthy balance of oils. Polyunsaturated fatty acids (PUFAs) are essential for health. As described in Chapter 5, they help to prevent OA. Both omega-3 and omega-6 fatty acids are essential for many biochemical pathways, including signaling molecules such as prostaglandins. But omega-6 fatty acids are much more common in the modern diet, because many vegetable oils used for cooking (the seed oils: canola, corn, cottonseed, safflower, soy) contain a robust amount. This might seem good, but these seed oils have a relative deficiency of omega-3 fatty acids. A diet with a low level of omega-3 compared with omega-6 fatty acids is linked with metabolic syndrome and inflammation.[242] And traditionally the diet contained more omega-3 fatty acids, in approximately a 1:1 ratio with omega-6 fatty acids.[243] For example, grass-fed beef contains higher levels of omega-3 fatty acids than grain-fed beef. Dark-green leafy vegetables such as collards, kale, and Swiss chard also contain more omega-3 than omega-6. To get a more healthy balance, it is best to use vegetable oils and spreads such as canola, corn, cottonseed, and soy only in moderate amounts, so that their high omega-6 content can be balanced by the more limited sources of omega-3 oils in the modern diet.[244]

Good sources of omega-3 fatty acids include flax meal and oil, walnuts, grass-fed eggs and meat, and fish oil.[245] To avoid heavy metals often present in large fish, eat fish low on the food chain, such as herring and sardines.[246] Wild-caught salmon are also low in heavy metals and have high levels of helpful omega-3 oils. Krill oil is an excellent source.[247] Because omega-3 oils go rancid quickly, they are often packaged in gelcaps that preserve the oil. However, it's important to make sure that the oil has been tested and does not contain heavy metals or other environmental toxins. Doses of omega-3 oils should be 1,000–4,000 mg per day. A combination of flax, walnut, and fish oils is recommended. For example, a tablespoon of flax seed meal with a 1,000 mg fish oil gelcap is a good choice.

POLYUNSATURATED VEGETABLE OILS SPOIL QUICKLY

Polyunsaturated omega-3 and omega-6 fatty acids (PUFAs) are essential for health. However, it's important to note that PUFA vegetable oils, including both omega-3 and omega-6 varieties (flax, walnut, canola, corn, cottonseed, safflower, soy, and so on) should not be used for cooking. They are readily oxidized by heat or bright light, and will go rancid in only a few minutes in a hot frying pan. Rancid oil can cause major oxidative stress to the body. It can cause age-related diseases such as cancer, heart disease, and arthritis. You can tell by the bad smell and taste whether an oil is going rancid in the container. Also, the smoke from oils heated to their smoke point temperature is bad for your health and like any other smoke is thought to cause cancer. Baked goods that contain a significant amount of omega-3 oil should be avoided because the heat from baking will turn the oil rancid. PUFAs or monounsaturated oils that have been heated and reused will go rancid faster than fresh oil. The reason is that free radicals in the oil generated by heating will quicken the oxidation to rancidity. Refined oils generally have a higher smoke point than unrefined oils, but if they contain PUFAs they can go rancid quickly.

Although PUFA oils typically contain a small amount of vitamin E as an antioxidant to prevent rancidity, after the bottle is opened the oil will start to go rancid even at room temperature. PUFAs such as canola, corn, or soy oil have a low omega-3 content and a high omega-6 content. After opening the bottle, they may go noticeably rancid at room temperature after six to twelve months. PUFA oils are widely used with high heat for conditioning cast-iron frying pans. The omega-3 and omega-6 content goes rancid quickly with high heat and polymerizes into varnish, which makes a nonstick surface. Although any rancid oil will cause oxidative stress, this conditioning process is generally not harmful as long as the pan is wiped clean and a more saturated fat (butter, peanut, or palm oil) is used for cooking.

A better alternative to PUFAs for cooking is to use butter (a saturated fat), or oils with a higher monounsaturated content and higher smoke point, such as peanut oil.[248] They don't go rancid as quickly. Peanut oil is good for high temperature cooking because it has a relatively high smoke point and doesn't go rancid as quickly as other oils. Olive oil with a higher monounsaturated content is good for low temperature cooking. It is considered better for cooking than sunflower oil, which also has a large monounsaturated component.[249] Virgin olive oils contain antioxidants that help to prevent oxidation when the oil is heated moderately.[250] Coconut oil is more saturated but has a relatively low smoke point and can be used for low temperature cooking. Palm oil is more saturated[251] and is widely used as a high temperature cooking oil because it doesn't go rancid as quickly and has a high smoke point. However, it is linked to forest destruction in tropical climates. Although we do not recommend large portions of fried or baked foods, if you do bake or cook with a frying pan, it's best to avoid the use of PUFAs.

Flax oil contains a very high content (53 percent) of alpha-linolenic acid, the only essential omega-3 fatty acid.[252] It will start to go rancid in a few weeks in a bottle kept at room temperature, and even faster if exposed to sunlight. When kept in the refrigerator or freezer it will stay fresh for several months. Flax oil is identical to linseed oil that for centuries was the base for oil paint. When heated it rapidly oxidizes, congeals, and makes varnish. Commercial boiled linseed oil is already partly oxidized (and is inedible), so it oxidizes faster than raw linseed oil. When absorbed into a crumpled paper towel (which has a large surface area in a small volume), will rapidly oxidize over several days. This releases heat that can actually start a fire. Flax oil in capsule form has a much longer shelf life and will stay fresh for six months or more. For the freshest flax oil, you can grind your own flax seed meal. The oil stays fresh inside the seeds, so they can be stored whole at room temperature for up to a year. You can then grind a small quantity into flax meal that you keep in the refrigerator for use within a few weeks.

For an excellent diet, we do not recommend large amounts of processed oils, because they contain many calories with few other nutrients. To get adequate omega-3 oils, we recommend flax meal, raw walnuts, and small oily fish such as sardines as good sources, along with large servings of dark-green leafy vegetables.

Calcium, Phosphorus, Magnesium

Calcium, phosphorus, and magnesium are essential for all cells in the body, especially bone and cartilage. An excellent diet including robust amounts of greens and other vegetables, moderate amounts of dairy products such as milk, cultured cheese, or yogurt, along with whole grains, beans and seeds, and moderate amounts of meat can supply adequate amounts of these minerals. Lecithin, derived from soybeans or other seeds, is a widely available and inexpensive source of phospholipids which are used throughout the body.

However, many older adults are deficient in calcium and magnesium. A calcium deficiency is common among those who don't eat dairy products or leafy green vegetables. Another common reason for calcium deficiency is inadequate vitamin D or magnesium, not a lack of calcium. Vitamin D plays an integral role in storing calcium, while magnesium influences the transport of calcium in tissues throughout the body including the bones.[1,203] Moreover, most people are deficient in magnesium, especially those who don't eat robust portions of greens, whole grains, beans, nuts, or seeds.[254] A common reason is that processed staple foods such as enriched flour, sugar, and white rice contain very little magnesium because it was removed in the processing steps.

A standard blood test cannot determine whether a magnesium deficiency exists, because the body keeps the magnesium level in the blood fairly constant. When inadequate magnesium is available in the diet, the body takes magnesium out of the bones for use by the tissues.[255] If the diet continues to be inadequate, a deficit of magnesium in the bones can build up over decades. Further, our absorption of magnesium from food typically drops as we age, so we need to consume larger amounts. Many people only get 200–300 mg of magnesium per day from their food, which is not enough for the body's needs. Calcium and magnesium should be taken along with vitamin D for the best absorption and effect.[256]

Magnesium balances the level of calcium in the blood in several ways.[257] It helps absorption of calcium into the bones, and it prevents excess excretion of calcium. For example, when too much protein is consumed without carbohydrates or fat, the metabolic products of protein will include uric acid which may cause calcium to be excreted. This is a common cause of a calcium deficiency. This can be prevented by taking extra magnesium, which takes the place of calcium in the urine.[258]

Supplements of calcium are often advised for older adults who simply aren't getting enough calcium in their diet. But supplements of calcium, when necessary, should be taken in moderation (200–600 mg per day in divided doses of a well-absorbed form) and should always be taken with magnesium, preferably in a 1:1

ratio.[259] Many antacid tablets contain calcium carbonate which can contribute to the total calcium intake. These should be considered as calcium supplements, but their use should be minimized. A proper diet will obviate the need for antacids. A recent concern about calcium supplements is that in excess they may raise the calcium level in the blood too high, causing calcification of the arteries, which is a leading cause of cardiovascular disease.[260] This can be prevented by several precautions. Avoid taking large amounts of calcium (1,000 mg or more) as a supplement, and avoid ingesting large amounts of dairy products that contain high levels of calcium.[261] Take calcium supplements in moderation, always with a corresponding amount of magnesium, and take supplements of vitamin K_2.[262]

Another related concern is that before taking calcium or magnesium supplements, it's important to make sure that the body can excrete any possible excess. If you have renal insufficiency (kidney failure) that prevents excretion of excess levels of these minerals, they can build up to an overdose over several days or weeks. Further, if you have myasthenia gravis (autoimmune neuromuscular weakness), a huge dose of magnesium (for example, an intravenous dose) might worsen muscle relaxation and prevent normal breathing. If you have an abnormally slow heart rate, magnesium's effect of relaxing the arteries and heart might excessively slow the heart rate.[263] And if you take a large oral dose of magnesium all at once, you're likely to get diarrhea. This is the body's natural way to rid itself of an overload. Take smaller doses throughout the day, as recommended for other essential nutrients such as niacin and vitamin C. It's always best to consult with your doctor before taking supplements of calcium and/or magnesium.

The Forms of Calcium and Magnesium for Best Absorption

An important concern with calcium and magnesium supplements is achieving good absorption. The most common forms of calcium and magnesium sold in inexpensive tablets are not well absorbed. Calcium carbonate is only about 30 percent absorbed, and magnesium oxide is only 5–10 percent absorbed in the gut.[264] Magnesium oxide is widely sold because it is inexpensive and contains more magnesium per unit volume compared to other magnesium compounds. This means that more magnesium is available in a smaller tablet, which makes it easier to swallow. But magnesium oxide is not well absorbed, so this widely available form isn't a very good buy. The unabsorbed magnesium oxide will tend to cause a laxative effect. Better choices are calcium lactate, malate, citrate, chelate, and orotate, and magnesium citrate, malate, chelate, and chloride. Magnesium chloride tablets are the best absorbed form of magnesium, virtually 100 percent, but some find its taste unpleasant and it costs a little more. Magnesium oil, which is just magnesium chloride dissolved in water, can be applied to the skin. It is readily absorbed and can be helpful in making up for a magnesium deficit. Magnesium chloride flakes are available to add to a bath and can function like Epsom salts (magnesium sulfate) to give you an extra dose.[265]

A good choice is a tablet containing 200 mg calcium and 100 mg magnesium in the chelate (amino acid) form, taken one to three times daily, along with an excellent diet. The chelate form is well absorbed. Magnesium citrate in tablets or powder form is a good buy but in large doses is often used as a laxative. Magnesium malate tablets (for instance, a 1,250 mg tablet that contains 146 mg of magnesium) are also a good buy and are also well absorbed.[266] Small amounts of magnesium and calcium are typically included in a multivitamin tablet, but these minerals take up too much volume to be included in an adequate amount.

Recovering from Magnesium Deficit

To recover from a deficit of calcium and/or magnesium, you can take supplements of 200–600 mg of calcium and 200–600 mg of magnesium per day in divided doses, along with an excellent diet including dairy products, green leafy vegetables, and other foods that are high in magnesium such as wheat germ. After a few months, you should lower the amount taken in supplements, staying with an excellent diet to maintain your levels of these essential minerals. Because magnesium deficit is generally more common than calcium deficit, it may be helpful to continue taking supplements of magnesium even after stopping calcium supplements.[267] To know for sure whether you're deficient in magnesium, the standard blood test that measures magnesium levels is inadequate because it does not register a deficit in the bones. A better choice is a magnesium challenge urine test, which registers the amount of magnesium that is absorbed from a specific dose.[268] However, rather than getting this time-consuming and cumbersome test, many people who suspect they are deficient prefer to simply increase their consumption of magnesium with supplements for several months. This should be done with the advice of a medical doctor.

Magnesium Sources in Food

Good sources of magnesium are wheat germ, buckwheat, millet, whole grains, chocolate, green leafy vegetables, tomatoes, yellow cornmeal, beans, legumes, and nuts. Remember, processed flour, even when enriched, contains very little of the magnesium originally contained in the whole grain. So to get the most magnesium from your diet, it's best to avoid white or "wheat" bread, white bagels, cookies, crackers, cake, and most pastas. If you do eat these foods, for example at a family, social, or professional event where you want to show solidarity, just remember to eat more vegetables or take supplements later that contain enough magnesium to make up the deficit.

Phytate, Oxalate, and Tannins

Several compounds in natural foods can bind to essential minerals, causing them to be eliminated instead of absorbed in the gut. Phytate (phytic acid, or IP6) in the hulls and bran of seeds such as wheat, rice, maize, and soy, can chelate (bind to) minerals such as calcium, magnesium, zinc, and iron. This is not usually a problem for most people who eat an excellent diet, because it provides more than enough minerals. However, when the levels of magnesium or calcium in the diet are inadequate, phytate can limit their uptake in the gut. This can be counteracted to some extent by vitamin C taken simultaneously.[269] However, phytate also has several benefits. It is helpful in binding and eliminating toxic heavy metals such as arsenic, cadmium, and lead that are sometimes found in high levels in some soils and foods. When taken on an empty stomach to prevent binding to minerals in food, phytate or IP6 can also help to remove calcium deposits in arteries. Phytate also has antioxidant and antitumor properties that can help prevent many diseases such as cancer and heart disease.[270]

Oxalate (in coffee, tea, spinach, rhubarb, beets, berries, and many other vegetables) can also bind to calcium, preventing both the calcium and oxalate from being absorbed. This can lower calcium absorption. However, eating foods that contain oxalate along with calcium-rich foods may be helpful in preventing kidney stones from an excess absorption of the oxalate. Creamed spinach is an example. Tannins found in black and green tea, especially bitter teas, bind to minerals and can limit the uptake of calcium and magnesium.[271]

To maximize intake of calcium and other minerals, the oxalate and phytate in many foods can be deactivated by cooking, sprouting, or soaking in water. As described above, the phytic acid in maize can be neutralized by soaking in an alkaline solution such as lime water, as native people in Central America have done for centuries. Soy products also contain a very high level of phytic acid, so in some regions of the world they are a major problem for uptake of minerals such as calcium and magnesium when these minerals are scarce. The phytic acid in soy is not removed well by extended cooking. Only fermented soy products, such as tempeh and miso, have lower levels of phytic acid. Soy milk and tofu can cause mineral deficiencies when taken in large amounts.[272] However, when the diet is excellent and contains adequate levels of calcium, magnesium, and iron (from greens, beans, nuts, seeds, whole grains, and meat), the oxalate and phytate content will usually not cause a deficiency of minerals.

Iron

For joint health and prevention and recovery from arthritis, an adequate amount of iron, but not too much, is essential.[273] To get an adequate but not excessive amount of iron, eat only moderate amounts of red meat (beef, pork, lamb, turkey, duck), because the absorption of its heme-bound iron is virtually complete and is not regulated in the gut. As an excellent alternative, many vegetables (green leafy vegetables, beans, legumes, whole grains) contain moderate amounts of iron.[274] Their advantage is that absorption of this "nonheme" form of iron is regulated according to the body's needs.[275] Therefore, vegetable sources of iron are generally more healthy. Another common source of iron is cooking in a cast-iron frying pan or pot, which with acid food (tomatoes, citrus) can leach 2–5 mg into a serving.[276]

There are several concerns about iron. One concern is that iron is toxic at high levels and causes oxidative stress in the body. It also tends to increase the risk of bacterial infection. High levels of iron can cause a deficiency of copper,[277] which is an essential cofactor in the production of collagen. A widely available blood test can tell you if your level of iron is too high or low. If your level is low, you should consider the sources of iron in your diet. As explained above, many common foods are good sources of iron. Enriched flour contains some iron, but we do not recommend enriched flour or foods containing it because they are missing several essential nutrients that are found in whole-grain flour. If you do not eat foods containing enough iron, you can take a multivitamin tablet that contains iron. Typical doses in multivitamin tablets are between 5 and 25 mg per day. Women of childbearing age may need doses of iron in the range of 10–20 mg per day. Multivitamin tablets for men often have no iron, which is reasonable for men who eat moderate amounts of meat and generous amounts of vegetables. If your blood level is too high, you can lower it by avoiding sources of "heme" iron such as meat and eggs, avoid eating food cooked in cast-iron pans, and let your body regulate its iron absorption from your vegetable intake. You should talk to your doctor before taking supplements containing iron.

Zinc, Copper, Selenium, and Trace Elements

These are essential minerals commonly deficient in people who do not eat an adequate diet. Zinc and selenium are antioxidants helpful in preventing oxidative stress. They are important for the immune system and a variety of biochemical reactions in the body.[278] Copper and selenium are necessary for many functions in the body, including synthesis of the extracellular matrix of collagen in cartilage. Arthritis patients are often deficient in zinc and other trace elements. Copper is toxic at doses much higher than a few milligrams per day, and an adequate dose can usually be supplied by an excellent diet, so a copper supplement is usually not necessary.[279] However, when a large dose of zinc is taken as a supplement, it can deplete the body of copper, so zinc supplements of 50 mg or greater commonly contain 2 mg of copper.[280] Selenium is toxic at doses higher than several hundred mcg per day. At high levels it can cause nails to crack and hair to break. This is fairly common among those eating large amounts of Brazil nuts, for just six nuts can contain as much as 500 mcg of selenium.[281] It may be helpful to limit your intake of Brazil nuts, especially if you are taking a multivitamin tablet with more than 50 mcg. Many multivitamin tablets contain 15 mg of zinc and 20–100 mcg of selenium. However, it is helpful to take zinc at a higher dose, typically 50 mg per day, along with 1–2 mg of copper.

Other important trace elements are chromium, iodine, manganese, and molybdenum.[282] They are thought to be necessary as cofactors for enzymes and are needed in only trace amounts that are usually supplied by an excellent diet. Ultratrace elements thought to be essential or helpful include arsenic, boron, fluoride, nickel, silicon, and vanadium. Several of these are helpful in bone and cartilage growth and maintenance.[283] To get adequate doses of these trace elements, use sea salt along with an excellent diet. Seaweed extracts or supplements are also an excellent source. Also, many multivitamin supplements contain all the essential trace elements.

Multivitamin Tablets

Most people are deficient in one or more of the essential nutrients. As we age, lower levels of nutrients are absorbed, even from an excellent diet. A good way to get most of the nutrients you need for optimal joint health is a high-dose multivitamin tablet. A variety of daily multivitamin tablets are available at low cost. The best ones include all the vitamins (A, B_1-B_{12}, C, D, E, K) as well as essential minerals (calcium, magnesium, zinc, iron, selenium, iodine) and other important nutrients. An excellent choice is a "mega" multivitamin tablet that has high doses of B vitamins (50–100 mg of B_1, B_2, B_3, B_5, B_6), as well as 400 mcg of folic acid, 100 mcg of biotin, and 100 mcg of B_{12}. These are water soluble and do not accumulate in the body, so it is best to take a robust dose every day. These doses are safe for most individuals. However, note that although doses of vitamin A included in most multivitamins are safe at the dose indicated on the package, a toxic level can build up if the daily suggested dose is exceeded or combined with large portions of foods that contain high levels of vitamin A, such as liver. To lower the dose of vitamin A they contain, many multivitamin tablets contain a moderate dose of vitamin A along with additional beta-carotene. Then the body can make additional vitamin A when required.

However, due to the compromise necessary to limit the size of the pill, it's impossible for multivitamin tablets to contain adequate levels of all essential nutrients. A daily dose of vitamin C considered barely adequate, 1,000 mg, comprises a large tablet. The same applies to vitamin E, because even a moderate dose (400 IU) would add too much volume to a multivitamin. And the calcium and magnesium required by most individuals takes a much larger volume, equivalent to several large tablets. Further, most mega-multivitamin tablets don't have an adequate amount of vitamin D, which should be in the range of 3,000–10,000 IU per day for most adults. Practically, this means that at a minimum you will need to purchase tablets with vitamin C, D, E, calcium, and magnesium for a complete supplement. Many of these mega-multivitamin tablets come in two versions, one with a dose of iron adequate for women of childbearing age (15–25 mg per day), and another without iron for other individuals who do not need additional iron. A good plan is to purchase both versions of the tablet, and routinely take the tablet without iron. Then, when you've not eaten meat or other foods containing adequate iron (eggs, leafy dark-green vegetables, beans, etc.) during the past few days, take the tablet that contains iron. Always remember that a multivitamin is not a panacea for not eating well. It's best to eat an excellent diet, and consider a multivitamin tablet in the context of this healthy combination of foods. Although we take multivitamins, we prefer to eat carrots.

Sulfate in Amino Acids

To boost your sulfate levels, you can eat foods high in sulfate such as dark-green leafy vegetables, cabbage, broccoli, and onions, and you can take supplements containing methionine and/or cysteine. The recommended (average adult) dose is 1,000 mg per day. The compound N-acetyl-cysteine contains sulfate and has been shown to suppress arthritis in mice.[284] Another way to boost your sulfate is to take an Epsom salt bath. This can boost your levels of both sulfate and magnesium by absorption through the skin, which can prevent a deficiency of magnesium and/or sulfate often found in OA and RA patients.[285] Both the magnesium and the sulfate in Epsom salts are essential nutrients, and are also helpful for pain relief and relaxation.[286] They are widely utilized and very safe when used in a bath. It is likely that after an Epsom salt bath, the level of sulfate in your joints is higher than possible through ingestion, for large amounts of Epsom salts taken orally are a laxative. Epsom salts are available in many grocery stores. A good starting dose for Epsom salts in a regular size bath is about 600 grams (about 1.3 pounds).

N-Acetyl-Cysteine and Alpha Lipoic Acid

These powerful antioxidants are not essential vitamins, but are helpful in preventing damage to joints caused by oxidative stress. N-acetyl-cysteine (NAC) is a precursor for glutathione and is well absorbed in the gut. As explained above, NAC also contains sulfate, which is necessary for regrowth and maintenance of cartilage. Alpha-lipoic acid (ALA) is also well absorbed. Supplements of NAC and ALA are widely available. Doses of 100–500 mg per day are commonly taken along with vitamins C and E. A liposomal preparation of glutathione is also available that gives excellent absorption in the gut. This form is supposed to be more effective than NAC at increasing levels of glutathione. It is a viscous oily liquid and can be taken by stirring it into water or juice.

ORTHOMOLECULAR DOSES OF NUTRIENTS TO PREVENT ARTHRITIS

It is helpful to take large doses of essential nutrients as supplements for preventing and reversing arthritis. For most nutrients the body can function better with higher levels than with the minimum daily requirement. Individuals vary in their nutritional needs, and older individuals may need higher doses. A typical daily supplement and foods focused on preventing or reversing arthritis for an average adult would include:

RECOMMENDED DAILY DOSES OF NUTRIENTS	
NUTRIENT	**RECOMMENDED DOSE**
Vitamin A	5,000–10,000 international units (IU)
Beta-carotene	10–20 milligrams (mg)
Thiamine (B_1)	50–100 mg
Riboflavin (B_2)	50–100 mg
Niacin (B_3)	400–2,000 mg, divided doses, replace with niacinamide to prevent flush
Pantothenate (B_5)	50–100 mg
Pyridoxine (B_6)	50–100 mg
Biotin (B_7)	50–100 micrograms (mcg)
Folate (B_9)	400–800 mcg
Cobalamin (B_{12})	10–100 mcg, methylcobalamin
Vitamin C	2,000–10,000 mg (20–50 mg/pound/day, divided doses, to bowel tolerance)
Vitamin D	2,000–10,000 IU (20–50 IU/pound/day), or direct summer midday sun (see text)
Vitamin E	400–1,200 IU mixed tocopherols and tocotrienols, including gamma-tocopherol.
Vitamin K_1	1,000 mcg (phylloquinone or phytonadione), when diet is inadequate
Vitamin K_2	1–15 mg of MK-4 (menaquinone-4 or menatetranone), or 100 mcg of MK-7
Calcium	200–600 mg (1.5–3 mg/pound/day), or 50–75 percent less if adequate in diet
Magnesium	200–600 mg (1.5–3 mg/pound/day), or 50–75 percent less if adequate in diet
Iron	0–20 mg, depending on need according to blood test, see text
Zinc	20–50 mg
Copper	2 mg, taken with 50 mg of zinc.
Manganese	1–10 mg

NUTRIENT	RECOMMENDED DOSE
Selenium	50–200 mcg
Iodine	150–400 mcg, found in seaweed, fish, eggs, yogurt
Omega-3 oils	1,000–3,000 mg (1–2 teaspoons flax seed oil; 1–3 tablespoons flax seed meal; 1–2 teaspoons fish oil)
Alpha-lipoic acid	100–500 mg
N-acetyl-cysteine	100–500 mg, divided doses
Coenzyme Q10	100–200 mg
Trace elements	Sea salt, multivitamin tablet

FOOD SOURCES FOR NUTRIENTS

FOOD	SERVING SIZE
Cherries	8–16 ounces cherry juice, 1–2 cups cherries, or $^1/_2$ cup dried cherries, divided doses
Ginger	$^1/_4$–$^1/_2$ cup chopped or minced, add to meals
Turmeric	Use liberally for sauces
Green tea	1–4 cups per day according to preference
Quercetin	200–1,000 mg, or eat plenty of grapes, apples, onions
Lycopene	10–20 mg, or eat plenty of tomatoes
Probiotics, yogurt	4 ounces yogurt and 1 probiotic tablet, twice per day.

IMPORTANT SUPPLEMENTS FOR TREATING ARTHRITIS

SUPPLEMENT	RECOMMENDED DOSE
Glucosamine sulfate	500–1,500 mg
Chondroitin sulfate	500–1,500 mg
MSM	1,000–3,000 mg, methyl-sulfonyl-methane, divided doses
SAM	500–1,000 mg, S-adenosyl-methionine, divided doses
ASU	500–1,000 mg, Avocado and soybean unsaponifiables

SUPPLEMENT	RECOMMENDED DOSE
Hydrolyzed collagen	1,000–3,000 mg hydrolyzed collagen type 2, divided doses
Undenatured collagen	1,000–3,000 mg, undenatured collagen type 2, divided doses
Resveratrol	100–500 mg, divided doses
PABA	100 mcg, para-aminobenzoic acid

TO BOOST STEM CELLS, HELPFUL IN TREATING ARTHRITIS

NUTRIENT	RECOMMENDED DOSE
Vitamin C	1,000 mg every hour for four to eight hours taken before stem cell therapy, to bowel tolerance.
Niacin (flush)	slowly build up from 25 mg once per day, to 500 mg taken four to six times daily.
Niacinamide (nonflush)	250 mg sixteen times daily; take at regular intervals, for example, every hour while awake.
Thiamine	1,000 mg, taken three times daily.
Beta 1,3 glucan	500 mg taken five times daily.

These doses are meant as total daily doses for the average adult. They are higher than available in most one-a-day multivitamin supplement tablets. Some doses depend on body weight. For children or small adults, the doses should be smaller, and for large adults the doses should be larger. You may need more or less than these doses. For the fat-soluble nutrients such as vitamins A, D, E and omega-3 oils, you can take a larger dose less often. For example, a dose of 20,000 IU of vitamin D taken once a week is roughly equivalent to 3,000 IU per day, because the level in the body rises and falls slowly. For the same reason, exposure over two days per week (for instance, Saturday and Sunday) to 20 to 120 minutes (depending on skin color) of summer midday sunlight will provide up to 20,000 IU, which also is roughly equivalent to the same dose of 3,000 IU per day. The skin will stop making vitamin D from sunlight when you've gotten enough. Of course, it may be better to take these vitamins in daily doses to make it easier to remember. The B vitamins are all water soluble and should be taken daily. Vitamin C and niacin should be taken in divided doses throughout the day, for their level drops quickly, in a matter of minutes to hours.

Many of these food supplements, including all of the vitamins, minerals, and some of the helpful nutrients mentioned above can be found in an excellent diet that includes plenty of leafy green vegatables, along with other colored vegetables such as carrots, tomatoes, sweet potatoes, winter squash, berries, and fruits. As we've emphasized above, taking these supplements is not an excuse to eat poorly. They are helpful to provide adequate amounts of essential nutrients that the modern diet, for one reason or another, so often lacks. They should be taken along with an excellent diet consisting of lots of dark-colored vegetables and fruits. You should maintain this excellent diet with supplements long term. The best time to start is before you have arthritis symptoms. But any time is a good time to start.

Easy Supplement Plan

Many people have asked, what is the simplest way to implement a supplement plan for preventing arthritis? An easy way is to take a mega-multivitamin tablet that contains most of the vitamins and minerals, and then take additional tablets for niacin, vitamins C, D, and E, calcium and magnesium, and omega-3 oils.

It's very important to take vitamin C and niacin (B_3) in divided doses throughout the day. Many people find their bowel tolerance for vitamin C is in the range of 2,000–6,000 mg per day when they are healthy and without much stress. For best results, you should take vitamin C in small divided doses: 500 mg, four times daily; or 1,000 mg, two times daily, working up to 1,000 mg, eight to ten times daily. If you have difficulty with these doses of vitamin C as tablet, try vitamin C powder in juice, or buffered vitamin C powder (sodium ascorbate). When you're sick or continue to have joint pain your bowel tolerance may go up, so you should try taking doses more often (1,000 mg every few hours, gradually decreasing the time span between doses to every 60 minutes, and down to every 20 minutes). To simplify the niacin supplements, you may want to take niacinamide instead of niacin. Niacinamide in large doses does not give a niacin flush, but it is best to start with small divided doses (25 mg, one time per day, then two times, then four times daily), and gradually build up to larger doses (100 mg two times per day, 200 mg, four times per day, and so on) up to a total of 2,000 mg per day or more to achieve a therapeutic effect. You will get more absorption with small doses taken frequently, such as every two to three hours. Remember, it's always best to discuss high-dose niacin (and niacinamide) with your doctor before proceeding. It's also helpful to take calcium and magnesium supplements in divided doses, for example, 200–400 mg, morning and night. But remember that for the strongest healing effect, these supplements are most effective when you're eating an excellent diet.

For specific help in preventing and reversing the symptoms of arthritis, you can include food supplements that are known to help prevent inflammation such as cherries and other dark berries, ginger, turmeric, resveratrol, and probiotics. They are not essential but have been shown to help prevent pain, inflammation, stiffness, and other symptoms of arthritis. Supplements of tamarind, chrysanthemum, and boswellia are widely available and are anti-inflammatory. You may also want to try other food supplements with a specific focus on arthritis such as glucosamine, chondroitin, and hydrolyzed collagen, MSM, and SAM. The idea is to try them for several weeks or months, at appropriate doses dependent on the form of the supplement, to to determine if they ameliorate your arthritis symptoms. Often glucosamine, chondroitin, and hydrolyzed collagen type II are taken together, and MSM and SAM are taken together. You may also want to include in your diet other food supplements such as the antioxidants alpha-lipoic acid, N-acetyl-cysteine, and resveratrol. With a variation on the elimination-challenge diet (see Chapter 5), you can test different combinations of supplements and foods to discover which are the most effective. Many allergies and food sensitivities can be prevented with adequate doses of vitamin C.[287]

Avoid Inflammation

As explained above, much of the tendency towards resorption of bone and degradation of cartilage at joints originates in inflammation that occurs throughout the body from a variety of sources. OA and RA are both known to be associated with inflammation. To recover from OA and RA it is imperative to remove or deal with all sources of oxidative stress and inflammation. That includes any type of bacterial or viral infection, infected teeth, a diet that includes a lot of sugar, inflammatory foods such as seed oils that contain a large proportion of omega-6 oils, rancid PUFA oils, lengthy constipation, smoking, environmental toxins, and damage to the joints.[288] Avoid eating large amounts of processed seed oils, for example, as are commonly found in in salad dressing, and make sure that any amount of processed oil that you eat is not rancid. Foods fried, broiled, or roasted at high temperature such as potatoes, chips, or nuts tend to cause oxidative stress and should be eaten in moderation. Nuts are best mildly roasted. If you suspect a food sensitivity or allergy, try to determine which foods cause it using an elimination-challenge diet.

If you eat an excellent diet with a large quantity of raw foods, you will get plenty of essential nutrients and antioxidants along with sufficient fiber. Juicing and sprouting are excellent ways to prepare food that prevents inflammation. Supplement your diet with vitamin C (3,000–10,000 mg per day or more, in divided doses, to bowel tolerance), niacin (400–2,000 mg per day in divided doses), and take mixed tocopherols and tocotrienols for the best protection against oxidative stress.

COOKING FOODS

Cooking is a huge and important topic. We rely on cooking to kill bacteria, viruses, and other pathological organisms, and to partially hydrolyze (break down) long-chain carbohydrates so they can be more fully digested and absorbed in the gut. Cooking also inactivates some harmful substances such as the trypsin inhibitor in soy, and phytic and oxalic acids in many vegetables.[289] Boiling, blanching, and steaming (to a lesser degree), also can significantly reduce the level of oxalate in many vegetables.[290] Oxalate is high in the skin of vegetables, and blanching reduces this oxalate that might otherwise migrate inwards during cooking.[291] The cooking methods that utilize water tend to lose some nutrients as well as oxalate into the cooking water.

However, cooking has some disadvantages. It can reduce the level of some nutrients, and can increase the level of toxic compounds. Vegetable oils with a large amount of polyunsaturated fatty acids (PUFAs), a category of seed oils (canola, corn, cottonseed, safflower, soy), should not be used for cooking because they quickly become oxidized (rancid), which can cause oxidative stress. Butter, and peanut and palm oil are safer for high temperature cooking. Olive oil has a high level of monounsaturated fatty acids and is good for cooking at low temperatures. Cholesterol is readily oxidized by oxygen when heated, which can cause oxidative stress and contribute to heart disease and arthritis. For this reason, boiled or poached eggs that are cooked with an unbroken yolk are likely more healthy than scrambled.[292] Avoid roasted walnuts because the heat causes their high content of omega-3 and omega-6 fatty acids to go rancid within a few weeks.

Advanced glycation end products ("AGEs") are formed in many foods when they are cooked at high temperatures. AGEs can damage tissues throughout the body, especially articular cartilage in joints. Fried chicken, French fried potatoes, potato chips, and other fried foods cooked without water tend to have high levels of AGEs. Browning foods by heating in a frying pan starts the reactions towards AGEs and reduces nutrient levels.[293]

Another problem recently discovered is that high temperature cooking of foods containing carbohydrates can generate acrylamide, a known toxin and carcinogen. Fried potatoes, chips, roasted cereals, and crackers contain high levels of acrylamide.[294] Boiling or steaming generates less acrylamide than frying or microwaving at high temperatures.[295] Acidity in the food tends to slow acrylamide formation during cooking. Almonds roasted at a high temperature (above 250 degrees Fahrenheit) to a medium brown color can also contain acrylamide. The amount of acrylamide increases during roasting, and is correlated with the resulting darkness in color.[296] It is also inversely correlated with the moisture content, because moisture keeps the temperature lower during roasting. The formation of acrylamide is more dependent on high temperature than the browning reaction, so roasting for a longer time at lower temperatures can produce browning with less acrylamide.[297]

Cooking at high temperature (such as broiling or frying) degrades vitamin C and thiamine, and can damage some amino acids in meat. Vitamin C is only partially degraded by boiling for a few minutes. Boiling vegetables in water can leach out much of their potassium and magnesium. Steaming leaches these minerals to a lesser degree. Iodine is lost by evaporation from food when cooked, so if you use iodized salt to obtain iodine it is better to salt food after it is cooked.[298] Heating foods with a microwave oven is convenient but can oxidize PUFAs and damage some amino acids, causing toxicity. Avoid the use of aluminum cookware with acid foods such as tomatoes because they can leach aluminum, which is thought to be associated with osteoporosis and Alzheimer's disease.[299]

SUMMARY: PREVENTING ARTHRITIS, STOPPING PAIN, AND FINDING AN EVENTUAL CURE

As we've seen, most types of arthritis are due to poor nutrition that causes deficiencies of essential nutrients. For OA, the best prevention is eating well starting early in adult life, avoiding injury to joints, maintaining excellent dietary habits, and watching out for and correcting deficiencies. Damage to the joints that occurs over decades is often unnoticed because articular cartilage contains no nerves to sense pain. When severe arthritis pain is evident, considerable damage has already occurred and recovery is slower and more difficult. As we all know, timing of the response after an acute injury is critical. To best manage the pain for a quick recovery from arthritis, it is necessary to empower the immune system and push the balance of the joints toward regrowth. This can best be achieved through a combination of vitamins, minerals, and soothing, nutritious anti-inflammatory foods that will speed up recovery. To lessen pain and recover from acute injury quickly, it's helpful to take megadoses of vitamin C and niacin along with appropriate doses of other B vitamins.

However, the joints take time to recover. Because articular cartilage contains no blood vessels, it takes longer to recover than other tissues. The sooner you start eating an excellent diet, making up deficiencies of essential nutrients, the better. The process of changing the balance towards regrowth can take several months to several years. It is a matter of making several important changes in your life: maintaining an excellent diet, taking supplements that prevent deficiencies, getting regular amounts of moderate exercise, and being sure to get adequate regular sleep.

The Overall Effect of an Excellent Diet

The diet and supplement plan we recommend will improve health in many ways, not limited to preventing and reversing arthritis.[300] This plan is similar to other diets that provide excellent nutrition known to prevent other age-related progressive diseases, such as heart disease,[301] cancer,[302] eye disease,[303] and diabetes.[304] You may find that you feel more energized, recover more quickly from physical and mental stress, have fewer bouts of colds or flu,[305] lessened asthma,[306] and have better mental function, such as more ability to focus and remember. You may find that supplements of magnesium alone will ameliorate asthma and cold hands and feet and drop high blood pressure, and have a host of other beneficial effects. The major cause of heart disease, as with arthritis, is malnutrition in one form or another.[307] The recommended doses of niacin and vitamins C, D, and

E along with an excellent diet will prevent most forms of cardiovascular disease, including atherosclerosis and strokes. Not only will your joints be healthier, you'll live longer too!

Learning Excellent Nutrition

Although doctors have long used nutrition to cure age-related diseases such as arthritis, over the last century most doctors' practices have been taken over by the pharmaceutical culture. However, as the science of nutrition science has matured and the biochemical pathways involved in age-related disease are becoming clarified, many doctors are considering the use of nutrition for preventative care as well as standard acute therapy. In recent years, supplements of vitamin D and magnesium have come into wide use. Millions of Americans, about half the population, take some form of vitamin supplements. Many doctors now realize they don't need to rely on drugs, which are unnatural for the body. There are many excellent books written by doctors about healing with nutrition.[308] A recent medical reference book with more than 1,300 pages is an excellent buy, because it covers the entire field of nutritional medicine.[309] And a new book, *The Orthomolecular Treatment of Chronic Disease,* explains how to cure many chronic diseases with nutrition.[310] Unfortunately, many doctors haven't caught on to this, and continue to deny the utility of supplements of essential nutrients.

The food you eat is directly responsible for your health. You are what you eat, and your recovery from arthritis depends on it. This knowledge is powerful because it can help you push the balance from resorption of bone and cartilage towards renewal and regrowth. It's not enough to rely on cultural traditions for the optimal foods to eat, for our ancestors grew up in a different world. The whole-grain unprocessed foods available two centuries ago contained more nutrients than the processed foods substituted for us today. A century ago, our grandparents grew up with "modern" processing and white flour and sugar that cause the age-related diseases we suffer from today. They substituted the processed foods into their cultural food traditions. It's up to us to revise the traditions again, using unprocessed foods to establish a new culture of healthy food.

Moreover, everyone has different nutritional requirements. Two people with arthritis may need very different doses of essential nutrients. For this reason it's imperative to understand, at a minimum, the basic functions of the essential nutrients, their different forms, and which foods and supplements contain them. It's also important for each individual to learn how to determine their optimal dose. As we've explained, it is crucial to get adequate doses of essential nutrients to avoid age-related disease as one gets older. You may benefit by discussing the recommendations provided in this book with your doctor. But you should rely on your knowledge and personal experience about how to tip the balance towards recovery. Finding the right balance of foods that provide excellent nutrition is a lifelong learning experience.

CONCLUSION

Throughout this book, we have emphasized the importance of knowledge about essential nutrients and learning which ones your body needs. An excellent diet that provides adequate amounts of these nutrients can keep you healthy. The scientific references we provide are current and up-to-date, but science is not static. The scientific method is continually testing new hypotheses. Research continues to learn more about nutrients in foods and how they affect us.[311] While there is overwhelming evidence that arthritis and other age-related disease is caused by dietary deficiencies, scientific knowledge will continue to progress and evolve. Certainly nutrition research will continue to make important discoveries. We hope that you do, too, concerning your nutritional needs. It seems possible, even likely, that several more essential nutrients will be added to the existing list of vitamins and minerals. Yet with our current knowledge of nutrition, we already know enough to prevent and reverse arthritis.

APPENDIX

Favorite Recipes

The following example recipes are simple, convenient, and provide excellent nutrition. They are inexpensive and provide robust amounts of essential nutrients. They can be elaborated upon to fit into any cultural tradition.

Frequently Used Ingredients

Wheat Germ: Wheat germ is part of the kernel discarded in refining white flour. It is packed with nutrients and is excellent added to breakfast cereals, sandwiches, soups, sauces, and stews.An opened package of wheat germ will remain fresh at room temperature for several days, but it should be stored in the refrigerator over longer periods to prevent it from going rancid. Although raw wheat germ is less expensive and may be healthier when fresh, many people prefer the toasted variety. You can tell by the smell if it's fresh.

Oats: Oats have the highest level of protein of any whole grain cereal, and make an excellent breakfast.Oats can be purchased on sale at most supermarkets every few months. The shelf life of rolled oats is several months to more than a year, so stock up during sales. However, note that oats can go rancid because of their relatively high fatty acid content (7 percent). It's best to store them in a cool dry place.

Flax Meal: Flax meal is sold in organic food supermarkets. Although the commercial variety is supposed to be packaged with an inert gas to prevent oxidation, it is often partly rancid. Some organic markets and food coops sell freshly ground flax meal. It should smell nutty. Many people prefer to purchase regular brown flax seeds and then grind new supply of flax meal every couple of weeks to prevent rancidity. Inexpensive flax seed mills are available online.

Lecithin: Lecithin granules contain phospholipids and essential fatty acids (omega-3, omega-6) which are used throughout the body.[1]

Brewer's Yeast: Brewer's yeast is packed full of nutrients and adds a nutty flavor. It is available in powder or flakes.

Nutritional Yeast: Nutritional yeast is similar to brewer's yeast but has a cheesy taste. It is widely available in powder or flakes. It is often used by vegetarians because most varieties contain more vitamin B_{12} than brewer's yeast.

Oats and Wheat Germ Granola

This is a nutritious and inexpensive granola type breakfast. Rolled oats are 100 percent whole-grain and contain high levels of protein, PUFAs, and other nutrients. They do not need to be cooked, for they are precooked quickly by steam heated rollers during the rolling process. This processing does not affect their nutrient content much, but makes them readily digestible. They remain a bit crunchy after absorbing some liquid, so it's important to chew them well. If you have difficulty digesting raw five-minute oats at first, use only raw one-minute oats for the first few weeks. This recipe is an excellent alternative to commercial breakfast cereal because it contains a robust amount of protein, less sugar, more magnesium and vitamins, and costs less. Rather than purchasing a commercial cereal enriched with vitamins, it is less expensive to take a multivitamin tablet separately.

MAKES $1^2/_3$ CUPS CEREAL MIX;
ONE ADULT SERVING.

1 cup rolled oats, 1-minute or 5-minute

$^1/_4$ cup (4 tablespoons) toasted wheat germ

1 teaspoon flax seed meal, freshly ground

1 teaspoon unsweetened ground coconut

$^1/_4$ cup blueberries,
(optional; frozen or fresh in season)

1 teaspoon lecithin granules

1 teaspoon brewer's yeast flakes

$^1/_2$ teaspoon brown sugar, to taste

$^1/_8$ teaspoon sea salt, to taste

sprinkle cinnamon, to taste

1 cup low-fat or skim milk, or water or juice

Mix the dry ingredients in a bowl. Slowly pour in the milk, and wait a minute for it to be absorbed before eating. When traveling or camping, you can utilize powdered milk. For convenience, it can be added into a premixed version of this recipe. Then only water needs to be added. For those who don't tolerate milk well, water or juice are good alternatives. Regular finely powdered brewer's yeast tends to cake up when the milk is added, but brewer's yeast flakes do not, and only cost a little more.

If your palate or stomach can't deal with the coconut, flax meal, lecithin or brewer's yeast right away, reduce their amounts or leave some or all of these out and focus on the oats and wheat germ. Experiment with adding different ingredients such as nuts, dried fruit, and spices.

Quick Sandwich Lunch

This is a classic peanut-buttter and jam sandwich lunch that is nutritious, inexpensive, and easy to make. The idea is to replace crackers, cookies, cake, donuts and similar processed foods with unprocessed healthy foods that are readily available.

1 SERVING

2 slices whole-wheat bread

1 tablespoon unsalted natural/organic peanut butter,*

1 tablespoon low sugar berry jam or preserves, no added fruit juice, high-fructose corn syrup, or artificial sweeteners

1 teaspoon brewer's yeast

Sprinkle of sea salt

8 cherry or grape tomatoes

1 carrot, cut into medium pieces

1/2 apple, pear, or peach, cut into medium pieces

3/4 cup cherries or grapes, or 1/2 cup raisins or dried cherries

1/2 cup nuts (peanuts, walnuts, almonds, pumpkin, and/or sunflower seeds)

**Keep in refrigerator; microwave for 10 seconds to a spreadable consistency. For those who can't tolerate peanut butter, substitute almond butter, available at most health food stores.*

Spread a thin layer of peanut butter on one slice of bread, sprinkle with sea salt and brewer's yeast. Spread a thin layer of jam on the other slice of bread, fold together to make a sandwich. Place in waxed paper bag. Wash and cut the carrot and fruit. Place the sandwich, carrot, tomatoes, nuts, and fruit into a lunch container or bag. In season, cherries are excellent for their anti-inflammatory properties.

Nutritious Pita Lunch

If you want to learn more about growing your own sprouts, many books and websites online explain how.[2] *Finish off this lunch with 1 cup cherries, blueberries, blackberries, or other fresh fruit.*

1 SERVING

2 whole-wheat pita bread rounds

2 slices Parmesan cheese

1 cup alfalfa sprouts

1/2 cup lentil, mung, or radish sprouts

2 leaves mustard greens

1 medium tomato, sliced, or 6 cherry or grape tomatoes

2 teaspoons flax seed meal

1/2 teaspoon brewer's yeast

1/2 cup walnuts and/or sunflower seeds

Cut each pita in half. Add the alfalfa sprouts, flax meal, and nuts to 2 of the pita halves. Add a slice of cheese to each of the other pita halves, and add lentil, mung, or radish sprouts. Add the tomato and mustard greens to all of the pita halves. Sprinkle on the brewer's yeast.

Green Smoothies

This is a complete meal. It contains a robust amount of fiber, which can be difficult at first for some to tolerate. The walnuts add omega-3 oil, and other nuts are also excellent. Experiment with different proportions and ingredients. The collards or kale are best grown in your backyard garden or purchased from a local supplier you can talk to. Then you'll be sure that they are grown without pesticides.

MAKES 3–4 CUPS

1 cup water

$^1/_2$ cup juice (orange, vegetable, pomegranate, cherry, without added sugar)

or $^1/_2$ apple, or ripe peach or pear

3–5 large leaves of collards or kale (more if leaves are smaller)

1–2 leaves mustard or radish greens, optional; for some zip

1 carrot, cut into 4–6 pieces, optional

5 cherry tomatoes, optional

2–4 tablespoons walnuts or other nuts, optional

Other vegetables, optional

Pour the water and juice into a blender. Add 1 collard leaf, replace the top of the blender, and blend or puree the mixture on high speed. Put in the next leaf and puree before adding the next one. Blending each leaf separately prevents the leaves from getting stuck above the blades without getting blended. Add the carrot, tomatoes, apple, and any other ingredients, and blend. The mustard or radish greens add some zip to the flavor.

Slow-Cooked Greens

For convenient snacks, scoop cooked greens into ice cube tray and freeze. Break open blocks of vegetables and eat throughout the day after microwaving. You can also pack the blocks to take for lunch.

MAKES 2–3 CUPS, OR 15–20 CUBES

2 cups collards and/or kale or broccoli

$^1/_2$ cup turnips, chopped

1 teaspoon butter

Pinch sea salt

Optional ingredients:

2 teaspoon ginger, finely chopped

1 clove garlic

1–2 cups mixed vegetables
(carrots, beans, peas, cauliflower)

Steam the kale and/or collards slowly with butter, ginger (if used), and turnips for 1–8 hours. The butter helps to extract the vitamin A and K. Puree in a blender to get maximum vitamin K and sulfur to help regrow cartilage. Save and add the cooking water to other foods, for it contains minerals leached from the greens.

Simple Beef Stew

Serve a small portion of stew (for instance, 3 heaping tablespoons per person) with a fresh salad (minimal dressing) and a generous serving of cooked greens (such as collards, kale, swiss chard, spinach, Brussels sprouts, beet or dandelion).

MAKES 8 CUPS OF STEW

1/2 pound beef, preferably grass-fed organic, cut into 3/4-inch chunks
3 small potatoes, cut into 3/4-inch chunks
3 carrots, chopped
1 stalk celery, finely chopped
1 medium onion, chopped
4 mushrooms, cut into pieces
8 teaspoons nutritional yeast
2 teaspoons brewer's yeast
1 vegetarian bouillon cube, no salt
1/4 teaspoon peanut butter, stirred in; optional
1/2 teaspoon sea salt
1 teaspoon spices, Italian mix
(basil, marjoram, oregano, rosemary, thyme)
1/2 teaspoon turmeric, optional
3 bay leaves
3 cups water (to cover)

1/2 cup quinoa
1/4 cup buckwheat kernels

Place all items except last two into a slow cooker and simmer for 8 hours. Stir in the quinoa and buckwheat and simmer for another 30 minutes to soak up the liquid and thicken the mixture.

Simple and Quick Bean Stew

Serve this bean stew with fresh tomatoes in season and freshly steamed green vegetables such as green beans, Brussels sprouts, broccoli, spinach, Swiss chard, collards, or kale. This makes a very nutritious and inexpensive meal. A small piece of cooked hamburger or Parmesan cheese goes well with the stew and vegetables.

MAKES 8 CUPS OF STEW

1/2 cup dry soybeans
1 1/2 cups of dry bean mixture*
1/4 cup millet, optional
1/4 cup wild brown rice, optional
1 vegetable unsalted bouillon cube
3 tablespoons nutritional yeast
1 tablespoons brewer's yeast
1 medium onion, chopped into small pieces
1 carrot, chopped into small pieces
1 stalk celery, chopped into small pieces
1/2 teaspoon sea salt
1 teaspoon spices, Italian mix (basil, marjoram oregano, rosemary, thyme)
1/2 teaspoon turmeric, optional
4–5 cups water (to cover)

1/2 cup quinoa**
1/4 cup buckwheat kernels**

Fast cooking method: Cook in a pressure cooker (standard 15 pound pressure), which greatly shortens the cooking time. Prepare the beans by soaking them in hot water for 15–30 minutes or overnight in cold water. Discard the soaking water to avoid gas-causing undigestible carbohydrates, or save for future use. Start by pressure cooking the soybeans in 2 cups of water for 30 minutes.

While waiting, chop up the onion, carrot and celery. Pressure down by cooling the top of the cooker with cold water before opening it. Add the dry bean mix, millet, wild rice, onion, carrot, celery, nutritional and brewer's yeast, spices, sea salt, and bouillon along with 3 cups of water, then cook at pressure for another 15 minutes.

Pressure down the cooker again and stir in the quinoa and buckwheat kernels, depending upon the desired thickness of the stew. Then close the lid and apply heat and pressure for 1 minute, or simmer in the open pot for 20 minutes to thicken.

The whole process from dry beans to fully cooked takes about 2 hours (or 1 hour without presoaking, or 30 minutes without soybeans.

Note: Occasionally the soybean coats will clog the pressure cooker vent, and the hissing sound will stop. If this happens, turn off the heat, pull the weight off the vent, and stick an unbent paperclip into the vent to unclog it. Immediately replace the weight to avoid losing much pressure.

Alternate slow cooking method: Simmer soybeans in 2 cups of water for 4 to 7 hours or until tender in a pot or slow cooker. Add the other items except quinoa and buckwheat, bring to boil again (if it can be removed from its base unit, heat the slow cooker pot in the microwave), and lower the heat. Simmer for another hour. Add the quinoa and buckwheat to absorb excess water, and simmer another 20 minutes.

*Typical beans included in mixtures (not including soybeans, which are cooked ahead separately) include baby limas, great northern, kidney, split peas, lentils, pigeon peas, black-eyed peas, adzuki beans, flageolet beans, and pinto beans. You can use just a few types or even just one type; elaborate or substitute according to preference. Pick over the beans before using to remove any small pebbles that may be present.

**As an alternate, substitute millet for the quinoa and/or the buckwheat. It is almost as nutritious.

Simple Raw and Steamed Vegetable Meal

All of the vegetables in this recipe can be grown in a back yard garden or purchased inexpensively. With one of the desserts listed below this makes a complete meal in 15 minutes

MAKES 2 SERVINGS

1 pound green beans

2 cups collards or kale greens, cut into 2-inch squares

1/4 medium butternut squash, peeled and cut into 3/4-inch chunks

1/2 onion, chopped into small pieces

1 carrot, cut into strips

1 stalk celery, cut into strips

1/2 green and/or red pepper, cut into strips

10 cherry or grape tomatoes

2 slices Parmesan cheese

3 teaspoon brewer's yeast

1/4 tsp spices, Italian mix (basil, marjoram, oregano, rosemary, thyme)

1/2 cup water

Add the green beans, collards or kale, squash, onion, and water to a large pot. Sprinkle on the spices and steam for 5–8 minutes, until the beans are tender (just past bright green) and the squash is getting soft.

While the vegetables are steaming, wash the carrot, celery, and pepper, and cut into strips for finger food. Serve the raw carrot, celery, pepper, and tomatoes with the brewer's yeast for dipping.

When the steamed vegetables are ready, serve immediately with the cheese.

Leftover Veggies with Savory Protein

This is a quick complete winter meal that can be prepared, eaten, and washed up in 15 minutes. If you have no leftovers, fresh greens can be steamed in 5 minutes. Substitute ingredients according to your taste!

1 SERVING

1 cup leftover steamed collards or kale

1 cup leftover steamed green beans (or any other green, yellow, or orange veggie)

1/2 cup leftover cooked winter squash chunks

1 sprinkle spices, Italian mix (basil, marjoram, oregano, rosemary, thyme)

1 thin slice Parmesan cheese

1 raw carrot, cut into strips

1 raw stalk celery, cut into strips

1/2 raw pepper, cut into strips

5 cherry or grape tomatoes

1/2 teaspoon brewer's yeast

1 sardine

1/2 hard-boiled egg

Place the leftover vegetables on a microwaveable plate. Cut the cheese into several pieces and place it on top of leftover beans and kale with a sprinkle of spices. Microwave for 1–2 minutes, until the cheese is partly melted.

Alternate: steam the vegetables for 2 minutes to heat them.

While the food is heating, wash and cut the raw carrot, celery, and pepper. Dip them and the tomatoes in the brewer's yeast, and eat.

Serve the vegetables hot with the cheese, egg, and sardine.

Pasta with Vegetables Dinner

Serve a large portion of raw vegetables (carrots, celery, peppers, tomatoes, pea pods, and so on) before this vegetable-tomato-sauce pasta. Serve the pasta with a large portion of greens (steamed or slow-cooked leafy green vegetables, or lettuce) on the side, and follow with the yogurt and fruit dessert.

MAKES 2–4 SERVINGS

1 carrot, chopped

1 stalk celery, chopped

1 green pepper, chopped

1 sweet red pepper, chopped

1 onion, chopped

$^1/_2$ cup sprouts (alfalfa, lentils, mung beans, radish seeds, and such)

$^1/_4$ clove garlic, chopped

$^1/_2$ cup tomato paste

2–4 tablespoons water

1 cup tomatoes, fresh or canned, chopped

1 teaspoon saturated fat cooking oil (peanut, palm, coconut or butter)

Other chopped vegetables such as peas, green beans, eggplant, leeks, bok choi, optional

$^1/_2$ teaspoon spices, Italian mix (basil, marjoram, oregano, rosemary, thyme)

$^1/_2$ cup grated Parmesan cheese

$^1/_4$ teaspoon sea salt, to taste

$^1/_2$ pound dry whole-wheat pasta

Water to cover

Saute the onion pieces to a light brown in a wok, cast-iron, or stainless frying pan using the cooking oil. Stir in the chopped vegetables and sprouts, tomato paste, and 2–4 tablespoons of water to make a consistent texture, cook for 10–20 minutes. Boil pasta in water with a pinch of salt until just tender, and drain. Serve the vegetable-tomato sauce over the pasta.

Vegetarian Chili

MAKES 8 CUPS

1/2 cup dry kidney beans, or 1 15-ounce can, drained

1/2 cup dry garbanzo beans, or 1 15-ounce can, drained

1/2 cup dry black beans, or 1 15-ounce can, drained

3 cups water

1/2 cup buckwheat groats

1/2 cup quinoa

2 cups water

2 stalks celery, chopped

2 green bell peppers, chopped

1 medium onion, chopped

1 tablespoon olive oil

2 bay leaves

1/2 teaspoon ground cumin

2 tablespoon spices, Italian mix
(basil, marjoram, oregano, rosemary, thyme)

3 cloves garlic, chopped

1/4 cup chili powder

1/2 tablespoon ground black pepper

1 teaspoon sea salt

1/2 cup water

For traditional taste:

8 medium (3-inch) tomatoes, peeled and sectioned,
or 1 28-ounce can whole peeled tomatoes, crushed

Alternate taste:

2 large carrots, chopped

6 tablespoons nutritional yeast

$^1/_2$ teaspoon brewer's yeast

1 cube unsalted vegetarian bouillon

1 teaspoon turmeric

$^1/_4$ teaspoon cinnamon

$^1/_4$ cup ginger, chopped or minced

$^1/_2$ teaspoon peanut butter, stirred in

For extra zip:

2 jalapeno peppers, chopped

2 green chile peppers, chopped, or 2 4-ounce cans, drained

Heat the beans in 3 cups water to a boil, then lower the heat and simmer for 60 minutes. Add the buckwheat and quinoa and an additional 2 cups of water. Raise the mixture to a boil again and lower the heat and simmer for another 20 minutes.

In a separate pan, sauté (cook in large pot or frying pan, stirring constantly) the onion in the olive oil with the spices and salt until the onion is tender. Mix in the remaining ingredients (depending upon which version you have selected) and $^1/_2$ cup water. When these vegetables are tender, reduce heat, cover the pan, and simmer for another 10 minutes. Add the cooked beans and simmer for another 5 minutes.

Serve the chili by itself or on whole-wheat pasta or bread, with a robust portion of greens.

To avoid the nightshade family, leave out the peppers and tomatoes.

DESSERTS

The idea for dessert is to have a little yogurt and some fresh fruit when in season, along with nuts to fill up.

Dessert with Fresh Fruit and Nuts

This dessert is the best option when fresh fruit is available.

MAKES 1 SERVING

1 cup cherries (in season)

1/2 cup fresh fruit or berries (blackberries, strawberries, blueberries, currants, or in season: ripe peach, pear, or apple)

1/2 cup blackberry, blueberry, or strawberry jam (in winter)

1/2 cup nuts (mixed peanuts, almonds, walnuts, pistachios, and sunflower or pumpkin seeds)

1/2 cup low or nonfat yogurt, unsweetened

Mix in or top the yogurt with the fruit and nuts.

Blueberry and Yogurt Dessert

This dessert is a good option in winter or when fresh fruit is unavailable.

MAKES 1 SERVING

1/2 cup nonfat yogurt

1/2 cup blueberries (fresh or frozen)

1/2 teaspoon brown sugar or jam (optional, to taste)

1 teaspoon lecithin granules

3 teaspoon toasted wheat germ

Mix the yogurt with a small amount of berry jam or brown sugar and the lecithin, wheat germ, and frozen berries.

REFERENCES

Chapter 1. Responsibility for Learning about Health: Your Role

1. Saul, A. *Doctor Yourself: Natural Healing That Works.* 2nd edition. Laguna Beach, CA: Basic Health Publications, 2012. www.doctoryourself.com.

2. Centers for Disease Control (CDC). "Arthritis: The Nation's Most Common Cause of Disability." www.cdc.gov/chronicdisease/resources/publications/aag/arthritis.htm (accessed Jan 2014).

3. Bland, J.H. "The Reversibility of Osteoarthritis: A Review." *Am J Med* 74(6A) (Jun 14, 1983):16–26.

4. Centers for Disease Control (CDC). "Prevalence of Arthritis." www.cdc.gov/arthritis/data_statistics/arthritis_related_stats.htm (accessed Jan 2014).

5. Claes, S., et al. "Is Osteoarthritis an Inevitable Consequence of Anterior Cruciate Ligament Reconstruction? A Meta-Analysis." *Knee Surg Sports Traumatol Arthrosc* 21(9) (Sep 21 2013):1967–76.

6. Hogervorst et al., "Hip ontogenesis: how evolution, genes, and load history shape hip morphotype and cartilotype. Clin Orthop Relat Res. 470(12) (Dec 2012):3284–96.

7. Doghramji, P.P., R.L. Wortmann. "Hyperuricemia and Gout: New Concepts in Diagnosis and Management." *Postgrad Med* 124(6) (Nov 2012):98–109.

8. Bottiglieri, S., et al. "Gemcitabine-Induced Gouty Arthritis Attacks." *J Oncol Pharm Pract* 19(3) (Sep 2013):284–8.

9. Ramírez, A.S., et al. "Relationship between Rheumatoid Arthritis and Mycoplasma Pneumoniae: A Case-Control Study." *Rheumatology (Oxford)* 44(7) (Jul 2005):912–4. Rivera, A., et al. "Experimental Arthritis Induced by a Clinical Mycoplasma Fermentans Isolate." *BMC Musculoskelet Disord* 3(15) (2002). DiCarlo, E.F., L.B. Kahn. "Inflammatory Diseases of the Bones and Joints." *Semin Diagn Pathol* 28(1) (Feb 2011):53–64. Murray, T.S., E.D. Shapiro. "Lyme Disease." *Clin Lab Med* 30(1) (Mar 2010):311–328. Gaby, A.R. *Nutritional Medicine.* Concord, NH: Fritz Perlberg Pub, 2011. Smith, B.G., et al. "Lyme Disease and the Orthopaedic Implications of Lyme Arthritis." *J Am Acad Orthop Surg* 19(2) (Feb 2011):91–100.

10. Gaby, A.R. *Nutritional Medicine.* Concord, NH: Fritz Perlberg Pub, 2011.

11. Deschner, J., et al. "Signal Transduction by Mechanical Strain in Chondrocytes." *Curr Opin Clin Nutr Metab Care* 6(3) (May 2003):289–293. Fransen, M., S. McConnell. "Exercise for Osteoarthritis of the Knee." *Cochrane Database Syst Rev* (4) (Oct 8, 2008):

CD004376. doi: 10.1002/14651858.CD004376.pub2. Chen, H., K. Onishi. "Effect of Home Exercise Program Performance in Patients with Osteoarthritis of the Knee or the Spine on the Visual Analog Scale After Discharge from Physical Therapy." *Int J Rehabil Res* 35(3) (Sep 2012):275–277. Garrison, D. "Osteoarthritis, Osteoporosis, and Exercise." *Workplace Health Saf* 60(9) (Sep 2012):381–3. Musumeci, G., et al. "The Effects of Physical Activity on Apoptosis and Lubricin Expression in Articular Cartilage in Rats with Glucocorticoid-Induced Osteoporosis." *J Bone Miner Metab* 31(3) (May 2013):274–284. Bergman, J. *How to Reverse Arthritis Naturally.* CreateSpace Independent Publishing. ISBN-13: 978–1482701524.

12. Miller, et al. "Why Don't Most Runners Get Knee Osteoarthritis? A Case for Per-Unit-Distance Loads." *Med Sci Sports Exerc* (Sep 12, 2013) [Epub ahead of print].

13. Gaby, A.R. *Nutritional Medicine.* Concord, NH: Fritz Perlberg Pub, 2011.

14. Hinson, J.A., D.W. Roberts, L.P. James. "Mechanisms of Acetaminophen-Induced Liver Necrosis." *Handb Exp Pharmacol* (196) (2010):369–405. U.S. Food and Drug Administration (FDA). "Acetaminophen and Liver Injury: Q & A for Consumers." www.fda.gov/forconsumers/consumerupdates/ucm168830.htm (accessed Jan 2014).

15. Brandt, K.D. "Nonsteroidal Antiinflammatory Drugs and Articular Cartilage." *J Rheumatol* 14 Spec No (May 1987):132–3. Brandt, K.D. "Effects of Nonsteroidal Anti-Inflammatory Drugs on Chondrocyte Metabolism in Vitro and in Vivo." *Am J Med* 83(5A) (Nov 1987):29–34. Rashad, S. et al. "Effect of Non-steroidal Anti-Inflammatory Drugs on the Course of Osteoarthritis." *Lancet* 2(8662) (Sep 2, 1989):519–22.

16. PubMed Health. "Osteoarthritis." www.ncbi.nlm.nih.gov/pubmedhealth/PMH0001460 (accessed Jan 2014).

17. Richette, P., C. Roux. "Impact of Treatments for Osteoporosis on Cartilage on Biomarkers in Humans." *Osteoporos Int* (23 Suppl 8) (Dec 2012):877–80.

18. International Lyme and Associated Diseases Society (ILADS). "What You Should Know About Lyme Disease." IGenex, Inc., (July 2002) www.ilads.org/lyme_research/lyme_articles6.html (accessed Jan 2014).

19. Devin, C.J., et al. "Hip-Spine Syndrome." *J Am Acad Orthop Surg* 20(7) (July 2012):434–42.

20. Egoscue, P., R. Gittines. *Pain Free: A Revolutionary Method for Stopping Chronic Pain.* New York: Bantam, 2000. Gokhale, E., S. Adams. *8 Steps to a Pain-Free Back: Natural Posture Solutions for Pain in the Back, Neck, Shoulder, Hip, Knee and Foot.* Stanford, CA: Pendo Press, 2008. McKenzie, R.A. *Treat Your Own Back.* 9th edition. Minneapolis, MN: Orthopedic Physical Therapy Products (OPTP), 2011. Hjorth, H.B. *Natural Back Pain Relief* [Kindle Edition]. Blazing Bolt Media, 2013.

21. Spahn, G., G.O. Hofmann, H.M. Klinger. "The Effects of Arthroscopic Joint Debridement in the Knee Osteoarthritis: Results of a Meta-Analysis." *Knee Surg Sports Traumatol Arthrosc* 21(7) (Jul 2013):1553–61.

22. Burr, D.B., M.A. Gallant. "Bone Remodelling in Osteoarthritis." *Nat Rev Rheumatol* 8(11) (Nov 2012):665–673.

23. Lalmohamed, A., et al. "Timing of Acute Myocardial Infarction in Patients Undergoing Total Hip or Knee Replacement: A Nationwide Cohort Study." Arch Intern Med 172(16) (Sep 10, 2012):1229–35.

24. Frech, T.M., D.O. Clegg. "The Utility of Nutraceuticals in the Treatment of Osteoarthritis." *Curr Rheumatol Rep* 9(1) (Apr 2007):25–30. Molnar-Kimber, K.L.

Rheumatoid-Arthritis-Decisions.com www.rheumatoid-arthritis-decisions.com (accessed Jan 2014).

25. Saul, A. *Doctor Yourself: Natural Healing That Works.* 2nd edition. Laguna Beach, CA: Basic Health Publications, 2012. www.doctoryourself.com.

26. Gaby, A.R. *Nutritional Medicine.* Concord, NH: Fritz Perlberg Pub, 2011.

27. Hyman, M. "Paradigm Shift: The End of "Normal Science" in Medicine. Understanding Function in Nutrition, Health, and Disease." *Altern Ther Health Med* 10 (5) (Sep-Oct 2004):10–5, 90–4.

28. Campbell, T.C. *Whole: Rethinking the Science of Nutrition.* Dallas, TX: BenBella Books, 2013.

29. Campbell, T.C. *Whole: Rethinking the Science of Nutrition.* Dallas, TX: BenBella Books, 2013. Angell M. The Truth About the Drug Companies: How They Deceive us and what to do about it. Random House, 2005.

30. Saul, A. *Doctor Yourself: Natural Healing That Works.* 2nd edition. Laguna Beach, CA: Basic Health Publications, 2012. www.doctoryourself.com.

31. Davis, A. *Let's Eat Right to Keep Fit.* rev edition. New York: Harcourt, Brace, Jovanovich, 1970.

32. Pauling, L. *Vitamin C and the Common Cold.* San Francisco: W. H. Freeman, 1970. Pauling, L. *How to Live Longer and Feel Better.* Corvallis, OR: Oregon State University Press, 1986, 2006.

33. Lappé, F.M. *Diet for a Small Planet.* 20th anniv edition. New York: Ballantine Books, 1971, 1985.

34. Pauling, L. *How to Live Longer and Feel Better.* Corvallis, OR: Oregon State University Press, 1986, 2006. Orthomolecular News Service (OMNS). "Vitamin C Slows Cancer Down. And, Doctors Say, Can Reverse It as Well." Oct 31, 2008. www.orthomolecular.org/resources/omns/v04n19.shtml (accessed Jan 2014). Orthomolecular News Service (OMNS). "About 'Objections' to Vitamin C Therapy." Oct 12, 2010. www.orthomolecular.org/resources/omns/v06n24.shtml (accessed Jan 2014). Orthomolecular News Service (OMNS). "Two Vitamin C Tablets Every Day Could Save 200,000 Lives Every Year: Ascorbate Supplementation Reduces Heart Failure." Nov 22, 2011. www.orthomolecular.org/resources/omns/v06n24.shtml (accessed Jan 2014). Smith, R.G. "Toxic Sugar." Orthomolecular News Service (OMNS). Editorial. Apr 24, 2012. www.orthomolecular.org/resources/omns/v08n14.shtml (accessed Jan 2014). Smith, R.G. "Daily Multivitamin Reduces Cancer Risk: Even Low-Dose Supplementation Would Save 48,000 Lives Annually." Orthomolecular News Service (OMNS). Oct 26, 2012. www.orthomolecular.org/resources/omns/v08n32.shtml (accessed Jan 2014). Orthomolecular News Service (OMNS). "What Really Causes Kidney Stones (And Why Vitamin C Does Not)." Feb 11, 2013. www.orthomolecular.org/resources/omns/v09n05.shtml (accessed Jan 2014). Hefti, R. "Anti-Vitamin Publications: Misinformation Presented As Truth" Orthomolecular News Service (OMNS). Jul 18, 2013. http://orthomolecular.org/resources/omns/v09n14.shtml (accessed Apr 2014).

35. Pauling, L. "Molecular Architecture and Biological Reactions." *Chem. Eng News* 24(10) (1946):1375–1377. Blomberg, R., et al. "Precision Is Essential for Efficient Catalysis in an Evolved Kemp Eliminase." *Nature* 503(7476) (Nov 21, 2013):418–21.

36. Crick, F. "The Impact of Linux Pauling on Molecular Biology. The Pauling Symposium." Oregon State University, 1995. http://oregonstate.edu/dept/Special_Collections/subpages/ahp/1995symposium/crick.html. (accessed Jan 2014).

37. Dean, C. *The Magnesium Miracle.* New York: Ballantine, 2007. Hickey, S, A.W. Saul. *Vitamin C: The Real Story, the Remarkable and Controversial Healing Factor.* Laguna Beach, CA: Basic Health Publications, 2008. Hoffer, A., A.W. Saul. *Orthomolecular Medicine for Everyone: Megavitamin Therapeutics for Families and Physicians.* Laguna Beach, CA: Basic Health Publications, 2008. Khalsa, S. *The Vitamin D Revolution: How the Power of This Amazing Vitamin Can Change Your Life.* Hay House, 2009.

38. Smith, R.G. *The Vitamin Cure for Eye Disease.* Laguna Beach, CA: Basic Health Publications, 2012.

39. Pearson, D., S. Shaw. *Life Extension: A Practical Scientific Approach.* New York: Warner Books, 1982.

40. Penberthy, W.T., J.B. Kirkland. "Niacin." In: *Present Knowledge in Nutrition.* Erdman, J.W. et al. 10th edition. Ames, IA: International Life Sciences Institute, 2012. p 293–306. Penberthy, W.T. "Niacin, Riboflavin, and Thiamine." In: *Biochemical, Physiological, and Molecular Aspects of Human Nutrition* M.H. Stipanuk and M.A. Caudill, eds. 3rd edition. St. Louis, MO: Saunders, 2012. p 540–564.

41. Kaufman, W. *Common Form of Niacin Amide Deficiency Disease: Aniacinamidosis.* Yale University Press, 1943. Kaufman, W. *The Common Form of Joint Dysfunction: Its Incidence and Treatment.* Brattleboro, VT: E.L. Hildreth, 1949.

42. U.S. National Library of Medicine. PubMed Health Database. (2013) www.ncbi.nlm.nih.gov/pubmedhealth/ (accessed Jan 2014).

43. Van Noorden, R. "Half of 2011 Papers Now Free to Read." *Nature* 500(7463) (Aug 20, 2013):386–387.

Chapter 2. Essential Nutrients and How They Were Discovered

1. Campbell, T.C., T.M. Campbell, II. *The China Study: The Most Comprehensive Study of Nutrition Ever Conducted and Startling Implications for Diet, Weight Loss, and Long-Term Health.* Dallas, TX: BenBella Books, 2006. Esselstyn, C.B. *Prevent and Reverse Heart Disease: The Revolutionary, Scientifically Proven, Nutrition-Based Cure.* New York: Avery, 2008. Pollan, M. *In Defense of Food: An Eater's Manifesto.* New York: Penguin, 2009. Campbell, T.C. *Whole: Rethinking the Science of Nutrition.* Dallas, TX: BenBella Books, 2013.

2. Pollan, M. *In Defense of Food: An Eater's Manifesto.* New York: Penguin, 2009.

3. Pollan, M. *In Defense of Food: An Eater's Manifesto.* New York: Penguin, 2009. Campbell, T.C. *Whole: Rethinking the Science of Nutrition.* Dallas, TX: BenBella Books, 2013.

4. Bell, R.R., C.A. Heller. "Nutrition Studies: An Appraisal of the Modern Northern Alaskan Eskimo Diet." in: Jamison, P.L., S.L. Zegura, F.A. Milan, eds. *Eskimos of Northwestern Alaska: A Biological Perspective.* Stroudsburg, PA: Dowden, Hutchinson and Ross, 1978:145–156. Draper, H.H. "Nutrition of Alaskan Natives." *Am J Clin Nutr* 57(5) (May 1993):698–699. Gadsby, P. "The Inuit Paradox: How Can People Who Gorge on Fat and Rarely See a Vegetable Be Healthier Than We Are?" *Discover Mag* (Oct 1, 2004). Bersamin, A., et al. "Nutrient Intakes Are Associated with Adherence to a Traditional Diet among Yup'ik Eskimos Living in Remote Alaska Native Communities: The CANHR Study." *Int J Circumpolar Health* 66(1) (2007):62–70.

5. Pollan, M. *In Defense of Food: An Eater's Manifesto.* New York: Penguin, 2009. Campbell, T.C., T.M. Campbell, II. *The China Study: The Most Comprehensive Study of Nutrition Ever Conducted and Startling Implications for Diet, Weight Loss, and Long-Term Health.* Dallas, TX: Ben-Bella Books, 2006.

6. Gropper, S.S., J.L. Smith. *Advanced Nutrition and Human Metabolism,* 6th edition. New York: Cengage Learning, 2013.

7. Ibid.

8. Jukes, T.H. "The Prevention and Conquest of Scurvy, Beri-Beri, and Pellagra." *Prev Med* 18(6) (Nov 1989):877–83.

9. Giovannoni, S.J."Vitamins in the Sea." *Proc Natl Acad Sci USA.* 109(35) (Aug 28, 2012):13888–13889. doi: 10.1073/pnas.121172210. Helliwell, K.E., G.L. Wheeler, A.G. Smith. "Widespread Decay of Vitamin-Related Pathways: Coincidence or Consequence?" *Trends Genet* 29(8) (Aug 29, 2013):469–78. Sañudo-Wilhelmy, S.A., et al. "The Role of B Vitamins in Marine Biogeochemistry." *Ann Rev Mar Sci* 6 (2014): 339–67.

10. Pauling, L. "Evolution and the Need for Ascorbic Acid." *Proc Natl Acad Sci USA* 67(4) (Dev 1970):1643–1648. Pauling, L. *Vitamin C and the Common Cold.* San Francisco: W. H. Freeman, 1970. Pauling, L. *How to Live Longer and Feel Better.* Corvallis, OR: Oregon State University Press, 1986, 2006. Drouin, G., J.R. Godin, B. Pagé. "The Genetics of Vitamin C Loss in Vertebrates." *Curr Genomics* 12(5) (Aug 12, 2011):371–8. Helliwell, K.E., G.L. Wheeler, A.G. Smith. "Widespread Decay of Vitamin-Related Pathways: Coincidence or Consequence?" *Trends Genet* 29(8) (Aug 29, 2013):469–78.

11. Pauling, L. *How to Live Longer and Feel Better.* Corvallis, OR: Oregon State University Press, 1986, 2006.

12. Mawer, E.B., et al. "The Metabolism of Isotopically Labelled Vitamin D_3 in Man: The Influence of the State of Vitamin D Nutrition." *Clin Sci* 40(1) (Jan 1971):39–53. Jones, G. "Pharmacokinetics of Vitamin D Toxicity." *Am J Clin Nutr* 88(2) (Aug 2008):582S-586S.

13. Hickey, S, A.W. Saul. *Vitamin C: The Real Story, the Remarkable and Controversial Healing Factor.* Laguna Beach, CA: Basic Health Publications, 2008.

14. Williams, R.J. *Biochemical Individuality.* New Canaan, CT: Keats Publishing, 1998.

15. Ibid.

16. Dean, C. *The Magnesium Miracle.* New York: Ballantine, 2007.

17. Kirkwood, T.B. "Understanding the Odd Science of Aging." *Cell* 120(4) (Feb 25, 2005):437–47.

18. Kirkwood, T.B. "Understanding Ageing from an Evolutionary Perspective." *J Intern Med* 263(2) (Feb 2008):117–127.

19. Ibid.

20. Kirkwood, T.B., A. Kowald. "The Free-Radical Theory of Ageing—Older, Wiser and Still Alive: Modelling Positional Effects of the Primary Targets of ROS Reveals New Support." *Bioessays* 34(8) (Aug 2012):692–700.

21. Paul, L. "Diet, Nutrition and Telomere Length." *J Nutr Biochem* 22(10) (Oct 2011):895–901.

22. Dean, C. *The Magnesium Miracle.* New York: Ballantine, 2007.

23. Hoffer, A., A.W. Saul. *Orthomolecular Medicine for Everyone: Megavitamin Therapeutics for Families and Physicians.* Laguna Beach, CA: Basic Health Publications, 2008.

24. Dean, C. *The Magnesium Miracle.* New York: Ballantine, 2007.

25. Levy, T.E. *Stop America's #1 Killer: Reversible Vitamin Deficiency Found to be Origin of All Coronary Heart Disease.* Henderson, NV: Livon Books, 2006. Levy, T.E. *Primal*

Panacea. Henderson, NV: MedFox Publishing, 2011. Levy, T.E. *Death by Calcium*. Henderson, NV: MedFox Publishing, 2013.

26. Hickey, S, A.W. Saul. *Vitamin C: The Real Story, the Remarkable and Controversial Healing Factor.* Laguna Beach, CA: Basic Health Publications, 2008. Hoffer, A., A.W. Saul. *Orthomolecular Medicine for Everyone: Megavitamin Therapeutics for Families and Physicians.* Laguna Beach, CA: Basic Health Publications, 2008. Levy, T.E. *Primal Panacea.* Henderson, NV: MedFox Publishing, 2011.

27. Harper, A.E. "Defining the Essentiality of Nutrients." Chapter 1 in *Modern Nutrition in Health and Disease,* editors Shils, M.E., et al., 9th edition. Baltimore: Williams and Wilkins, 1999. p 3–10.

28. McCollum, E.V. "Diet and Nutrition: Better Nutrition as a Health Measure." *Can Med Assoc J* 40(4) (Apr 1939):393–5. Harper, A.E. "Defining the Essentiality of Nutrients." Chapter 1 in *Modern Nutrition in Health and Disease,* editors Shils, M.E., et al., 9th edition. Baltimore: Williams and Wilkins, 1999. p 3–10.

29. Jukes, T.H. "The Prevention and Conquest of Scurvy, Beri-Beri, and Pellagra." *Prev Med* 18(6) (Nov 1989):877–83.

30. Crawford, E.M. "Scurvy in Ireland during the Great Famine." *Soc Hist Med* 1(3) (1988):281–300. Carpenter, K.J. *The History of Scurvy and Vitamin C.* Cambridge: Cambridge Univ. Press, 1988.

31. Lind, J. *A Treatise on the Scurvy.* London: Kincaid & Donaldson, 1753. Lind, J. *A Treatise on the Scurvy.* 3rd edition. London: Crowder. 1772. (available on Google Books.)

32. Lind, J. *A Treatise on the Scurvy.* 3rd edition. London: Crowder. 1772. (available on Google Books.). Bartholomew, M. "James Lind's Treatise of the Scurvy (1753)." *Postgrad Med J* 78(925) (Nov 2002):695–6.

33. Cook, J. "The Method Taken for Preserving the Health of the Crew of His Majesty's Ship the Resolution during Her Late Voyage Round the World." *Phil Trans R Soc Lond* 66 (Jan 1, 1776):402–406.

34. Carpenter, K.J. *The History of Scurvy and Vitamin C.* Cambridge: Cambridge Univ. Press, 1988. Baron, J.H. "Sailors' Scurvy before and after James Lind—A Reassessment." *Nutr Rev* 67(6) (Jun 2009):315–32.

35. Carpenter, K.J. *The History of Scurvy and Vitamin C.* Cambridge: Cambridge Univ. Press, 1988.

36. Bartholomew, M. "James Lind's Treatise of the Scurvy (1753)." *Postgrad Med J* 78(925) (Nov 2002):695–6.

37. Carpenter, K.J. *The History of Scurvy and Vitamin C.* Cambridge: Cambridge Univ. Press, 1988. Baron, J.H. "Sailors' Scurvy before and after James Lind—A Reassessment." *Nutr Rev* 67(6) (Jun 2009):315–32.

38. Carpenter, K.J. *The History of Scurvy and Vitamin C.* Cambridge: Cambridge Univ. Press, 1988.

39. Carter, K.C. "The Germ Theory, Beriberi, and the Deficiency Theory of Disease." *Med Hist.* 21(2) (Apr 1977): 119–136. Carpenter, K.J. *The History of Scurvy and Vitamin C.* Cambridge: Cambridge Univ. Press, 1988. Baron, J.H. "Sailors' Scurvy before and after James Lind—A Reassessment." *Nutr Rev* 67(6) (Jun 2009):315–32.

40. Carter, K.C. "The Germ Theory, Beriberi, and the Deficiency Theory of Disease." *Med Hist.* 21(2) (Apr 1977): 119–136. Carpenter, K.J. *The History of Scurvy and Vitamin C.* Cambridge: Cambridge Univ. Press, 1988.

41. Carter, K.C. "The Germ Theory, Beriberi, and the Deficiency Theory of Disease." *Med Hist.* 21(2) (Apr 1977): 119–136.

42. Hyman, M. "Paradigm Shift: The End of "Normal Science" in Medicine. Understanding Function in Nutrition, Health, and Disease." *Altern Ther Health Med* 10(5) (Sep-Oct 2004):10–5, 90–4. Hickey, S., H. Roberts. *Tarnished Gold: The Sickness of Evidence-based Medicine.* CreateSpace Independent Publishing, 2011. Heaney, R.P. "The Nutrient Problem." *Nutr Rev* 70(3) (Mar 2012):165–69.

43. Hill, A.B. "The Environment and Disease: Association or Causation?" Proc R Soc Med. 58(5) (May 1965):295–300. Carpenter, K.J. *The History of Scurvy and Vitamin C.* Cambridge: Cambridge Univ. Press, 1988. Attia, P. "Is the Obesity Crisis Hiding a Bigger Problem?" TED Talks: TED Partner Series video. 2013 www.ted.com/talks/peter_attia_what_if_we_re_wrong_about_diabetes.html (accessed Jan 2014).

44. Matthews, J.N.S. *Introduction to Randomized Controlled Clinical Trials,* 2nd edition. Boca Raton, FL: Chapman & Hall/CRC, 2006. Hickey, S., H. Roberts. *Tarnished Gold: The Sickness of Evidence-based Medicine.* CreateSpace Independent Publishing, 2011. Smith, R.G. *The Vitamin Cure for Eye Disease.* Laguna Beach, CA: Basic Health Publications, 2012.

45. Hickey, S., H. Roberts. *Tarnished Gold: The Sickness of Evidence-based Medicine.* CreateSpace Independent Publishing, 2011.

46. Ibid.

47. Heaney, R.P. "The Nutrient Problem." *Nutr Rev* 70(3) (Mar 2012):165–69.

48. Hickey, S., H. Roberts. *Tarnished Gold: The Sickness of Evidence-based Medicine.* CreateSpace Independent Publishing, 2011.

49. Rossini, M., et al. (2013) "Regional Differences of Vitamin D Deficiency in Rheumatoid Arthritis Patients in Italy." *Reumatismo* 65(3) (Jul 23, 2013):113–120.

50. Mister, S., J. Hathcock. "Review of Supplements Ignores Evidence-Based Nutrition to Promote Tighter Regulation." *J Parenter Enteral Nutr* 36(3) (May 2012):265.

51. Hathcock, J.N. "Vitamins and Minerals: Efficacy and Safety." *Am J Clin Nutr.* 66(2) (May 1997):427–437. Hoffer, A., A.W. Saul. *Orthomolecular Medicine for Everyone: Megavitamin Therapeutics for Families and Physicians.* Laguna Beach, CA: Basic Health Publications, 2008.

52. Potischman, N., D.L. Weed. "Causal Criteria in Nutritional Epidemiology." *Am J Clin Nutr.* 69(6) (Jun 1999):1309S-1314S. Hickey, S., H. Roberts. *Tarnished Gold: The Sickness of Evidence-based Medicine.* CreateSpace Independent Publishing, 2011.

53. Goodwin, J.S., M.R. Tangum. "Battling Quackery: Attitudes about Micronutrient Supplements in American Academic Medicine." *Arch Intern Med* 158(20) (Nov 9, 1998): 2187–2191.

54. Hathcock, J.N. "Vitamins and Minerals: Efficacy and Safety." *Am J Clin Nutr.* 66(2) (May 1997):427–437. Hyman, M. "Paradigm Shift: The End of "Normal Science" in Medicine. Understanding Function in Nutrition, Health, and Disease." *Altern Ther Health Med* 10 (5) (Sep-Oct 2004):10–5, 90–4. Heaney, R.P. "The Nutrient Problem." *Nutr Rev* 70(3) (Mar 2012):165–69. Mister, S., J. Hathcock. "Review of Supplements Ignores Evidence-Based Nutrition to Promote Tighter Regulation." *J Parenter Enteral Nutr* 36(3) (May 2012):265.

55. Tann, J., R.G. Jones. "Technology and Transformation: The Diffusion of the Roller Mill in the British Flour Milling Industry, 1870–1907." *Technol Cult* 37(1) (Jan 1996):36–69. Also at: www.jstor.org/stable/3107201 (accessed Jan 2014).

56. Babcock, J.W. *Prevalence of Pellagra.* U.S. Government Printing Office, 1911. (available on Google Books).

57. Buecker, T.R. (2001) "Flour Milling in Nebraska." Nebraska State Historical Society, www.usgennet.org/usa/ne/topic/resources/NSHS/EDLFT/edlft17.html (accessed Jan 2014). Tann, J., R.G. Jones. "Technology and Transformation: The Diffusion of the Roller Mill in the British Flour Milling Industry, 1870–1907." *Technol Cult* 37(1) (Jan 1996):36–69. Also at: www.jstor.org/stable/3107201 (accessed Jan 2014).

58. Hall, H. *America's Successful Men of Affairs: The United States at Large.* Volume 2 in *America's Successful Men of Affairs,* New York: New York Tribune, 1896. (Available on Google Books, www.dromo.info/pillsburybio.htm (accessed Jan 2014).

59. Tann, J., R.G. Jones. "Technology and Transformation: The Diffusion of the Roller Mill in the British Flour Milling Industry, 1870–1907." *Technol Cult* 37(1) (Jan 1996):36–69. Also at: www.jstor.org/stable/3107201 (accessed Jan 2014).

60. Babcock, J.W. *Prevalence of Pellagra.* U.S. Government Printing Office, 1911. (available on Google Books).

61. Brenton, B.P. "Pellagra, Sex and Gender: Biocultural Perspectives on Differential Diets and Health". *Nutr Anth* 23(1) (Spring 2000):20–24.

62. Lanska, D.J. "Historical Aspects of the Major Neurological Vitamin Deficiency Disorders: The Water-Soluble B Vitamins." Chapter 30 in: *Handb Clin Neurol.* 95 (2010): 445–76.

63. Carter, K.C. "The Germ Theory, Beriberi, and the Deficiency Theory of Disease." *Med Hist.* 21(2) (Apr 1977): 119–136. Pauling, L. *How to Live Longer and Feel Better.* Corvallis, OR: Oregon State University Press, 1986, 2006.

64. Crellin, J.K. *Home Medicine: The Newfoundland Experience.* Montreal; Buffalo: McGill-Queen's University Press, 1994.

65. Ibid.

66. Brooke, C.L. "Enrichment and Fortification of Cereals and Cereal Products with Vitamins and Minerals." J. Agric. Food Chem. 16(2) (1968):163–167. Bishai, D., R. Nalubola. "The History of Food Fortification in the United States: Its Relevance for current Fortification Efforts in Developing Countries." *Econ Dev Cult Change* 51(1) (Oct 2002):37–53. www.jstor.org/stable/10.1086/345 (accessed Jan 2014).

67. Bishai, D., R. Nalubola. "The History of Food Fortification in the United States: Its Relevance for current Fortification Efforts in Developing Countries." *Econ Dev Cult Change* 51(1) (Oct 2002):37–53. www.jstor.org/stable/10.1086/345 (accessed Jan 2014).

68. Ibid.

69. Park, Y.K., et al. "History of Cereal-Grain Product Fortification in the United States." *Nutr Today* 36(3) (Apr 2001):124–37.

70. Kaufman, W. *The Common Form of Joint Dysfunction: Its Incidence and Treatment.* Brattleboro, VT: E.L. Hildreth, 1949.

71. McCollum, E.V. "Bread "Enrichment"." *Science* 102(2642) (Aug 17, 1945):181–2.

72. Blanck, F.C,, E.V. McCollum, D.B. Jones. "Cereals and Their Products : Report of the Committee." *Am J Public Health Nations Health* 19(4) (Apr 1929):410–3.

73. Nobelprize.org. "The Nobel Prize in Physiology or Medicine 1929." www.nobelprize.org/nobel_prizes/medicine/laureates/1929/

74. Hopkins, F.G. "Feeding Experiments Illustrating the Importance of Accessory Factors

in Normal Dietaries." *J Physiol* 44(5–6) (Jul 15, 2012):425–460. Funk, C., H.E. Dubin. *The Vitamines.* Williams & Wilkins, 1922. Modern duplicate available from Cornell University Library ISBN 781112241376 or RareBooksClub.com, 2012. ISBN-13: 978–1232102885. Williams, R.R. *Toward the Conquest of Beriberi.* Literary Licensing, LLC., 2011. Bémeur, C., R.F. Butterworth. "Thiamin." Chapter 21 in *Modern Nutrition in Health and Disease,* editors A.C. Ross, et al., 11th ed. Baltimore: Lippincott Williams & Wilkins, 2012.

75. Penberthy, W.T., J.B. Kirkland. "Niacin." In: *Present Knowledge in Nutrition.* Erdman, J.W. et al. 10th edition. Ames, IA: International Life Sciences Institute, 2012. p 293–306.

76. Brenton, B.P. "Pellagra, Sex and Gender: Biocultural Perspectives on Differential Diets and Health". *Nutr Anth* 23(1) (Spring 2000):20–24.

77. Food and Agriculture Organization of the United Nations (FAO). *Maize in Human Nutrition.* 1992. www.fao.org/docrep/T0395E/t0395e/t0395e00.htm. (see Chapter 5, "Lime-Treated Maize, part II." www.fao.org/docrep/t0395e/T0395E07.htm#Lime-treated%20maize%20%28part%20II%29

78. Goldberger, J., et al. "A Study of the Blacktongue-Preventive Action of 16 Foodstuffs, with Special Reference to the Identity of Blacktongue of Dogs and Pellagra of Man." *Pub Hlth Rep* 43(23) (Jun 8, 1928):1385.

79. Elvehjem, C.A., et al. "Relation of Nicotinic Acid and Nicotinic Acid Amide to Canine Black Tongue." *J Am Chem Soc* 59(9) (1937):1767–1768.

80. Jukes, T.H. "The Prevention and Conquest of Scurvy, Beri-Beri, and Pellagra." *Prev Med* 18(6) (Nov 1989):877–83.

81. Jukes, T.H. "The Prevention and Conquest of Scurvy, Beri-Beri, and Pellagra." *Prev Med* 18(6) (Nov 1989):877–83. Kirkland, J.B. "Niacin." Chapter 23 in *Modern Nutrition in Health and Disease,* editors A.C. Ross, et al., 11th ed. Baltimore: Lippincott Williams & Wilkins, 2012.

82. Babcock, J.W. *Prevalence of Pellagra.* U.S. Government Printing Office, 1911. (available on Google Books).

83. Funk, C., H.E. Dubin. *The Vitamines.* Williams & Wilkins, 1922. Modern duplicate available from Cornell University Library ISBN 781112241376 or RareBooksClub.com, 2012. ISBN-13: 978–1232102885. McCollum, E.V. "The Paths to the Discovery of Vitamins A and D." *J Nutr* 91(2 Suppl 1) (Feb 1, 1967):11–6. Carter, K.C. "The Germ Theory, Beriberi, and the Deficiency Theory of Disease." *Med Hist.* 21(2) (Apr 1977): 119–136.

84. Carpenter, K.J. "The Discovery of Vitamin C." *Ann Nutr Metab* 61(3) (2012):259–64. Nobel Prize in Physiology or Medicine, 1937. www.nobelprize.org/nobel_prizes/chemistry/laureates/1937.

85. LegalForce Trademarks. Hoffman-La Roche, Inc.: Redoxon, (Patent issued 1934) www.trademarkia.com/redoxon-71350953.html

86. McCollum, E.V. "Diet and Nutrition: Better Nutrition as a Health Measure." *Can Med Assoc J* 40(4) (Apr 1939):393–5. Harper, A.E. "Defining the Essentiality of Nutrients." Chapter 1 in *Modern Nutrition in Health and Disease,* editors Shils, M.E., et al., 9th edition. Baltimore: Williams and Wilkins, 1999. p 3–10.

87. Hyman, M. "Paradigm Shift: The End of "Normal Science" in Medicine. Understanding Function in Nutrition, Health, and Disease." *Altern Ther Health Med* 10 (5) (Sep-Oct 2004):10–5, 90–4.

88. Hickey, S, A.W. Saul. *Vitamin C: The Real Story, the Remarkable and Controversial Healing Factor.* Laguna Beach, CA: Basic Health Publications, 2008.

89. Hoffer, A., A.W. Saul. *Orthomolecular Medicine for Everyone: Megavitamin Therapeutics for Families and Physicians.* Laguna Beach, CA: Basic Health Publications, 2008.

90. Pauling, L. *How to Live Longer and Feel Better.* Corvallis, OR: Oregon State University Press, 1986, 2006.

91. Heaney, R.P. "The Nutrient Problem." *Nutr Rev* 70(3) (Mar 2012):165–69.

92. Williams, R.J. *Biochemical Individuality.* New Canaan, CT: Keats Publishing, 1998. Hoffer, A., A.W. Saul. *Orthomolecular Medicine for Everyone: Megavitamin Therapeutics for Families and Physicians.* Laguna Beach, CA: Basic Health Publications, 2008.

93. Kaufman, W. *The Common Form of Joint Dysfunction: Its Incidence and Treatment.* Brattleboro, VT: E.L. Hildreth, 1949.

94. Williams, R.J. *Biochemical Individuality.* New Canaan, CT: Keats Publishing, 1998.

95. Ashtari, M., et al. "The Human Visual Cortex Responds to Gene Therapy-Mediated Recovery of Retinal Function." *J Clin Invest* 121(6) (Jun 2011):2160–8. Maguire, A.M., et al. "Safety and Efficacy of Gene Transfer for Leber's Congenital Amaurosis." *N Engl J Med* 358(21) (May 22: 2008)2240–8.

96. Stattin, E.L., et al. "A Missense Mutation in the Aggrecan C-Type Lectin Domain Disrupts Extracellular Matrix Interactions and Causes Dominant Familial Osteochondritis Dissecans." *Am J Hum Genet* 86(2) (Feb 12, 2010):126–137.

97. Kirkwood, T.B., A. Kowald. "The Free-Radical Theory of Ageing—Older, Wiser and Still Alive: Modelling Positional Effects of the Primary Targets of ROS Reveals New Support." *Bioessays* 34(8) (Aug 2012):692–700.

98. Kirkwood, T.B. "Understanding the Odd Science of Aging." *Cell* 120(4) (Feb 25, 2005):437–47.

99. Williams, R.J. *Biochemical Individuality.* New Canaan, CT: Keats Publishing, 1998. Dean, C. *The Magnesium Miracle.* New York: Ballantine, 2007. Roberts, H., S. Hickey. *The Vitamin Cure for Heart Disease: How to Prevent and Treat Heart Disease Using Nutrition and Vitamin Supplementation.* Laguna Beach, CA: Basic Health Publications, 2011. Brighthope, I.E. *The Vitamin Cure for Diabetes: Prevent and Treat Diabetes Using Nutrition and Vitamin Supplementation.* Laguna Beach, CA: Basic Health Publications, 2012. Saul, A. *Doctor Yourself: Natural Healing That Works.* 2nd edition. Laguna Beach, CA: Basic Health Publications, 2012. www.doctoryourself.com. Smith, R.G. *The Vitamin Cure for Eye Disease.* Laguna Beach, CA: Basic Health Publications, 2012.

100. Ames, B.N. "Low Micronutrient Intake May Accelerate the Degenerative Diseases of Aging through Allocation of Scarce Micronutrients by Triage." *Proc Natl Acad Sci USA.* 103(47) (Nov 21, 2006):17589–94. Kirkwood, T.B. "Understanding Ageing from an Evolutionary Perspective." *J Intern Med* 263(2) (Feb 2008):117–127. McCann, J.C., B.N. Ames. "Vitamin K, An Example of Triage Theory: Is Micronutrient Inadequacy Linked to Diseases of Aging?" *Am J Clin Nutr* 90(4) (Oct 2009):889–907. McCann, J.C., B.N. Ames. "Adaptive Dysfunction of Selenoproteins from the Perspective of the Triage Theory: Why Modest Selenium Deficiency May Increase Risk of Diseases of Aging." *FASEB J* 25(6) (Jun 2011):1793–814.

101. Ames, B.N. "Low Micronutrient Intake May Accelerate the Degenerative Diseases of Aging through Allocation of Scarce Micronutrients by Triage." *Proc Natl Acad Sci USA* 103(47) (Nov 21, 2006):17589–94. Kirkwood, T.B. "Understanding Ageing from an Evolutionary Perspective." *J Intern Med* 263(2) (Feb 2008):117–127. McCann, J.C., B.N.

Ames. "Vitamin K, An Example of Triage Theory: Is Micronutrient Inadequacy Linked to Diseases of Aging?" *Am J Clin Nutr* 90(4) (Oct 2009):889–907. Theuwissen, E., E. Smit, C. Vermeer. "The Role of Vitamin K in Soft-Tissue Calcification." *Adv Nutr* 3(2) (Mar 2012):166–173.

102. Iserson, K.V., J.C. Moskop. "Triage in Medicine, Part I: Concept, History, and Types." *Ann Emerg Med* 49(3) (Mar 2007):275–281.

103. Ames, B.N. "Low Micronutrient Intake May Accelerate the Degenerative Diseases of Aging through Allocation of Scarce Micronutrients by Triage." *Proc Natl Acad Sci USA.* 103(47) (Nov 21, 2006):17589–94. Ames, B.N. "Optimal Micronutrients Delay Mitochondrial Decay and Age-Associated Diseases." *Mech Ageing Dev* 131(7–8) (Jul-Aug 2010):473–479. Ames, B.N. "Prevention of Mutation, Cancer, and Other Age-Associated Diseases by Optimizing Micronutrient Intake." *J Nucleic Acids* (Sep 22, 2010). pii:725071.

104. Hyman, M. "Paradigm Shift: The End of "Normal Science" in Medicine. Understanding Function in Nutrition, Health, and Disease." *Altern Ther Health Med* 10 (5) (Sep-Oct 2004):10–5, 90–4.

105. Kirkwood, T.B., A. Kowald. "The Free-Radical Theory of Ageing—Older, Wiser and Still Alive: Modelling Positional Effects of the Primary Targets of ROS Reveals New Support." *Bioessays* 34(8) (Aug 2012):692–700.

106. Ames, B.N. "Optimal Micronutrients Delay Mitochondrial Decay and Age-Associated Diseases." *Mech Ageing Dev* 131(7–8) (Jul-Aug 2010):473–479. Ames, B.N. "Prevention of Mutation, Cancer, and Other Age-Associated Diseases by Optimizing Micronutrient Intake." *J Nucleic Acids* (Sep 22, 2010). pii:725071.

107. McCann, J.C., B.N. Ames. "Vitamin K, An Example of Triage Theory: Is Micronutrient Inadequacy Linked to Diseases of Aging?" *Am J Clin Nutr* 90(4) (Oct 2009):889–907. Theuwissen, E., E. Smit, C. Vermeer. "The Role of Vitamin K in Soft-Tissue Calcification." *Adv Nutr* 3(2) (Mar 2012):166–173.

108. Pauling, L. *How to Live Longer and Feel Better.* Corvallis, OR: Oregon State University Press, 1986, 2006. McCann, J.C., B.N. Ames. "Vitamin K, An Example of Triage Theory: Is Micronutrient Inadequacy Linked to Diseases of Aging?" *Am J Clin Nutr* 90(4) (Oct 2009):889–907. Ames, B.N. "Optimal Micronutrients Delay Mitochondrial Decay and Age-Associated Diseases." *Mech Ageing Dev* 131(7–8) (Jul-Aug 2010):473–479.

109. Szilard, L. "On the Nature of the Aging Process." *Proc Natl Acad Sci USA* 45(1) (Jan 1959):30–45. Kirkwood, T.B., A. Kowald. "The Free-Radical Theory of Ageing—Older, Wiser and Still Alive: Modelling Positional Effects of the Primary Targets of ROS Reveals New Support." *Bioessays* 34(8) (Aug 2012):692–700.

110. Kirkwood, T.B., A. Kowald. "The Free-Radical Theory of Ageing—Older, Wiser and Still Alive: Modelling Positional Effects of the Primary Targets of ROS Reveals New Support." *Bioessays* 34(8) (Aug 2012):692–700. Levy, T.E. *Stop America's #1 Killer: Reversible Vitamin Deficiency Found to be Origin of All Coronary Heart Disease.* Henderson, NV: Livon Books, 2006. Levy, T.E. *Primal Panacea.* Henderson, NV: MedFox Publishing, 2011.

111. Schectman, G., J.C. Byrd, H.W. Gruchow. "The Influence of Smoking on Vitamin C Status in Adults." *Am J Public Health* 79(2) (Feb 1989):158–62. Handelman, G.J., L. Packer, C.E. Cross. "Destruction of Tocopherols, Carotenoids, and Retinol in Human Plasma by Cigarette Smoke. *Am J Clin Nutr* 63(4) (Apr 1996):559–65. Frikke-Schmidt, et al. "High Dietary Fat and Cholesterol Exacerbates Chronic Vitamin C Deficiency in Guinea Pigs." *Br J Nutr* 105(1) (Jan 2011):54–61.

112. Levy, T.E. *Stop America's #1 Killer: Reversible Vitamin Deficiency Found to be Ori-*

gin of All Coronary Heart Disease. Henderson, NV: Livon Books, 2006. Levy, T.E. *Death by Calcium*. Henderson, NV: MedFox Publishing, 2013.

113. Levy, T.E. *Death by Calcium*. Henderson, NV: MedFox Publishing, 2013.

114. Kirkwood, T.B., A. Kowald. "The Free-Radical Theory of Ageing—Older, Wiser and Still Alive: Modelling Positional Effects of the Primary Targets of ROS Reveals New Support." *Bioessays* 34(8) (Aug 2012):692–700.

115. Watson, J. "Oxidants, Antioxidants and the Current Incurability of Metastatic Cancers." *Open Biol* 3(1) (Jan 8, 2013):120144. http://rsob.royalsocietypublishing.org/content/3/1/120144.full (accessed Feb 2014).

116. Kotsias, F., et al. "Reactive Oxygen Species Production in the Phagosome: Impact on Antigen Presentation in Dendritic Cells." *Antioxid Redox Signal* 18(6) (Feb 20, 2013):714–29.

117. Chen, Y., et al. "Oral N-acetylcysteine Rescues Lethality of Hepatocyte-Specific Gclc-Knockout Mice, Providing a Model for Hepatic Cirrhosis." *J Hepatol* 53(6) (Dec 2010):1085–94.

118. Lu, S.C. "Glutathione Synthesis." *Biochim Biophys Acta* 1830(5) (May 2013):3143–53.

119. Schafer, F.Q., G.R. Buettner. "Redox Environment of the Cell As Viewed through the Redox State of the Glutathione Disulfide/Glutathione Couple." *Free Radic Biol Med.* 30(11) (Jun 1, 2001):1191–212.

120. Johnson, W.M., A.L. Wilson-Delfosse, J.J. Mieyal. "Dysregulation of Glutathione Homeostasis in Neurodegenerative Diseases." *Nutrients.* 4(10) (Oct 9, 2012):1399–440. Lu, S.C. "Glutathione Synthesis." *Biochim Biophys Acta* 1830(5) (May 2013):3143–53.

121. Lu, S.C. "Glutathione Synthesis." *Biochim Biophys Acta* 1830(5) (May 2013):3143–53.

122. Comar, J.F., et al. "Oxidative State of the Liver of Rats with Adjuvant-Induced Arthritis." *Free Radic Biol Med* (May 2013)58:144–53.

123. Johnson, W.M., A.L. Wilson-Delfosse, J.J. Mieyal. "Dysregulation of Glutathione Homeostasis in Neurodegenerative Diseases." *Nutrients.* 4(10) (Oct 9, 2012):1399–440.

124. Al-Qudah, K.M., Z.B. Ismail. "The Relationship between Serum Biotin and Oxidant/Antioxidant Activities in Bovine Lameness." *Res Vet Sci.* 92(1) (Feb 2012):138–141.

125. Pauling, L. "Evolution and the Need for Ascorbic Acid." *PNAS* 67(4) (Dec 1, 1970):1643–48. Pauling, L. *Vitamin C and the Common Cold.* San Francisco: W. H. Freeman, 1970. Pauling, L. *How to Live Longer and Feel Better.* Corvallis, OR: Oregon State University Press, 1986, 2006.

126. Bourne, G.H. "Vitamin C and Immunity." *Brit J Nutr* 2(4) (Dec 1949):341–347.

127. Drouin, G., J.R. Godin, B. Pagé. "The Genetics of Vitamin C Loss in Vertebrates." *Curr Genomics* 12(5) (Aug 12, 2011):371–8.

128. Pauling, L. *How to Live Longer and Feel Better.* Corvallis, OR: Oregon State University Press, 1986, 2006.

129. Graumlich, J.F., et al. "Pharmacokinetic Model of Ascorbic Acid in Healthy Male Volunteers During Depletion and Repletion." *Pharm Res* 14(9) (Sep 1997):1133–9.

130. Pauling, L. *How to Live Longer and Feel Better.* Corvallis, OR: Oregon State University Press, 1986, 2006.

131. Stone, I." Homo Sapiens Ascorbicus, a Biochemically Corrected Robust Human Mutant." *Med Hypotheses* 5(6) (Jun 1979):711–21. Pauling, L. *How to Live Longer and Feel Better.* Corvallis, OR: Oregon State University Press, 1986, 2006. Drouin, G., J.R. Godin, B. Pagé. "The Genetics of Vitamin C Loss in Vertebrates." *Curr Genomics* 12(5) (Aug 12, 2011):371–8.

132. Drouin, G., J.R. Godin, B. Pagé. "The Genetics of Vitamin C Loss in Vertebrates." *Curr Genomics* 12(5) (Aug 12, 2011):371–8.

133. Ibid.

134. Helliwell, K.E., G.L. Wheeler, A.G. Smith. "Widespread Decay of Vitamin-Related Pathways: Coincidence or Consequence?" *Trends Genet* 29(8) (Aug 29, 2013):469–78.

135. Drouin, G., J.R. Godin, B. Pagé. "The Genetics of Vitamin C Loss in Vertebrates." *Curr Genomics* 12(5) (Aug 12, 2011):371–8.

136. Williams, R.J. *Biochemical Individuality.* New Canaan, CT: Keats Publishing, 1998. Levy, T.E. *Primal Panacea.* Henderson, NV: MedFox Publishing, 2011.

137. Richmond, R.L., J. Law, F. Kaylambkin. "Morbidity Profiles and Lifetime Health of Australian Centenarians." *Australas J Ageing* 31(4) (Dec 2012):227–32.

138. Rivas, C.I., et al. "Vitamin C Transporters." *J Physiol Biochem* 64(4) (Dec 2008):357–75.

139. Lindblad, M., P. Tveden-Nyborg, J. Lykkesfeldt. "Regulation of Vitamin C homeostasis During Deficiency." *Nutrients.* 5(8) (Aug 2013):2860–79.

140. Mendiratta, S., Z.C. Qu, J.M. May. "Erythrocyte Ascorbate Recycling: Antioxidant Effects in Blood." *Free Radic Biol Med* 24(5) (Mar 15, 1998):789–97. Lindblad, M., P. Tveden-Nyborg, J. Lykkesfeldt. "Regulation of Vitamin C homeostasis During Deficiency." *Nutrients.* 5(8) (Aug 2013):2860–79.

141. Mann, G.V., P. Newton. "The Membrane Transport of Ascorbic Acid." *Ann N Y Acad Sci* 258 (Sep 30, 1975):243–52.

142. Montel-Hagen, A., M. Sitbon, N. Taylor. "Erythroid Glucose Transporters." *Curr Opin Hematol* 16(3) (May 2009):165–72.

143. Li, X., C.E. Cobb, J.M. May. "Mitochondrial Recycling of Ascorbic Acid from Dehydroascorbic Acid: Dependence on the Electron Transport Chain." *Arch Biochem Biophys* 403(1) (Jul 2002):103–10.

144. Root-Bernstein, R." An Insulin-Like Modular Basis for the Evolution of Glucose Transporters (GLUT) with Implications for Diabetes." *Evol Bioinform Online* 3 (Oct 15, 2007):317–31.

145. Hickey, S, A.W. Saul. *Vitamin C: The Real Story, the Remarkable and Controversial Healing Factor.* Laguna Beach, CA: Basic Health Publications, 2008. Berger, M.M. "Vitamin C Requirements in Parenteral Nutrition." *Gastroenterology* 137(5 Suppl) (Nov 2009):S70–8.

146. Pauling, L. *How to Live Longer and Feel Better.* Corvallis, OR: Oregon State University Press, 1986, 2006. Cathcart, R.F. "A Unique Function for Ascorbate." *Med Hypotheses* 35(1) (May 1991):32–7. Hickey, S, A.W. Saul. *Vitamin C: The Real Story, the Remarkable and Controversial Healing Factor.* Laguna Beach, CA: Basic Health Publications, 2008. Hoffer, A., A.W. Saul. *Orthomolecular Medicine for Everyone: Megavitamin Therapeutics for Families and Physicians.* Laguna Beach, CA: Basic Health Publications, 2008.

147. Panda. K., et al. "Vitamin C Prevents Cigarette Smoke Induced Oxidative Damage

of Proteins and Increased Proteolysis." *Free Radic Biol Med* 27(9–10) (Nov 1999): 1064–79. Panda, K, et al. "Vitamin C Prevents Cigarette Smoke-Induced Oxidative Damage in Vivo." *Free Radic Biol Med* 29(2) (Jul 15, 2000):115–24.

148. Schectman, G., J.C. Byrd, H.W. Gruchow. "The Influence of Smoking on Vitamin C Status in Adults." *Am J Public Health* 79(2) (Feb 1989):158–62. Handelman, G.J., L. Packer, C.E. Cross. "Destruction of Tocopherols, Carotenoids, and Retinol in Human Plasma by Cigarette Smoke. *Am J Clin Nutr* 63(4) (Apr 1996):559–65. Berger, M.M. "Vitamin C Requirements in Parenteral Nutrition." *Gastroenterology* 137(5 Suppl) (Nov 2009):S70–8. Ichim, T.E., et al. "Intravenous ascorbic acid to prevent and treat cancer-associated sepsis?" *J Transl Med* 9 (Mar 4, 2011):25.

149. Berger, M.M. "Vitamin C Requirements in Parenteral Nutrition." *Gastroenterology* 137(5 Suppl) (Nov 2009):S70–8.

150. Nathens, A.B,, et al. "Randomized, Prospective Trial of Antioxidant Supplementation in Critically Ill Surgical Patients." *Ann Surg* 236(6) (Dec 2002):814–22. Berger, M.M. "Vitamin C Requirements in Parenteral Nutrition." *Gastroenterology* 137(5 Suppl) (Nov 2009):S70–8. Berger, M.M. "Vitamin C Requirements in Parenteral Nutrition." *Gastroenterology* 137(5 Suppl) (Nov 2009):S70–8.

151. Hickey, S, A.W. Saul. *Vitamin C: The Real Story, the Remarkable and Controversial Healing Factor.* Laguna Beach, CA: Basic Health Publications, 2008.

152. Padayatty, S.J., et al. "Vitamin C Pharmacokinetics: Implications for Oral and Intravenous Use." *Ann Intern Med* 140(7) (Apr 6, 2004):533–7.

153. Hickey, S., H. Roberts. *Ascorbate: The Science of Vitamin C.* Lulu, 2004. Hickey, S, A.W. Saul. *Vitamin C: The Real Story, the Remarkable and Controversial Healing Factor.* Laguna Beach, CA: Basic Health Publications, 2008. Berger, M.M. "Vitamin C Requirements in Parenteral Nutrition." *Gastroenterology* 137(5 Suppl) (Nov 2009):S70–8.

154. Hickey, S, A.W. Saul. *Vitamin C: The Real Story, the Remarkable and Controversial Healing Factor.* Laguna Beach, CA: Basic Health Publications, 2008. Traber, M.G., J.F. Stevens. "Vitamins C and E: Beneficial Effects from a Mechanistic Perspective." *Free Radic Biol Med* 51(5) (Sep 1, 2011):1,000–13. Levine, M., S.J. Padayatty "Vitamin C." Chapter 29 in *Modern Nutrition in Health and Disease,* editors A.C. Ross, 11th ed. Baltimore: Lippincott Williams & Wilkins, 2012.

155. Stoyanovsky, D.A., et al. "Endogenous Ascorbate Regenerates Vitamin E in the Retina Directly and in Combination with Exogenous Dihydrolipoic Acid." *Curr Eye Res* 14 (Mar 1995):181–9. Papas, A. *The Vitamin E Factor: The Miraculous Antioxidant for the Prevention and Treatment of Heart Disease, Cancer, and Aging.* HarperCollins, 1999.

156. Hickey, S., H. Roberts. *Ascorbate: The Science of Vitamin C.* Lulu, 2004. Padayatty, S.J., et al. "Vitamin C Pharmacokinetics: Implications for Oral and Intravenous Use." *Ann Intern Med* 140(7) (Apr 6, 2004):533–7. Hickey, S, A.W. Saul. *Vitamin C: The Real Story, the Remarkable and Controversial Healing Factor.* Laguna Beach, CA: Basic Health Publications, 2008. Levine, M., S.J. Padayatty, M.G. Espey. "Vitamin C: A Concentration-Function Approach Yields Pharmacology and Therapeutic Discoveries." *Adv Nutr* 2(2) (Mar 2011):78–88.

157. Pauling, L. *How to Live Longer and Feel Better.* Corvallis, OR: Oregon State University Press, 1986, 2006. Levy, T.E. *Primal Panacea.* Henderson, NV: MedFox Publishing, 2011. Hickey, S, A.W. Saul. *Vitamin C: The Real Story, the Remarkable and Controversial Healing Factor.* Laguna Beach, CA: Basic Health Publications, 2008.

158. Enzymes, 2013. www.ebi.ac.uk/thornton-srv/databases/CoFactor/enzymes.php?cid =12 (accessed Feb 2014).

159. Bánhegyi, G., et al. "Role of Ascorbate in Oxidative Protein Folding." *Biofactors* 17(1–4) (2003):37–46.

160. Gropper, S.S., J.L. Smith. *Advanced Nutrition and Human Metabolism,* 6th Edition. New York: Cengage Learning, 2013.

161. Pauling, L. *How to Live Longer and Feel Better.* Corvallis, OR: Oregon State University Press, 1986, 2006.

162. Levy, T.E. *Primal Panacea.* Henderson, NV: MedFox Publishing, 2011. Levy, T.E. *Death by Calcium.* Henderson, NV: MedFox Publishing, 2013.

163. Yudoh, K., et al. "Potential Involvement of Oxidative Stress in Cartilage Senescence and Development of Osteoarthritis: Oxidative Stress Induces Chondrocyte Telomere Instability and Downregulation of Chondrocyte Function." *Arthritis Res Ther* 7(2) (2005):R380–91.

164. Levy, T.E. *Primal Panacea.* Henderson, NV: MedFox Publishing, 2011.

165. Hopkins, F.G., E.J. Morgan. "Some Relations between AscorbicAcid and Glutathione." *Biochem J* 30(8) (Aug 1936):1446–62.

166. Altindag, O., et al. "Increased Oxidative Stress and Its Relation with Collagen Metabolism in Knee Osteoarthritis." *Rheumatol Int* 27(4) (Feb 2007):339–44. Kotani, K., et al. "Levels of Reactive Oxygen Metabolites in Patients with Knee Osteoarthritis." *Australas J Ageing* 30(4) (Dec 2011):231–3.

167. Jones, G. "Vitamin D." Chapter 18 in *Modern Nutrition in Health and Disease,* editors A.C. Ross, et al., 11th ed. Baltimore: Lippincott Williams & Wilkins, 2012.

168. McCollum, E.V. "The Paths to the Discovery of Vitamins A and D." *J Nutr* 91(2 Suppl 1) (Feb 1, 1967):11–6.

169. Kwiecinski, G.G., et al. "Observations on Serum 25-Hydroxyvitamin D and Calcium Concentrations from Wild-Caught and Captive Neotropical Bats, Artibeus Jamaicensis." *Gen Comp Endocrinol* 122(2) (May 2001):225–31. Cavaleros, M., et al. "Vitamin D Metabolism in a Frugivorous Nocturnal Mammal, the Egyptian Fruit Bat (Rousettus Aegyptiacus)." *Gen Comp Endocrinol* 133(1) (Aug 2003):109–17.

170. Jones, G. "Vitamin D." Chapter 18 in *Modern Nutrition in Health and Disease,* editors A.C. Ross, et al., 11th ed. Baltimore: Lippincott Williams & Wilkins, 2012.

171. Reid, I.R., M.J. Bolland, A. Grey. "Effects of Vitamin D Supplements on Bone Mineral Density: A Systematic Review and Meta-Analysis." *Lancet* 383(9912) (Jan 11, 2014):146–55.

172. Rosen, C.J. "Vitamin D Supplementation: Bones of Contention." *Lancet* 383(9912) (Jan 11, 2014):108–10.

173. Norman, A.W. "The History of the Discovery of Vitamin D and Its Daughter Steroid Hormone." *Ann Nutr Metab* 61(3) (2012):199–206.

174. Jones, G. "Vitamin D." Chapter 18 in *Modern Nutrition in Health and Disease,* editors A.C. Ross, et al., 11th ed. Baltimore: Lippincott Williams & Wilkins, 2012.

175. Neve, A., A. Corrado, F.P. Cantatore. "Osteocalcin: Skeletal and Extra-Skeletal Effects." *J Cell Physiol.* 228(6) (Jun 2013):1149–53.

176. Jones, G. "Vitamin D." Chapter 18 in *Modern Nutrition in Health and Disease,* editors A.C. Ross, et al., 11th ed. Baltimore: Lippincott Williams & Wilkins, 2012.

177. Khalsa, S. *The Vitamin D Revolution: How the Power of This Amazing Vitamin Can Change Your Life.* Hay House, 2009. Madrid, E. *Vitamin D Prescription: The Healing*

Power of the Sun & How It Can Save Your Life. BookSurge Publishing, 2009. Holick M.F. *The Vitamin D Solution: A 3-Step Strategy to Cure Our Most Common Health Problems.* New York: Penguin Group USA, 2011. Jones, G. "Vitamin D." Chapter 18 in *Modern Nutrition in Health and Disease,* editors A.C. Ross, et al., 11th ed. Baltimore: Lippincott Williams & Wilkins, 2012.

178. Holick M.F. *The Vitamin D Solution: A 3-Step Strategy to Cure Our Most Common Health Problems.* New York: Penguin Group USA, 2011. Jones, G. "Vitamin D." Chapter 18 in *Modern Nutrition in Health and Disease,* editors A.C. Ross, et al., 11th ed. Baltimore: Lippincott Williams & Wilkins, 2012.

179. Jones, G. "Vitamin D." Chapter 18 in *Modern Nutrition in Health and Disease,* editors A.C. Ross, et al., 11th ed. Baltimore: Lippincott Williams & Wilkins, 2012.

180. Sen, D., P. Ranganathan. "Vitamin D in Rheumatoid Arthritis: Panacea or Placebo?" *Discov Med* 14(78) (Nov 2012):311–19.

181. Papas, A. *The Vitamin E Factor: The Miraculous Antioxidant for the Prevention and Treatment of Heart Disease, Cancer, and Aging.* HarperCollins, 1999. Traber, M.G. "Vitamin E." Chapter 19 in *Modern Nutrition in Health and Disease,* editors A.C. Ross, et al., 11th ed. Baltimore: Lippincott Williams & Wilkins, 2012. Niki, E, M.G. Traber. "A History of Vitamin E." *Ann Nutr Metab* 61(3) (2012):207–12.

182. Papas, A. *The Vitamin E Factor: The Miraculous Antioxidant for the Prevention and Treatment of Heart Disease, Cancer, and Aging.* HarperCollins, 1999. Traber, M.G. "Vitamin E." Chapter 19 in *Modern Nutrition in Health and Disease,* editors A.C. Ross, et al., 11th ed. Baltimore: Lippincott Williams & Wilkins, 2012.

183. Evans, H.M., K.S. Bishop. "On the Existence of a Hitherto Unrecognized Dietary Factor Essential for Reproduction." *Science* 56(1458) (Dec 8, 1922):650–51.

184. Papas, A. *The Vitamin E Factor: The Miraculous Antioxidant for the Prevention and Treatment of Heart Disease, Cancer, and Aging.* HarperCollins, 1999. Traber, M.G. "Vitamin E." Chapter 19 in *Modern Nutrition in Health and Disease,* editors A.C. Ross, et al., 11th ed. Baltimore: Lippincott Williams & Wilkins, 2012. Sen, C.K., C. Rink, S. Khanna. "Palm Oil-Derived Natural Vitamin E alpha-Tocotrienol in Brain Health and Disease." *J Am Coll Nutr* 29(3 Suppl) (Jun 2010):314S-323S. Wong, R.S., A.K. Radhakrishnan. "Tocotrienol Research: Past into Present." *Nutr Rev* 70(9) (Sep 2012):483–90.

185. Wong, R.S., A.K. Radhakrishnan. "Tocotrienol Research: Past into Present." *Nutr Rev* 70(9) (Sep 2012):483–90.

186. Niki, E, M.G. Traber. "A History of Vitamin E." *Ann Nutr Metab* 61(3) (2012): 207–12.

187. Papas, A. *The Vitamin E Factor: The Miraculous Antioxidant for the Prevention and Treatment of Heart Disease, Cancer, and Aging.* HarperCollins, 1999. Traber, M.G. "Vitamin E." Chapter 19 in *Modern Nutrition in Health and Disease,* editors A.C. Ross, et al., 11th ed. Baltimore: Lippincott Williams & Wilkins, 2012. Azzi, A. "Molecular Mechanism of Alpha-Tocopherol Action." *Free Radic Biol Med* 43(1) (Jul 1, 2007):16–21. Wang, Y., et al. "Vitamin E Forms Inhibit IL-13/STAT6-Induced Eotaxin-3 Secretion by Up-Regulation of PAR4, an Endogenous Inhibitor of Atypical PKC in Human Lung Epithelial Cells." *J Nutr Biochem* 23(6) (Jun 2012):602–8. Wong, R.S., A.K. Radhakrishnan. "Tocotrienol Research: Past into Present." *Nutr Rev* 70(9) (Sep 2012):483–90.

188. Raju, T.N. "The Nobel Chronicles. 1943: Henrik Carl Peter Dam (1895–1976); and Edward Adelbert Doisy (1893–1986)." *Lancet* 353(9154) (Feb 27, 1999):761.

189. Russo, G.L. "Dietary n-6 and n-3 Polyunsaturated Fatty Acids: from Biochemistry to

Clinical Implications in Cardiovascular Prevention." *Biochem Pharmacol* 77(6) (Mar 15 2009):937–46. Gropper, S.S., J.L. Smith. *Advanced Nutrition and Human Metabolism,* 6th Edition. New York: Cengage Learning, 2013.

190. Russo, G.L. "Dietary n-6 and n-3 Polyunsaturated Fatty Acids: from Biochemistry to Clinical Implications in Cardiovascular Prevention." *Biochem Pharmacol* 77(6) (Mar 15 2009):937–46.

191. Burr, G.O. "The Essential Fatty Acids Fifty Years Ago." *Prog Lipid Res* 20 (1981):xxvii-xxix.

192. Ibid.

193. Burr, G.O., M.M. Burr. "On the Nature and Role of the Fatty Acids Essential in Nutrition." *J. Biol. Chem* 86 (1930):587–621.

194. Russell, F.D., C.S. Bürgin-Maunder. "Distinguishing Health Benefits of Eicosapentaenoic and Docosahexaenoic Acids." *Mar Drugs* 10(11) (Nov 2012):2535–59.

195. Cunnane, S.C., P. Guesnet. "Linoleic Acid Recommendations—A House of Ccards." *Prostaglandins Leukot Essent Fatty Acids* 85(6) (Dec 2011):399–402. National Institutes of Health. Office of Dietary Supplements. "Omega-3 Fatty Acids and Health." http://ods.od.nih.gov/factsheets/Omega3FattyAcidsandHealth-HealthProfessional/ (accessed Feb. 2014).

196. Weaver, C.M., R.P. Heaney. "Calcium" Chapter 7 in *Modern Nutrition in Health and Disease,* editors A.C. Ross, et al., 11th ed. Baltimore: Lippincott Williams & Wilkins, 2012.

197. Potter, J.D., S.P. Robertson, J.D. Johnson. "Magnesium and the Regulation of Muscle Contraction." *Fed Proc* 40(12) (Oct 1981):2653–6.

198. Rude, R.K. "Magnesium" Chapter 9 in *Modern Nutrition in Health and Disease,* editors A.C. Ross, et al., 11th ed. Baltimore: Lippincott Williams & Wilkins, 2012.

199. Bergstrom, W.H., E.H. Bell. "Bone Magnesium Content in Normal and Acidotic Rats." *J Bone Joint Surg Am* 42-A (May 1960):437–8. Carqué, O. *Vital Facts About Foods: A Guide to Health and Longevity.* Health Research, 1974

200. Dean, C. *The Magnesium Miracle.* New York: Ballantine, 2007.

201. Saggese, G., et al. "Bone Demineralization and Impaired Mineral Metabolism in Insulin-Dependent Diabetes Mellitus. A possible Role of Magnesium Deficiency." *Helv Paediatr Acta* 43(5–6) (Jun 1989):405–14. Dean, C. *The Magnesium Miracle.* New York: Ballantine, 2007.

202. Zofková, I., R.L. Kancheva. "The Relationship between Magnesium and Calciotropic Hormones." *Magnes Res* 8(1) (Mar 1995):77–84. Carpenter, T.O. "Disturbances of Vitamin D Metabolism and Action During Clinical and Experimental Magnesium Deficiency." *Magnes Res* 1(3–4) (Dec 1988):131–9.

203. Dean, C. *The Magnesium Miracle.* New York: Ballantine, 2007.

204. Zofková, I., R.L. Kancheva. "The Relationship between Magnesium and Calciotropic Hormones." *Magnes Res* 8(1) (Mar 1995):77–84..

205. Dean, C. *The Magnesium Miracle.* New York: Ballantine, 2007.

206. Penido, M.G., U.S. Alon. "Phosphate Homeostasis and Its Role in Bone Health." *Pediatr Nephrol* 27(11) (Nov 2012):2039–48.

207. Ibid.

208. Dean, C. *The Magnesium Miracle.* New York: Ballantine, 2007.

209–213. Ibid.

214. Agricultural Research Service, United States Department of Agriculture (USDA). "Nutrient Database for Standard Reference," National Nutrient Database for Standard Reference. Release 26 v.1.3.1, 2011. http://ndb.nal.usda.gov/ndb/nutrients/index (accessed Apr 2014).

215. Gropper, S.S., J.L. Smith. *Advanced Nutrition and Human Metabolism,* 6th Edition. New York: Cengage Learning, 2013.

216. Penberthy, W.T., J.B. Kirkland. "Niacin." in: *Present Knowledge in Nutrition.* Erdman, J.W. et al. 10th edition. Ames, IA: International Life Sciences Institute, 2012. p. 293–306. Hoffer, A., A.W. Saul, H.D. Foster. *Niacin: The Real Story: Learn about the Wonderful Healing Properties of Niacin.* Laguna Beach, CA: Basic Health Publications, 2012.

217. Jukes, T.H. "The Prevention and Conquest of Scurvy, Beri-Beri, and Pellagra." *Prev Med* 18(6) (Nov 1989):877–83.

218. Brenton, B.P. "Pellagra, Sex and Gender: Biocultural Perspectives on Differential Diets and Health." *Nutr Anth* 23(1) (Spring 2000):20–24.

219. Ibid.

220. Hanson, J., et al. "Nicotinic Acid- and Monomethyl Fumarate-Induced Flushing Involves GPR109A Expressed by Keratinocytes and COX-2-Dependent Prostanoid Formation in Mice." *J Clin Invest* 120(8) (Aug 2010):2910–9.

221. Saul, A. *Doctor Yourself: Natural Healing That Works.* 2nd edition. Laguna Beach, CA: Basic Health Publications, 2012. www.doctoryourself.com.

222. Hanson, J., et al. "Nicotinic Acid- and Monomethyl Fumarate-Induced Flushing Involves GPR109A Expressed by Keratinocytes and COX-2-Dependent Prostanoid Formation in Mice." *J Clin Invest* 120(8) (Aug 2010):2910–9.

223. Altschul, R., A. Hoffer, J.G. Stephen. "Influence of Nicotinic Acid on Serum Cholesterol in Man." *Arch Biochem Biophys* 54(2) (Feb 1955):558–9. Hamoud, S., et al. "Niacin Administration Significantly Reduces Oxidative Stress in Patients with Hypercholesterolemia and Low Levels of High-Density Lipoprotein Cholesterol." *Am J Med Sci* 345(3) (Mar 2012):195–9.

224. Hoffer, A., A.W. Saul, H.D. Foster. *Niacin: The Real Story: Learn about the Wonderful Healing Properties of Niacin.* Laguna Beach, CA: Basic Health Publications, 2012. Penberthy, W.T., J.B. Kirkland. "Niacin." in: *Present Knowledge in Nutrition.* Erdman, J.W. et al. 10th edition. Ames, IA: International Life Sciences Institute, 2012. p. 293–306.

225. Hoffer, A., A.W. Saul, H.D. Foster. *Niacin: The Real Story: Learn about the Wonderful Healing Properties of Niacin.* Laguna Beach, CA: Basic Health Publications, 2012.

226. Kaufman, W. *Common Form of Niacin Amide Deficiency Disease: Aniacinamidosis.* Yale University Press, 1943. Kaufman, W. *The Common Form of Joint Dysfunction: Its Incidence and Treatment.* Brattleboro, VT: E.L. Hildreth, 1949.

227. Kaufman, W. "Niacinamide as a Therapeutic Agent: A Memoir." 2001. www.doctoryourself.com/kaufman12.html.

228. Ibid.

229–231. Kaufman, W. *The Common Form of Joint Dysfunction: Its Incidence and Treatment.* Brattleboro, VT: E.L. Hildreth, 1949.

Chapter 3. Joints: How They Work, and What Can Go Wrong

1. Brandt, K.D. "Osteoarthritis Clinical Trials Have Not Identified Efficacious Therapies because Traditional Imaging Outcome Measures Are Inadequate." *Arthritis Rheum* (Jul 9, 2013) doi: 10.1002/art.38084 [epub ahead of print].

2. Stein, T.P. "Weight, Muscle and Bone Loss during Space Flight: Another Perspective." *Eur J Appl Physiol* 113(9) (Sep 2013):2171–81.

3. Linus Pauling Institute, Oregon State University, 2012. http://lpi.oregonstate.edu/infocenter/bonehealth.html#overview (accessed Feb 2014).

4. Burr, D.B., M.A. Gallant. "Bone Remodelling in Osteoarthritis." *Nat Rev Rheumatol* 8(11) (Nov 2012):665–673.

5. Neve, A., A. Corrado, F.P. Cantatore. "Osteocalcin: Skeletal and Extra-Skeletal Effects." *J Cell Physiol.* 228(6) (Jun 2013):1149–53.

6. van Bezooijen, R.L., et al. "Control of Bone Formation by Osteocytes? Lessons from the Rare Skeletal Disorders Sclerosteosis and van Buchem Disease." *BoneKEy-Osteovision* (12) (Dec 2005):33–38

7. Ahmadieh, H, A. Arabi. "Vitamins and Bone Health: Beyond Calcium and Vitamin D." *Nutr Rev* 69(10) (Oct 2011):584–98.

8. Levy, T.E. *Death by Calcium.* Henderson, NV: MedFox Publishing, 2013.

9. Shier, D, J. Butler, R. Lewis. "Joints." Chapter 8 in *Hole's Human Anatomy & Physiology,* 12th edition. New York: McGraw-Hill, 2009.

10. Winter, D.A. "Human Balance and Posture Control during Standing and Walking." *Gait and Posture* 3(4) (Dec 1995):193–214.

11. Aspberg, A. "The Different Roles of Aggrecan Interaction Domains." *J Histochem Cytochem* 60(12) (Dec 2012):987–96.

12. Schumacher, B.L., et al. "A Novel Proteoglycan Synthesized and Secreted by Chondrocytes of the Superficial Zone of Articular Cartilage." *Arch Biochem Biophys.* 311(1) (May 15, 1994):144–52. Yoshida, M., et al. "Expression Analysis of Three Isoforms of Hyaluronan Synthase and Hyaluronidase in the Synovium of Knees in Osteoarthritis and Rheumatoid Arthritis by Quantitative Real-Time Reverse Transcriptase Polymerase Chain Reaction." *Arthritis Res Ther* 6(6) (2004):R514–20.

13. Yoshida, M., et al. "Expression Analysis of Three Isoforms of Hyaluronan Synthase and Hyaluronidase in the Synovium of Knees in Osteoarthritis and Rheumatoid Arthritis by Quantitative Real-Time Reverse Transcriptase Polymerase Chain Reaction." *Arthritis Res Ther* 6(6) (2004):R514–20.

14. Shiraev, T, S. Anderson, N. Hope. "Meniscal Tear—Presentation, Diagnosis and Management." *Aust Fam Physician* 41(4) (Apr 2012):182–7.

15. Ibid.

16. Lohmander, L.S., et al. "High Prevalence of Knee Osteoarthritis, Pain, and Functional Limitations in Female Soccer Players Twelve Years after Anterior Cruciate Ligament Injury." *Arthritis Rheum* 50(10) (Oct 2004):3145–52. Englund, M., L.S. Lohmander. "Risk Factors for Symptomatic Knee Osteoarthritis Fifteen to Twenty-Two Years after Meniscectomy." Arthritis Rheum. 50(9) (Sep 2004):2811–9.

17. Frech, T.M., D.O. Clegg. "The Utility of Nutraceuticals in the Treatment of Osteoarthritis." *Curr Rheumatol Rep* 9(1) (Apr 2007):25–30.

18. Frech, T.M., D.O. Clegg. "The Utility of Nutraceuticals in the Treatment of

Osteoarthritis." *Curr Rheumatol Rep* 9(1) (Apr 2007):25–30. Heiss, C., et. "Diagnosis of Osteoporosis with Vitamin K as a New Biochemical Marker." *Vitam Horm* 78 (2008):417–34. doi: 10.1016/S0083-6729(07)00017-9.

19. Darlington, L.G., T.W. Stone. "Antioxidants and Fatty Acids in the Amelioration of Rheumatoid Arthritis and Related Disorders." *Br J Nutr* 85(3) (Mar 2001):251–69.

20. Feldmann, M., F.M. Brennan, R.N. Maini. "Role of Cytokines in Rheumatoid Arthritis." *Ann Rev Immunol* 14 (1996):397–440. Hitchon, C.A, H.S. El-Gabalawy. "The Synovium in Rheumatoid Arthritis." *Open Rheumatol J* 5 (2011):107–14.

21. Müller-Ladner, U., et al. "Mechanisms of Disease: The Mmolecular and Cellular Basis of Joint Destruction in Rheumatoid Arthritis." *Nat Clin Pract Rheumatol* 1(2) (Dec 2005):102–10.

22. Darlington, L.G., T.W. Stone. "Antioxidants and Fatty Acids in the Amelioration of Rheumatoid Arthritis and Related Disorders." *Br J Nutr* 85(3) (Mar 2001):251–69.

23. Eckstein, F., et al. "Thickness of the Subchondral Mineralised Tissue Zone (SMZ) in Normal Male and Female and Pathological Human Patellae." *J Anat* 192(Part 1) (Jan 1998):81–90.

24. Wang, Y., A.E. Wluka, F.M. Cicuttini. "The Determinants of Change in Tibial Plateau Bone Area in Osteoarthritic Knees: A Cohort Study." *Arthritis Res Ther* 7(3) (2005): R687–93. Burr, D.B., M.A. Gallant. "Bone Remodelling in Osteoarthritis." *Nat Rev Rheumatol* 8(11) (Nov 2012):665–673.

25. Bay-Jensen, A.C., et al. "Which Elements are Involved in Reversible and Irreversible Cartilage Degradation in Osteoarthritis?" *Rheumatol Int* 30(4) (Feb 2010):435–42.

26. Chen-An, P., et al. "Investigation of Chondrocyte Hypertrophy and Cartilage Calcification in a Full-Depth Articular Cartilage Explants Model." *Rheumatol Int* 33(2) (Feb 2013):401–11.

27. Burr, D.B., M.A. Gallant. "Bone Remodelling in Osteoarthritis." *Nat Rev Rheumatol* 8(11) (Nov 2012):665–673.

28. Lee, A.S., et al. "A Current Review of Molecular Mechanisms Regarding Osteoarthritis and Pain." *Gene* 527(2) (Sep 25, 2013): 440–7.

29. Chen-An, P., et al. "Investigation of Chondrocyte Hypertrophy and Cartilage Calcification in a Full-Depth Articular Cartilage Explants Model." *Rheumatol Int* 33(2) (Feb 2013):401–11.

30. Mobasheri, A., et al. "Glucose Transport and Metabolism in Chondrocytes: A Key to Understanding Chondrogenesis, Skeletal Development and Cartilage Degradation in Osteoarthritis." *Histol Histopathol* 17(4) (Oct 2002):1239–67.

31. Bay-Jensen, A.C., et al. "Which Elements are involved in Reversible and Irreversible Cartilage Degradation in Osteoarthritis?" *Rheumatol Int* 30(4) (Feb 2010):435–42.

32. Bay-Jensen, A.C., et al. "Which Elements are involved in Reversible and Irreversible Cartilage Degradation in Osteoarthritis?" *Rheumatol Int* 30(4) (Feb 2010):435–42. Mahjoub, M., F. Berenbaum, X. Houard. "Why Subchondral Bone in Osteoarthritis? The Importance of the Cartilage Bone Interface in Osteoarthritis." *Osteoporos Int* (23 Suppl 8) (Dec 2012):841–6.

33. Stattin, E.L., et al. "A Missense Mutation in the Aggrecan C-Type Lectin Domain Disrupts Extracellular Matrix Interactions and Causes Dominant Familial Osteochondritis Dissecans." *Am J Hum Genet* 86(2) (Feb 12, 2010):126–137.

34. Mobasheri, A., et al. "Glucose Transport and Metabolism in Chondrocytes: A Key to Understanding Chondrogenesis, Skeletal Development and Cartilage Degradation in Osteoarthritis." *Histol Histopathol* 17(4) (Oct 2002):1239–67. Gropper, S.S., J.L. Smith. *Advanced Nutrition and Human Metabolism*, 6th edition. New York: Cengage Learning, 2013.

35. Dean, C. *The Magnesium Miracle*. New York: Ballantine, 2007.

36. Zhu, L.L., et al. "Vitamin C Prevents Hypogonadal Bone Loss." *PLoS One* 7(10) (2012):e47058. doi: 10.1371/journal.pone.0047058.

37. Yoshida, M., et al. "Expression Analysis of Three Isoforms of Hyaluronan Synthase and Hyaluronidase in the Synovium of Knees in Osteoarthritis and Rheumatoid Arthritis by Quantitative Real-Time Reverse Transcriptase Polymerase Chain Reaction." *Arthritis Res Ther* 6(6) (2004):R514–20.

38. Filaire, E., H. Toumi. "Reactive Oxygen Species and Exercise on Bone Metabolism: Friend or Enemy?" *Joint Bone Spine* 79(4) (Jul 2012):341–6.

39. Roosendaal, G., et al. "Blood-Induced Joint Damage: A Human In Vitro Study." *Arthritis Rheum* 42(5) (May 1999):1025–32.

40. Pritzker, K.P., et al. "Osteoarthritis Cartilage Histopathology: Grading and Staging." *Osteoarthritis Cartilage* 14(1) (Jan 2006):13–29. Bay-Jensen, A.C., et al. "Which Elements are involved in Reversible and Irreversible Cartilage Degradation in Osteoarthritis?" *Rheumatol Int* 30(4) (Feb 2010):435–42.

41. Bay-Jensen, A.C., et al. "Which Elements are involved in Reversible and Irreversible Cartilage Degradation in Osteoarthritis?" *Rheumatol Int* 30(4) (Feb 2010):435–42.

42. Richette, P., C. Roux. "Impact of Treatments for Osteoporosis on Cartilage on Biomarkers in Humans." *Osteoporos Int* (23 Suppl 8) (Dec 2012):877–80.

43. Peregoy, J., F.V. Wilder. "The Effects of Vitamin C Supplementation on Incident and Progressive Knee Osteoarthritis: A Longitudinal Study." *Public Health Nutrition* 14(4) (Apr 2011):709–15.

44. Darlington, L.G., T.W. Stone. "Antioxidants and Fatty Acids in the Amelioration of Rheumatoid Arthritis and Related Disorders." *Br J Nutr* 85(3) (Mar 2001):251–69. de Lange-Brokaar, B.J., et al. "Synovial Inflammation, Immune Cells and Their Cytokines in Osteoarthritis: A Review." *Osteoarthritis Cartilage* 20(12) (Dec 2012):1484–99.

45. Goldring, M.B., M. Otero. "Inflammation in Osteoarthritis." *Curr Opin Rheumatol* 23(5) (Sep 2011):471–8. Berenbaum, F. "Osteoarthritis as an Inflammatory Disease (Osteoarthritis Is Not Osteoarthrosis!). *Osteoarthritis Cartilage* 21(1) (Jan 2013):16–21. de Lange-Brokaar, B.J., et al. "Synovial Inflammation, Immune Cells and Their Cytokines in Osteoarthritis: A Review." *Osteoarthritis Cartilage* 20(12) (Dec 2012):1484–99.

46. Mobasheri, A, et al. "Scientific Evidence and Rationale for the Development of Curcumin and Resveratrol as Nutraceuticals for Joint Health." *Int J Mol Sci* 13(4) (2012):4202–32.

47. Berenbaum, F. "Osteoarthritis as an Inflammatory Disease (Osteoarthritis Is Not Osteoarthrosis!). *Osteoarthritis Cartilage* 21(1) (Jan 2013):16–21.

48. Rosenbloom, A.L., J.H. Silverstein. "Connective Tissue and Joint Disease in Diabetes Mellitus." *Endocrinol Metab Clin North Am* 25(2) (Jun 1996):473–83. Mobasheri, A. "Glucose: An Energy Currency and Structural Precursor in Articular Cartilage and Bone with Emerging Roles as an Extracellular Signaling Molecule and Metabolic Regulator." *Front Endocrinol* (*Lausanne*) 3 (Dec 17, 2012):153.

49. McAlindon, T.E., B.A. Biggee. "Nutritional Factors and Osteoarthritis: Recent Developments." *Curr Opin Rheumatol* (Sep 2005) 17(5):647–52.

50. Berenbaum, F. "Osteoarthritis as an Inflammatory Disease (Osteoarthritis Is Not Osteoarthrosis!). *Osteoarthritis Cartilage* 21(1) (Jan 2013):16–21. Berenbaum, F., F. Eymard, X. Houard. "Osteoarthritis, Inflammation and Obesity." *Curr Opin Rheumatol* 25(1) (Jan 2013):114–118. Goldring, M.B., M. Otero. "Inflammation in Osteoarthritis." *Curr Opin Rheumatol* 23(5) (Sep 2011):471–8.

51. Berenbaum, F., F. Eymard, X. Houard. "Osteoarthritis, Inflammation and Obesity." *Curr Opin Rheumatol* 25(1) (Jan 2013):114–118.

52. Berenbaum, F. "Osteoarthritis as an Inflammatory Disease (Osteoarthritis Is Not Osteoarthrosis!). *Osteoarthritis Cartilage* 21(1) (Jan 2013):16–21. Berenbaum, F., F. Eymard, X. Houard. "Osteoarthritis, Inflammation and Obesity." *Curr Opin Rheumatol* 25(1) (Jan 2013):114–118.

53. de Lange-Brokaar, B.J., et al. "Synovial Inflammation, Immune Cells and Their Cytokines in Osteoarthritis: A Review." *Osteoarthritis Cartilage* 20(12) (Dec 2012):1484–99.

54. Mobasheri, A. "Glucose: An Energy Currency and Structural Precursor in Articular Cartilage and Bone with Emerging Roles as an Extracellular Signaling Molecule and Metabolic Regulator." *Front Endocrinol (Lausanne)* 3 (Dec 17, 2012):153.

55. Rosa, S.C., et al. "Role of Glucose as a Modulator of Anabolic and Catabolic Gene Expression in Normal and Osteoarthritic Human Chondrocytes." *J Cell Biochem* 112(10) (Oct 2011):2813–24.

56. Robertson, L.T., J.R. Mitchell. "Benefits of Short-Term Dietary Restriction in Mammals." *Exp Gerontol* 48(10) (Oct 2013):1043–8.

57. O'Neill, L.A., D.G. Hardie. "Metabolism of Inflammation Limited by AMPK and Pseudo-Starvation." *Nature* 493(7432) (Jan 17 2013):346–55.

58. Chambers, A.P., D.A. Sandoval, R.J. Seeley. "Integration of Satiety Signals by the Central Nervous System." *Curr Biol* 23(9) (May 6, 2013):R379–88.

59. Ibid.

60. Ibid

61. Attia, P. "Is the Obesity Crisis Hiding a Bigger Problem?" TED Talks: TED Partner Series video. 2013 www.ted.com/talks/peter_attia_what_if_we_re_wrong_about_diabetes .html (accessed Jan 2014).

62. Dolgin, E. "Deprivation: A Wake-Up Call." *Nature* 497(7450) (May 23, 2013):S6–7.

63. Owens, B. "Obesity: Heavy Sleepers." *Nature* 497(7450) (May 23, 2013):S8–9.

64. Solarz, D.E., J.M. Mullington, H.K. Meier-Ewert. "Sleep, Inflammation and Cardiovascular Disease." *Front Biosci (Elite Ed)*. 4 (Jun 1, 2012):2490–501.

65. Möller-Levet, C.S., et al. "Effects of Insufficient Sleep on Circadian Rhythmicity and Expression Amplitude of the Human Blood Transcriptome." *Proc Natl Acad Sci USA* 110(12) (2013):E1132–41.

66. van Leeuwen, W.M., et al. "Sleep Restriction Increases the Risk of Developing Cardiovascular Diseases by Augmenting Proinflammatory Responses through IL-17 and CRP." *PLoS One* 4(2) (2009):e4589.

67. Killick, R., S. Banks, P.Y. Liu. "Implications of Sleep Restriction and Recovery on Metabolic Outcomes." *J Clin Endocrinol Metab* 97(11) (Nov 2012):3876–90. Owens, B., 2013.

68. Kouri, V.P., et al. "Circadian Timekeeping is Disturbed in Rheumatoid Arthritis at Molecular Level." *PLoS One* 8(1) (Jan 15, 2013):e54049.

69. Egermann, M., et al. "Pinealectomy Affects Bone Mineral Density and Structure—An Experimental Study in Sheep." *BMC Musculoskelet Disord* 12 (2011):271.

70. Gossan, N., et al. "The Circadian Clock in Chondrocytes Regulates Genes Controlling Key Aspects of Cartilage Homeostasis." Arthritis Rheum 65(9) (2013):2334–45.

71. Ibid.

72. Ibid.

73. Dolgin, E. "Deprivation: A Wake-Up Call." *Nature* 497(7450) (May 23, 2013):S6–7. Vijayan, V.K. "Morbidities Associated with Obstructive Sleep Apnea." *Expert Rev Respir Med* (Nov 2012) 6(5):557–66.

74. Czeisler, C.A. "Perspective: Casting Light on Sleep Deficiency." *Nature* 497(7450) (May 23, 2013):S13. Eisenstein, M. "Chronobiology: Stepping Out of Time." *Nature* 497(7450) (May 23, 2013):S10–2.

75. Czeisler, C.A. "Perspective: Casting Light on Sleep Deficiency." *Nature* 497(7450) (May 23, 2013):S13.

76. Miller, M.A., F.P. Cappuccio. "Inflammation, Sleep, Obesity and Cardiovascular Disease." *Curr Vasc Pharmacol* 5(2) (Apr 2007):93–102.

77. Lee, Y.C., et al. "The Role of Sleep Problems in Central Pain Processing in Rheumatoid Arthritis." *Arthritis Rheum* 65(1) (Jan 2013):59–68. Lee, A.S., et al. "A Current Review of Molecular Mechanisms Regarding Osteoarthritis and Pain." *Gene* 527(2) (Sep 25, 2013): 440–7.

78. Pattison, D.J., P.G. Winyard. "Dietary Antioxidants in Inflammatory Arthritis: Do They Have Any Role in Etiology or Therapy?" *Nat Clin Pract Rheumatol* 4(11) (Nov 4, 2008):590–6.

79. Hitchon, C.A, H.S. El-Gabalawy. "The Synovium in Rheumatoid Arthritis." *Open Rheumatol J* 5 (2011):107–14.

80. Yun, B.R., et al. "Glutathione S-transferase M1, T1, and P1 Genotypes and Rheumatoid Arthritis." *J Rheumatol* 32(6) (Jun 2005):992–7. Rohr, P., et al. "GSTT1, GSTM1 and GSTP1 Polymorphisms and Susceptibility to Juvenile Idiopathic Arthritis." *Clin Exp Rheumatol* 26(1) (Jan-Feb 2008):151–5.

81. Winyard, P.G., et al. "Measurement and Meaning of Markers of Reactive Species of Oxygen, Nitrogen and Sulfur in Healthy Human Subjects and Patients with Inflammatory Joint Disease." *Biochem Soc Trans* 39(5) (Oct 2011):1226–1232.

82. Strollo, R., et al. "Auto-Antibodies to Post Translationally Modified Type II Collagen as Potential Biomarkers for Rheumatoid Arthritis." *Arthritis Rheum* 65(7) (Jul 2013):1702–12.

83. Hitchon, C.A, H.S. El-Gabalawy. "The Synovium in Rheumatoid Arthritis." *Open Rheumatol J* 5 (2011):107–14.

84. Bazzichi, L., et al. "Impaired Glutathione Reductase Activity and Levels of Collagenase and Elastase in Synovial Fluid in Rheumatoid Arthritis." *Clin Exp Rheumatol* 20(6) (Nov-Dec 2002):761–6.

85. Hitchon, C.A., H.S. El-Gabalawy. "Oxidation in Rheumatoid Arthritis." *Arthritis Res Ther* 6(6) (2004):265–278; Molnar-Kimber, K.L., H.E. Buttram. "Evidence that Intravenous Administration of Glutathione and Vitamin C Relieved Acute Pain from Rheumatoid Arthritis Flare." *Townsend Letter* 304 (Nov 2008): 60–1.

86. Molnar-Kimber, K.L. Rheumatoid-Arthritis-Decisions.com. www.rheumatoid-arthritis-decisions.com (2013) (accessed Jan 2014).

87. Ibid.

88. Pattison, D.J., P.G. Winyard. "Dietary Antioxidants in Inflammatory Arthritis: Do They Have Any Role in Etiology or Therapy?" *Nat Clin Pract Rheumatol* 4(11) (Nov 4, 2008):590–6.

89. Molnar-Kimber, K.L., C.T. Kimber. "Each Type of Cause that Initiates Rheumatoid Arthritis or RA Flares Differentially Affects the Response to Therapy." *Med Hypotheses* 78(1) (Jan 2012):123–9.

90. Yun, B.R., et al. "Glutathione S-transferase M1, T1, and P1 Genotypes and Rheumatoid Arthritis." *J Rheumatol* 32(6) (Jun 2005):992–997. Rohr P, Veit TD, Scheibel I, Xavier RM, Brenol JC, Chies JA, et al. (2008) GSTT1, GSTM1 and GSTP1 polymorphisms and susceptibility to juvenile idiopathic arthritis. Clin Exp Rheumatol. 26:151–155.

91. Pattison, D.J., P.G. Winyard. "Dietary Antioxidants in Inflammatory Arthritis: Do They Have Any Role in Etiology or Therapy?" Nat Clin Pract Rheumatol 4(11) (Nov 4, 2008):590–6.

92. Molnar-Kimber, K.L. Rheumatoid-Arthritis-Decisions.com. www.rheumatoid-arthritis-decisions.com (2013) (accessed Jan 2014).

93. Gaby, A.R. *Nutritional Medicine.* Concord, NH: Fritz Perlberg Pub, 2011; Molnar-Kimber, K.L., C.T. Kimber. "Each Type of Cause that Initiates Rheumatoid Arthritis or RA Flares Differentially Affects the Response to Therapy." Med Hypotheses. 78(1) (Jan 2012):123–9.

94. Molnar-Kimber, K.L. "Will This New Rheumatoid Arthritis Medication or Alternative Therapy Relieve Your Arthritis? 10 Questions to Answer before Starting." Rheumatoid-Arthritis-Decisions.com. (2013) www.rheumatoid-arthritis-decisions.com/New-Rheumatoid-Arthritis-Medication-Questions-before.html (accessed March 2014).

96. Lahiri, M., et al. "Modifiable Risk Factors for RA: Prevention, Better than Cure?" *Rheumatology (Oxford)* 51(3) (Mar 2012):499–512.

96. Molnar-Kimber, K.L. Rheumatoid-Arthritis-Decisions.com. www.rheumatoid-arthritis-decisions.com (2013) (accessed Jan 2014).

97. Cerhan, J.R., et al. "Antioxidant Micronutrients and Risk of Rheumatoid Arthritis in a Cohort of Older Women." *Am J Epidemiol* 57(4) (Feb 15, 2003):345–54. Merlino, L.A., et al. "Vitamin D Intake is Inversely Associated with Rheumatoid Arthritis: Results from the Iowa Women's Health Study." Arthritis Rheum. 50(1) (Jan 2004):72–7.

98. Molnar-Kimber, K.L. Rheumatoid-Arthritis-Decisions.com. www.rheumatoid-arthritis-decisions.com (2013) (accessed Jan 2014).

99. Criswell, L.A., et al. "Smoking Interacts with Genetic Risk Factors in the Development of Rheumatoid Arthritis among Older Caucasian Women." *Ann Rheum Dis* 65(9) (Sep 2006):1163–7.

100. Leirisalo-Repo, M.. "Early Arthritis and Infection." *Curr Opin Rheumatol* 17(4) (Jul 2005):433–9.

101. Zhang, X., et al. "Enzyme Degradation and Proinflammatory Activity in Arthritogenic and Nonarthritogenic Eubacterium aerofaciens Cell Walls." *Infect Immun* 69(12) (Dec 2001):7277–84.

102. Lilea, G.C., et al. "Clinical Particularities and Response to the Anti-Inflammatory Effect of Antiviral Treatment in Patients with Chronic Hepatitis C and Rheumatoid Syn-

drome." *J Med Life* 5(4) (Dec 15, 2012):439–43. Almoallim, H., I. Jali, G. Wali. "Successful Use of Antitumor Necrosis Factor-Alpha Biological Therapy in Managing Human Immunodeficiency Virus-Associated Arthritis: Three Case Studies from Saudi Arabia." *Joint Bone Spine* 80(4) (Jul 2013):426–8. Vassilopoulos, D., L.H. Calabrese. "Viral Hepatitis: Review of Arthritic Complications and Therapy for Arthritis in the Presence of Active HBV/HCV." *Curr Rheumatol Rep* 15(4) (Apr2013):319.

103. Droz N, et al. "Kinetic Profiles and Management of Hepatitis B Virus Reactivation in Patients with Immune-Mediated Inflammatory Diseases." *Arthritis Care Res (Hoboken).* 65(9) (Sep 2013):1504–14.

104. Leirisalo-Repo, M. "Reactive Arthritis." *Scand J Rheumatol* 34(4) (2005):251–9.

105. Tuompo, R., et al. "Reactive Arthritis following Salmonella Infection: A Population-Based Study." *Scand J Rheumatol* 42(3) (2013):196–202.

106. Ogrendik, M. "Effects of Clarithromycin in Patients with Active Rheumatoid Arthritis." *Curr Med Res Opin* 23(Mar 2007):515–22. Ogrendik M. "Rheumatoid Arthritis is an Autoimmune Disease Caused by Periodontal Pathogens." *Int J Gen Med* 6 (2013):383–6.

107. Ogrendik M. "Rheumatoid Arthritis is an Autoimmune Disease Caused by Periodontal Pathogens." *Int J Gen Med* 6 (2013):383–6.

108. Ramírez, A.S., et al. "Relationship between Rheumatoid Arthritis and Mycoplasma Pneumoniae: A Case-Control Study." *Rheumatology (Oxford)* 44(7) (Jul 2005):912–4. Rivera, A., et al. "Experimental Arthritis Induced by a Clinical Mycoplasma Fermentans Isolate." *BMC Musculoskelet Disord* 3(15) (2002). Gil, C., et al. "Presence of Mycoplasma Fermentans in the Bloodstream of Mexican Patients with Rheumatoid Arthritis and IgM and IgG Antibodies against Whole Microorganism." *BMC Musculoskelet Disord* 10 (2009):97. Sato, H., et al. "Hypogammaglobulinemic Patient with Polyarthritis Mimicking Rheumatoid Arthritis Finally Diagnosed as Septic arthritis Caused by Mycoplasma Hominis." Intern Med. 51(4) (2012):425–9.

109. Handelman, G.J., L. Packer, C.E. Cross. "Destruction of Tocopherols, Carotenoids, and Retinol in Human Plasma by Cigarette Smoke. *Am J Clin Nutr* 63(4) (Apr 1996):559–65. Schectman, G., J.C. Byrd, H.W. Gruchow. "The Influence of Smoking on Vitamin C Status in Adults." *Am J Public Health* 79(2) (Feb 1989):158–62. Frikke-Schmidt, et al. "High Dietary Fat and Cholesterol Exacerbates Chronic Vitamin C Deficiency in Guinea Pigs." *Br J Nutr* 105(1) (Jan 2011):54–61.

110. Afridi, H.I., et al. "Interaction between Zinc, Cadmium, and Lead in Scalp Hair Samples of Pakistani and Irish Smokers Rheumatoid Arthritis Subjects in Relation to Controls." *Biol Trace Elem Res* 148(2) (Aug 2012):139–47.

111. Criswell, L.A., et al. "Smoking Interacts with Genetic Risk Factors in the Development of Rheumatoid Arthritis among Older Caucasian Women." *Ann Rheum Dis* 65(9) (Sep 2006):1163–7. Molnar-Kimber KL. "24 Ways to Help Rheumatoid Arthritis Patients Neutralize Toxic Substances, Decrease Exposure and Reduce Your Flares." Rheumatoid-Arthritis-Decisions.com (2013) www.rheumatoid-arthritis-decisions.com/rheumatoid-arthritis-toxic-substances.html. (accessed Mar 2014).

112. Jenkins M. *What's Gotten into Us?: Staying Healthy in a Toxic World.* New York: Random House, 2011.

113. Crinnion, W.J. "Toxic Effects of the Easily Avoidable Phthalates and Parabens." *Altern Med Rev* 15(3) (Sep 2010):190–6.

114. Crinnion, W.J. "Toxic Effects of the Easily Avoidable Phthalates and Parabens."

Altern Med Rev 15(3) (Sep 2010):190–6. Crinnion, W.J. "Do Environmental Toxicants Contribute to Allergy and Asthma?" *Altern Med Rev* 17(1) (Mar 2012):6–18.

115. Vandenberg, L.N., et al. "Human Exposure to Bisphenol A (BPA)." *Reprod Toxicol* 24(2) (Aug-Sep 2007):139–77. Vogt, R., et al. "Cancer and Non-Cancer Health Effects from Food Contaminant Exposures for Children and Adults in California: A Risk Assessment." *Environ Health* 11 (Nov 9, 2012):83.

116. Chun, Z., et al. "Most Plastic Products Release Estrogenic Chemicals: A Potential Health Problem That Can Be Solved." *Environ Health Perspect* 119(7) (2011):989–96.

117. Crinnion, W.J. "Do Environmental Toxicants Contribute to Allergy and Asthma?" *Altern Med Rev* 17(1) (Mar 2012):6–18.

118. Lee, H.G., J.H. Yang. "PCB126 Induces Apoptosis of Chondrocytes via ROS-Dependent Pathways." *Osteoarthritis Cartilage* 20(10) (Oct 2012):1179–85.

119. Crinnion, W.J. "Do Environmental Toxicants Contribute to Allergy and Asthma?" *Altern Med Rev* 17(1) (Mar 2012):6–18.

120. Jenkins M. *What's Gotten into Us? Staying Healthy in a Toxic World.* New York: Random House, 2011.

121. Markowitz, G., D. Rosner. *Lead Wars: The Politics of Science and the Fate of America's Children.* Berkeley, CA: University of California Press, 2013.

122. Madhavan, S., K.D. Rosenman, T. Shehata. "Lead in Soil: Recommended Maximum Permissible Levels." *Environ Res* 49(1) (Jun 1989):136–42.

123. Markowitz, G., D. Rosner. *Lead Wars: The Politics of Science and the Fate of America's Children.* Berkeley, CA: University of California Press, 2013.

124. Afridi, H.I., et al. "Interaction between Zinc, Cadmium, and Lead in Scalp Hair Samples of Pakistani and Irish Smokers Rheumatoid Arthritis Subjects in Relation to Controls." *Biol Trace Elem Res* 148(2) (Aug 2012):139–47. Afridi, H.I., et al. "Evaluation of Status of Arsenic, Cadmium, Lead and Zinc Levels in Biological Samples of Normal and Arthritis Patients of Age Groups (46–60) and (61–75) Years." *Clin Lab* 59(1–2) (2013):143–53.

125. Speck-Hernandez, C.A., G. Montoya-Ortiz. "Silicon, a Possible Link between Environmental Exposure and Autoimmune Diseases: The Case of Rheumatoid Arthritis." *Arthritis* 2012 (2012):604187. doi: 10.1155/2012/604187.

126. Crinnion, W. "Pinch Me, I Must Be Dreaming." *Altern Med Rev* 15(2) (2010): 188–189.

127. Vogt, R., et al. "Cancer and Non-Cancer Health Effects from Food Contaminant Exposures for Children and Adults in California: A Risk Assessment." Environ Health. 11 (Nov 9, 2012):83.

128. Carson, R. *Silent Spring*. 40th anniv ed. New York: Houghton Mifflin Harcourt, 2002. [Originally published 1962.]

129. Szpyrka, E., et al. "Consumer Exposure to Pesticide Residues in Apples from the Region of South-Eastern Poland." *Environ Monit Assess* 185(11) (Nov 2013):8873–8.

130. Kong, Z., et al. "Effect of Home Processing on the Distribution and Reduction of Pesticide Residues in Apples." *Food Addit Contam Part A Chem Anal Control Expo Risk Assess* 29(8) (Aug 2012):1280–7.

131. Fan, A.M., R.J. Jackson. "Pesticides and Food Safety." *Regul Toxicol Pharmacol* 9(2) (Apr 1989):158–74. Cross, P. "Pesticide Hazard Trends in Orchard Fruit Production in

Great Britain from 1992 to 2008: A Time-Series Analysis." *Pest Manag Sci* (Jun 2013) 69(6) (2013):768–74.

132. Vogt, R., et al. "Cancer and Non-Cancer Health Effects from Food Contaminant Exposures for Children and Adults in California: A Risk Assessment." *Environ Health* 11 (Nov 9, 2012):83.

133. Crinnion, W.J. "Polychlorinated Biphenyls: Persistent Pollutants with Immunological, Neurological, and Endocrinological Consequences." *Altern Med Rev* 16(1) (Mar 2011):5–13.

134. Cutler, G.C., C.D. Scott-Dupree, D.M. Drexler. "Honey Bees, Neonicotinoids and Bee Incident Reports: The Canadian Situation." *Pest Manag Sci* (Jul 19, 2013): doi: 10.1002/ps.3613. [Epub ahead of print]. Di Prisco, G., et al. "Neonicotinoid Clothianidin Adversely Affects Insect Immunity and Promotes Replication of a Viral Pathogen in Honey Bees." *Proc Natl Acad Sci USA* (Oct 21, 2013). [Epub ahead of print]. Pettis, J.S., et al. "Crop Pollination Exposes Honey Bees to Pesticides Which Alters Their Susceptibility to the Gut pathogen Nosema Ceranae." *PLoS One* 8(7) (Jul 24, 2013):e70182. doi: 10.1371/journal.pone.0070182.

135. Robbins, J. "The Year the Monarch Didn't Appear." *The New York Times Sunday Review* (Nov 24, 2013):SR9. www.nytimes.com/2013/1$^{1}/_{2}$4/sunday-review/the-year-the-monarch-didnt-appear.html (accessed Mar 2014).

136. Vogt, R., et al. "Cancer and Non-Cancer Health Effects from Food Contaminant Exposures for Children and Adults in California: A Risk Assessment." *Environ Health* 11 (Nov 9, 2012):83.

137. Séralini, G.E., et al. "Long Term Toxicity of a Roundup Herbicide and a Roundup-Tolerant Genetically Modified Maize." *Food Chem Toxicol* 50(11) (Nov 2012):4221–31.

138. Séralini, G.E., et al. "Answers to Critics: Why There is a Long Term Toxicity Due to a Roundup-Tolerant Genetically Modified Maize and to a Roundup Herbicide." *Food Chem Toxicol* 53 (2013):476–483.

139. Alliance for Natural Health. Demon Weeds and Human Health Impacts. (2013) www.anh-usa.org/gmo (accessed Mar 2014).

140. United States Department of Agriculture (USDA). Biotechnology Regulatory Services. "Okanagan Specialty Fruits Inc. Petition for Determination of Nonregulated Status: Arctic™ Apple (*Malus x domestica*) Events GD743 and GS784." (Jul 13, 2012) www.aphis.usda.gov/brs/aphisdocs/10_16101p.pdf (accessed Mar 2014). Arctic Apples. "USDA APHIS Open 2nd Comment Period for Arctic Apples." (Nov 8, 2013) www.arcticapples.com/blog/neal/usda-aphis-open-2nd-comment-period-arctic%C2%AE-apples (accessed Mar 2014).

141. Lewis, J. "The Birth of EPA." United States Environmental Protection Agency [*EPA Journal* Nov 1985] (2013) http://www2.epa.gov/aboutepa/birth-epa (accessed Mar 2014).

142. Vogt, R., et al. "Cancer and Non-Cancer Health Effects from Food Contaminant Exposures for Children and Adults in California: A Risk Assessment." *Environ Health* 11 (Nov 9, 2012):83.

143. Levy, T.E. *Primal Panacea.* Henderson, NV: MedFox Publishing, 2011.

144. Nebert, D.W., D.W. Russell. "Clinical Importance of the Cytochromes P450." *Lancet* 360(9340) (Oct 12, 2002):1155–62.

145. Gambhir, J.K., P. Lali, A.K. Jain. "Correlation between Blood Antioxidant Levels and Lipid Peroxidation in Rheumatoid Arthritis." *Clin Biochem* 30(4) (Jun 1997):351–5.

Hitchon, C.A., H.S. El-Gabalawy. "Oxidation in Rheumatoid Arthritis." *Arthritis Res Ther* 6(6) (2004):265–278. Valko, M., et al. "Free Radicals and Antioxidants in Normal Physiological Functions and Human Disease." *Int J Biochem Cell Biol* 39(1) (2007):44–84.

146. Dickinson, B.C., et al. "Nox2 redox signaling maintains essential cell populations in the brain." *Nat Chem Biol* 7(2) (Feb 2011):106–12.

147. Gelderman, K.A., et al. "T Cell Surface Redox Levels Determine T Cell Reactivity and Arthritis Susceptibility." *Proc Natl Acad Sci USA* 103(34) (Aug 22, 2006):12831–6. Hultqvist, M., et al. "A New Arthritis Therapy with Oxidative Burst Inducers." *PLoS Med* 3(9) (Sep 2006):e348.

148. Valko, M., H. Morris, M.T. Cronin. "Metals, Toxicity and Oxidative Stress." *Curr Med Chem* 12(10) (2005):1161–1208.

149. Biniecka, M., et al. "Hypoxia Induces Mitochondrial Mutagenesis and Dysfunction in Inflammatory Arthritis." *Arthritis Rheum* 63(8) (Aug 2011):2172–82.

150. Agency for Toxic Substances & Disease Registry (ATSDR). "Minimal Risk Levels List." (Jul 2013) www.atsdr.cdc.gov/mrls/mrllist.asp (accessed Mar 2014). Centers for Disease Control and Prevention (CDC). "Lead." (Dec 18, 2013) www.cdc.gov/nceh/lead (accessed Mar 2014).

151. Jenkins M. *What's Gotten into Us? Staying Healthy in a Toxic World.* New York: Random House, 2011.

152. Crinnion, W.J. "Do Environmental Toxicants Contribute to Allergy and Asthma?" *Altern Med Rev* 17(1) (Mar 2012):6–18.

153. Simelyte, E., D.L. Boyle, G.S. Firestein. "DNA Mismatch Repair Enzyme Expression in Synovial Tissue." *Ann Rheum Dis* 63(12) (Dec 2004):1695–9.

154. Crinnion, W.J. "Do Environmental Toxicants Contribute to Allergy and Asthma?" *Altern Med Rev* 17(1) (Mar 2012):6–18.

155. Schafer, F.Q., G.R. Buettner. "Redox Environment of the Cell As Viewed through the Redox State of the Glutathione Disulfide/Glutathione Couple." *Free Radic Biol Med.* 30(11) (Jun 1, 2001):1191–212. Valko, M., H. Morris, M.T. Cronin. "Metals, Toxicity and Oxidative Stress." *Curr Med Chem* 12(10) (2005):1161–1208.

156. Hassan, M.Q., et al. "The Glutathione Defense System in the Pathogenesis of Rheumatoid Arthritis." *J Appl Toxicol* 21(1) (Jan-Feb 2001):69–73. Jaswal, S., et al. "Antioxidant Status in Rheumatoid Arthritis and Role of Antioxidant Therapy." *Clin Chim Acta* 338(1–2) (Dec 2003):123–9. Kamanli, A., et al. "Plasma Lipid Peroxidation and Antioxidant Levels in Patients with Rheumatoid Arthritis." *Cell Biochem Funct* 22(1) (Jan-Feb 2004):53–57. Pedersen-Lane, J.H., R.B. Zurier, D.A. Lawrence. "Analysis of the Thiol Status of Peripheral Blood Leukocytes in Rheumatoid Arthritis Patients." *J Leukoc Biol* 81(4) (Apr 2007):934–41.

157. Jacobson, G.A., et al. "Plasma Glutathione Peroxidase (GSH-Px) Concentration Is Elevated in Rheumatoid Arthritis: A Case-Control Study." *Clin Rheumatol* 31(11) (Nov 2012):1543–7.

158. Hassan, M.Q., et al. "The Glutathione Defense System in the Pathogenesis of Rheumatoid Arthritis." *J Appl Toxicol* 21(1) (Jan-Feb 2001):69–73. Kamanli, A., et al. "Plasma Lipid Peroxidation and Antioxidant Levels in Patients with Rheumatoid Arthritis." *Cell Biochem Funct* 22(1) (Jan-Feb 2004):53–57. Sarban, S., et al. "Plasma Total Antioxidant Capacity, Lipid Peroxidation, and Erythrocyte Antioxidant Enzyme Activities in Patients with Rheumatoid Arthritis and Osteoarthritis." *Clin Biochem* 38(11) (Nov

2005):981–6. Seven, A., et al. "Lipid, Protein, DNA Oxidation and Antioxidant Status in Rheumatoid Arthritis." *Clin Biochem* 41(7–8) (May 2008):538–43.

159. Hassan, M.Q., et al. "The Glutathione Defense System in the Pathogenesis of Rheumatoid Arthritis." *J Appl Toxicol* 21(1) (Jan-Feb 2001):69–73. Pedersen-Lane, J.H., R.B. Zurier, D.A. Lawrence. "Analysis of the Thiol Status of Peripheral Blood Leukocytes in Rheumatoid Arthritis Patients." *J Leukoc Biol* 81(4) (Apr 2007):934–41.

160. Hassan, S.Z., et al. "Oxidative Stress in Systemic Lupus Erythematosus and Rheumatoid Arthritis Patients: Relationship to Disease Manifestations and Activity." *Int J Rheum Dis* 14(4) (Oct 2011):325–31.

161. Yu, D.H., et al. "Over-Expression of Extracellular Superoxide Dismutase in Mouse Synovial Tissue Attenuates the Inflammatory Arthritis." *Exp Mol Med* 44(9) (Sep 30, 2012):529–35.

162. Molnar-Kimber, K.L., H.E. Buttram. "Evidence that Intravenous Administration of Glutathione and Vitamin C Relieved Acute Pain from Rheumatoid Arthritis Flare." *Townsend Letter* 304 (Nov 2008): 60–1.

163. Karatas F, et al. "Antioxidant Status & Lipid Peroxidation in Patients with Rheumatoid Arthritis." *Indian J Med Res* 118 (Oct 2003):178–81.

164. Miao, X., et al. "Zinc Homeostasis in the Metabolic Syndrome and Diabetes." *Front Med* 7(1) (Mar 2013):31–52. doi: 10.1007/s11684-013-0251-9.

165. Afridi, H.I., et al. "Evaluation of Status of Arsenic, Cadmium, Lead and Zinc Levels in Biological Samples of Normal and Arthritis Patients of Age Groups (46–60) and (61–75) Years." *Clin Lab* 59(1–2) (2013):143–53.

166. Molnar-Kimber, K.L. Rheumatoid-Arthritis-Decisions.com. http:// www.rheumatoid-arthritis-decisions.com (2013) (accessed Jan 2014).

167. Aesoph, L.M. *How to Eat Away Arthritis: Gain Relief from the Pain and Discomfort of Arthritis Through Nature's Remedies.* New York: Prentice Hall Press, 1996. Allan, B. *Conquering Arthritis: What Doctors Don't Tell You Because They Don't Know (9 Secrets I Learned the Hard Way).* 2nd ed. Phoenix: Shining Prairie Flower Productions, 2009. Gerson, C. *Defeating Arthritis, Bone and Joint Diseases.* Carmel, CA: Gerson Health Media, 2011.

168. Boyce, J.A., et al. "Guidelines for the Diagnosis and Management of Food Allergy in the United States: Summary of the NIAID-Sponsored Expert Panel Report." *Nutrition* 27 (2011):253–67.

169. Peltonen, R., et al. "Faecal Microbial Flora and Disease Activity in Rheumatoid Arthritis During a Vegan Diet." *Br J Rheumatol* 36(1) (Jan 1997):64–8. Zhang, X., et al. "Enzyme Degradation and Proinflammatory Activity in Arthritogenic and Nonarthritogenic Eubacterium aerofaciens Cell Walls." *Infect Immun* 69(12) (Dec 2001):7277–84. Mandel, D.R., K. Eichas, J. Holmes. "Bacillus Coagulans: A Viable Adjunct Therapy for Relieving Symptoms of Rheumatoid Arthritis According to a Randomized, Controlled Trial." *BMC Complement Altern Med* 10 (Jan 12, 2010):1.

170. Mandel, D.R., K. Eichas, J. Holmes. "Bacillus Coagulans: A Viable Adjunct Therapy for Relieving Symptoms of Rheumatoid Arthritis According to a Randomized, Controlled Trial." *BMC Complement Altern Med* 10 (Jan 12, 2010):1.

171. Saul, A. *Doctor Yourself: Natural Healing That Works.* 2nd edition. Laguna Beach, CA: Basic Health Publications, 2012. www.doctoryourself.com.

172. Hagel, A.F., et al. "Intravenous Infusion of Ascorbic Acid Decreases Serum Histamine

Concentrations in Patients with Allergic and Non-Allergic Diseases." *Naunyn Schmiedebergs Arch Pharmacol* 386(9) (Sep 2013):789–93. Hemilä, H. "Vitamin C and Common Cold-Induced Asthma: A Systematic Review and Statistical Analysis." *Allergy Asthma Clin Immunol* 9(1) (Nov 26, 2013):9–46.

173. Buchanan, H.M., et al. "Is Diet Important in Rheumatoid Arthritis?" *Br J Rheumatol* 30(2) (Apr 1991):125–34. Denton, C. "The Elimination/Challenge Diet." *Minn Med* 98(12) (Dec 2012):43–4. www.minnesotamedicine.com/PastIssues/December2012/theeliminationchallengediet.aspx

174. Boyce, J.A., et al. "Guidelines for the Diagnosis and Management of Food Allergy in the United States: Summary of the NIAID-Sponsored Expert Panel Report." *Nutrition* 27 (2011):253–67. Skypala, I. "Adverse Food Reactions—An Emerging Issue for Adults." *J Am Diet Assoc* 111(12) (Dec 2011):1877–91.

175. Denton, C. "The Elimination/Challenge Diet." *Minn Med* 98(12) (Dec 2012):43–4. www.minnesotamedicine.com/PastIssues/December2012/theeliminationchallengediet.aspx. Molnar-Kimber, K.L. "Optimal Rheumatoid Arthritis Nutrition." Rheumatoid-Arthritis-Decisions.com (2013) www.rheumatoid-arthritis-decisions.com/rheumatoid-arthritis-nutrition.html (accessed Mar 2014).

176. Gaby, A.R. *Nutritional Medicine.* Concord, NH: Fritz Perlberg, 2011.

177. Ibid.

178. Denton, C. "The Elimination/Challenge Diet." *Minn Med* 98(12) (Dec 2012):43–4. www.minnesotamedicine.com/PastIssues/December2012/theeliminationchallengediet.aspx

179. Campbell, T.C., T.M. Campbell, II. *The China Study: The Most Comprehensive Study of Nutrition Ever Conducted and Startling Implications for Diet, Weight Loss, and Long-Term Health.* Dallas, TX: Ben-Bella Books, 2006. Esselstyn, C.B. *Prevent and Reverse Heart Disease: The Revolutionary, Scientifically Proven, Nutrition-Based Cure.* New York: Avery, 2008. Pollan, M. *In Defense of Food: An Eater's Manifesto.* New York: Penguin, 2009. Davis. W. *Wheat Belly: Lose the Wheat, Lose the Weight, and Find Your Path Back to Health.* Emmaus, PA: Rodale Books, 2011. Campbell, T.C. *Whole: Rethinking the Science of Nutrition.* Dallas, TX: BenBella Books, 2013. Perlmutter, D. *Grain Brain: The Surprising Truth about Wheat, Carbs, and Sugar—Your Brain's Silent Killers.* Boston, Little, Brown and Company, 2013.

180. Molnar-Kimber, K.L., C.T. Kimber. "Each Type of Cause that Initiates Rheumatoid Arthritis or RA Flares Differentially Affects the Response to Therapy." *Med Hypotheses* 78(1) (Jan 2012):123–9.

181. Lahiri, M., et al. "Modifiable Risk Factors for RA: Prevention, Better than Cure?" *Rheumatology (Oxford)* 51(3) (Mar 2012):499–512.

182. Molnar-Kimber KL. "24 Ways to Help Rheumatoid Arthritis Patients Neutralize Toxic Substances, Decrease Exposure and Reduce Your Flares." Rheumatoid-Arthritis-Decisions.com (2013) www.rheumatoid-arthritis-decisions.com/rheumatoid-arthritis-toxic-substances.html. (accessed Mar 2014).

183. Molnar-Kimber, K.L. Rheumatoid-Arthritis-Decisions.com. http:// www.rheumatoid-arthritis-decisions.com (2013) (accessed Jan 2014).

184. Nowlin, S.Y., M.J. Hammer, G. D'Eramo Melkus. "Diet, Inflammation, and Glycemic Control in Type 2 Diabetes: An Integrative Review of the Literature." *J Nutr Metab* 2012 (2012):542698. Solarz, D.E., J.M. Mullington, H.K. Meier-Ewert, 2012. Ong, K.L., et al. "Arthritis: Its Prevalence, Risk Factors, and Association with Cardiovascular Diseases in the United States, 1999 to 2008." *Ann Epidemiol* 23(2) (Feb 2013):80–6.

185. Levy, T.E. *Primal Panacea.* Henderson, NV: MedFox Publishing, 2011. Levy, T.E. *Death by Calcium.* Henderson, NV: MedFox Publishing, 2013. Pfister, R., et al. "Plasma Vitamin C Predicts Incident Heart Failure in Men and Women in European Prospective Investigation into Cancer and Nutrition-Norfolk Prospective Study." *Am Heart J* 162(2) (Aug 2011):246–53.

186. Ong, K.L., et al. "Arthritis: Its Prevalence, Risk Factors, and Association with Cardiovascular Diseases in the United States, 1999 to 2008." *Ann Epidemiol* 23(2) (Feb 2013):80–6.

187. Maradit-Kremers, H., et al. "Increased Unrecognized Coronary Heart Disease and Sudden Deaths in Rheumatoid Arthritis: A Population-Based Cohort Study." *Arthritis Rheum* 52(2) (Feb 2005):402–11. John, H., T.E. Toms, G.D. Kitas. "Rheumatoid Arthritis: Is It a Coronary Heart Disease Equivalent?" *Curr Opin Cardiol* 26(4) (Jul 2011):327–33. Ong, K.L., et al. "Arthritis: Its Prevalence, Risk Factors, and Association with Cardiovascular Diseases in the United States, 1999 to 2008." *Ann Epidemiol* 23(2) (Feb 2013):80–6.

188. Ong, K.L., et al. "Arthritis: Its Prevalence, Risk Factors, and Association with Cardiovascular Diseases in the United States, 1999 to 2008." *Ann Epidemiol* 23(2) (Feb 2013):80–6.

189. Addimanda, O., et al. "Clinical Associations in Patients with Hand Osteoarthritis." *Scand J Rheumatol* 41(4) (Aug 2012):310–3.

190. Suri, P., et al. "Vascular Disease is Associated with Facet Joint Osteoarthritis." *Osteoarthritis Cartilage* 18(9) (Sep 2010):1127–32.

191. Hickey, S., H. Roberts. *Tarnished Gold: The Sickness of Evidence-based Medicine.* CreateSpace Independent Publishing, 2011. Levy, T.E. *Primal Panacea.* Henderson, NV: MedFox Publishing, 2011.

192. Levy, T.E. *Stop America's #1 Killer: Reversible Vitamin Deficiency Found to be Origin of All Coronary Heart Disease.* Henderson, NV: Livon Books, 2006. Levy, T.E. *Primal Panacea.* Henderson, NV: MedFox Publishing, 2011.

193. Monin, J.K., et al. "Spouses' Cardiovascular Reactivity to Their Partners' Suffering." *J Gerontol B Psychol Sci Soc Sci* 65B(2) (Mar 2010):195–201.

194. Meadows, S. "The Boy with a Thorn in His Joints." *The New York Times Magazine* (Feb 1, 2013) www.nytimes.com/2013/02/03/magazine/the-boy-with-a-thorn-in-his-joints.html

195. Cordain, L., et al. "Modulation of Immune Function by Dietary Lectins in Rheumatoid Arthritis." *Br J Nutr* 83(3) (Mar 2000):207–17.

196. Debnath, T., H. Kim da, B.O. Lim. "Natural Products as a Source of Anti-Inflammatory Agents Associated with Inflammatory Bowel Disease." *Molecules* 18(6) (Jun 19, 2013):7253–70.

197. Barrett, J.S. "Extending Our Knowledge of Fermentable, Short-Chain Carbohydrates for Managing Gastrointestinal Symptoms." *Nutr Clin Pract* 28(3) (Jun 2013):300–6. Muir, J.G., P.R. Gibson. "The Low FODMAP Diet for Treatment of Irritable Bowel Syndrome and Other Gastrointestinal Disorders." *Gastroenterol Hepatol* (NY) 9(7) (Jul 2013):450–2.

198. Rashid, T., C. Wilson, A. Ebringer. "The Link between Ankylosing Spondylitis, Crohn's Disease, Klebsiella, and Starch Consumption." *Clin Dev Immunol* 2013 (2013):872632.

199. Cathcart, R.F. "Vitamin C, Titrating to Bowel Tolerance, Anascorbemia, and Acute Induced Scurvy." *Medical Hypotheses* 7(11) (Nov 1981):1359–76. Saul, A. *Doctor Your-*

self: Natural Healing That Works. 2nd edition. Laguna Beach, CA: Basic Health Publications, 2012. www.doctoryourself.com.

200. Cousins, N. *Anatomy of an Illness: As Perceived by the Patient.* Reprint ed. New York: W W Norton & Company; 1967, 2005.

201. Cathcart, R.F. "Vitamin C, Titrating to Bowel Tolerance, Anascorbemia, and Acute Induced Scurvy." *Medical Hypotheses* 7(11) (Nov 1981):1359–76.

202. Rashid, T., C. Wilson, A. Ebringer. "The Link between Ankylosing Spondylitis, Crohn's Disease, Klebsiella, and Starch Consumption." *Clin Dev Immunol* 2013 (2013):872632.

203. Ogrendik, M. "Treatment of Ankylosing Spondylitis with Moxifloxacin." *South Med J* 100(4) (Apr 2007):366–70.

204. Rashid, T., C. Wilson, A. Ebringer. "The Link between Ankylosing Spondylitis, Crohn's Disease, Klebsiella, and Starch Consumption." *Clin Dev Immunol* 2013 (2013):872632.

205. Richette, P., T. Bardin. "Gout." *Lancet* 375(9711) (Jan 23, 2010):318–28.

206. Weaver, A.L. "Epidemiology of Gout." *Cleve Clin J Med* 75 Suppl 5 (Jul 2008):S9–12. Zhu, Y., B.J. Pandya, H.K. Choi. "Prevalence of Gout and Hyperuricemia in the US General Population: The National Health and Nutrition Examination Survey 2007–2008." *Arthritis Rheum* 63(10) (Oct 2011):3136–41.

207. Richette, P., T. Bardin. "Gout." *Lancet* 375(9711) (Jan 23, 2010):318–28.

208. Harrold, L. "New Developments in Gout." *Curr Opin Rheumatol* 25(3) (May 2013):304–9.

209. Weaver, A.L. "Epidemiology of Gout." *Cleve Clin J Med* 75 Suppl 5 (Jul 2008):S9–12.

210. Richette, P., T. Bardin. "Gout." *Lancet* 375(9711) (Jan 23, 2010):318–28. Bottiglieri, S., et al. "Gemcitabine-Induced Gouty Arthritis Attacks." *J Oncol Pharm Pract* 19(3) (Sep 2013):284–8.

211. Marickar, Y.M. "Calcium Oxalate Stone and Gout." *Urol Res* 37(6) (Dec 2009):345–7. Gaby, A.R. *Nutritional Medicine.* Concord, NH: Fritz Perlberg Pub, 2011.

212. Richette, P., T. Bardin. "Gout." *Lancet* 375(9711) (Jan 23, 2010):318–28.

213. DiCarlo, E.F., L.B. Kahn. "Inflammatory Diseases of the Bones and Joints." *Semin Diagn Pathol* 28(1) (Feb 2011):53–64.

214. Burrascano, J.J. "Advanced Topics in Lyme Disease: Diagnostic Hints and Treatment Guidelines for Lyme and Other Tick Borne Illneses." 16th ed. (Oct 2008) www.lymenet.org/BurrGuide200810.pdf (accessed Mar 2014).

215. Pollack, R.J., S.R. Telford 3rd, A. Spielman. "Standardization of Medium for Culturing Lyme Disease Spirochetes." *J Clin Microbiol* 31(5) (May 1993):1251–5.

216. Burrascano, J.J. "Advanced Topics in Lyme Disease: Diagnostic Hints and Treatment Guidelines for Lyme and Other Tick Borne Illneses." 16th ed. (Oct 2008) www.lymenet.org/BurrGuide200810.pdf (accessed Mar 2014).

217. IGeneX. "A Reference Laboratory Specializing in State of the Art Clinical and Research Testing for Lyme Disease and Associated Tick-Borne Diseases." (2013) http://igenex.com (accessed Mar 2014). International Lyme and Associated Diseases Society (ILADS). "What You Should Know About Lyme Disease." IGenex, Inc., (July 2002) www.ilads.org/lyme_research/lyme_articles6.html (accessed Jan 2014). Lyme Disease Asso-

ciation of Southeastern Pennsylvania (LDASEPA) http://lympa.org/index.html (accessed Mar 2014).

218. Burrascano, J.J. "Advanced Topics in Lyme Disease: Diagnostic Hints and Treatment Guidelines for Lyme and Other Tick Borne Illneses." 16th ed. (Oct 2008) www.lymenet.org/BurrGuide200810.pdf (accessed Mar 2014).

219. Rivera, A., et al. "Experimental Arthritis Induced by a Clinical Mycoplasma Fermentans Isolate." *BMC Musculoskelet Disord* 3(15) (2002). Ramírez, A.S., et al. "Relationship between Rheumatoid Arthritis and Mycoplasma Pneumoniae: A Case-Control Study." *Rheumatology* (*Oxford*) 44(7) (Jul 2005):912–4. Nicolson, G.L. "Chronic Bacterial and Viral Infections in Neurodegenerative and Neurobehavioral Diseases." *Lab Med* 39(5) (2008):291–9. Nicolson, G.L., J. Haier. "Role of Chronic Bacterial and Viral Infections in Neurodegenerative, Neurobehavioural, Psychiatric, Autoimmune and Fatiguing Illnesses: Part 2." *BJMP* 3(1) (2010):301. Smith, B.G., et al. "Lyme Disease and the Orthopaedic Implications of Lyme Arthritis." *J Am Acad Orthop Surg* 19(2) (Feb 2011):91–100.

220. Smith, B.G., et al. "Lyme Disease and the Orthopaedic Implications of Lyme Arthritis." *J Am Acad Orthop Surg* 19(2) (Feb 2011):91–100.

221. Zhang, Q.C., Y. Zhang. *Lyme Disease and Modern Chinese Medicine.* Sino-Med Research Institute, 2006.

222. Singleton, K.B. *The Lyme Disease Solution.* Dallas: BookSurge Publishing, 2008. Strasheim, C. *Insights Into Lyme Disease Treatment: 13 Lyme-Literate Health Care Practitioners Share Their Healing Strategies.* BioMed Publishing Group, 2009.

223. Burrascano, J.J. "Advanced Topics in Lyme Disease: Diagnostic Hints and Treatment Guidelines for Lyme and Other Tick Borne Illneses." 16th ed. (Oct 2008) www.lymenet.org/BurrGuide200810.pdf (accessed Mar 2014).

224. Embers, M.E., S. Narasimhan. "Vaccination Against Lyme Disease: Past, Present, and Future." *Front Cell Infect Microbiol* 3 (2013): 6. Centers for Disease Control (CDC). "CDC Provides Estimate of Americans Diagnosed with Lyme Disease Each Year." (Aug 19, 2013): www.cdc.gov/media/releases/2013/p0819-lyme-disease.html (accessed Apr 2014).

225. European Concerted Action on Lyme Borreliosis (EUCALB) 2013. www.eucalb.com (accessed Mar 2014).

226. IGeneX. "A Reference Laboratory Specializing in State of the Art Clinical and Research Testing for Lyme Disease and Associated Tick-Borne Diseases." (2013) http://igenex.com (accessed Mar 2014). International Lyme and Associated Diseases Society (ILADS). "What You Should Know About Lyme Disease." IGenex, Inc., (July 2002) www.ilads.org/lyme_research/lyme_articles6.html (accessed Jan 2014). Lyme Disease Association of Southeastern Pennsylvania (LDASEPA) http://lympa.org/index.html (accessed Mar 2014).

Chapter 4. What Genetics Can Teach Us about Arthritis

1. U.S. Department of Health & Human Services. NIH Research Portfolio Online Reporting Tools (RePORT). "Estimates of Funding for Various Research, Condition, and Disease Categories. (RCDC)." (Mar 7, 2014): http://report.nih.gov/categorical_spending.aspx (accessed Apr 2014).

2. U.S. National Library of Medicine. "PubMed Health Database." (2013) www.ncbi.nlm.nih.gov/pubmedhealth/ (accessed Apr 2014).

3. OMIM. Online Mendelian Inheritance in Man (2014) www.ncbi.nlm.nih.gov/omim. (accessed Apr 2014).

4. Ibid.

5. Hefti, R. "Anti-Vitamin Publications: Misinformation Presented As Truth" Orthomolecular News Service (OMNS). Jul 18, 2013. http://orthomolecular.org/resources/omns/v09n14.shtml (accessed Apr 2014).

6. Lazarou, J., B. Pomeranz, P.N. Corey. "Incidence of Adverse Drug Reactions in Hospitalized Patients: A Meta-Analysis of Prospective Studies." *JAMA* 279(15) (Apr 15, 1998):1200–5. Institute of Medicine (IOM): Committee on Quality of Health Care in America. "To Err is Human: Building a Safer Health System." Washington, DC: National Academy Press; 2000. Available at: www.nap.edu/openbook.php?isbn=0309068371. Starfield, B. "Is US Health Really the Best in the World?" *JAMA*. 284(4) (Jul 26, 2000):483–5. Centers for Disease Control (CDC). "Drug Overdose in the United States: Fact Sheet."(2013): www.cdc.gov/homeandrecreationalsafety/overdose/facts.html. (accessed Apr 2014). U.S. Food and Drug Administration (FDA). "Preventable Adverse Drug Reactions: A Focus on Drug Interactions. (2013): www.fda.gov/drugs/developmentapprovalprocess/developmentresources/druginteractionslabeling/ucm110632.htm. (accessed Apr 2014).

7. OMIM. Online Mendelian Inheritance in Man (2014) www.ncbi.nlm.nih.gov/omim. (accessed Apr 2014).

8. see also Reynard, L.N., J. Loughlin. "The Genetics and Functional Analysis of Pprimary Osteoarthritis Susceptibility." *Expert Rev Mol Med* 15 (Feb 18, 2013):e2. doi: 10.1017/erm.2013.4.

9. Gropper, S.S., J.L. Smith. *Advanced Nutrition and Human Metabolism,* 6th edition. New York: Cengage Learning, 2013.

10. Chen, C.G., et al. "Chondrocyte-Intrinsic Smad3 Represses Runx2-Inducible Matrix Metalloproteinase 13 Expression to Maintain Articular Cartilage and PreventOsteoarthritis." *Arthritis Rheum* 64(10) (Oct 2012):3278–89.

11. Li, J., et al. "Resveratrol Inhibits Renal Fibrosis in the Obstructed Kidney: Potential Role in Deacetylation of Smad3." *Am J Pathol* 177(3) (Sep 2010):1065–71.

12. Parcell, S. "Sulfur in Human Nutrition and Applications in Medicine." *Altern Med Rev* 7(1) (Feb 2002):22–44.

13. Vanhees, K., et al. "You Are What You Eat, and So Are Your Children: The Impact of Micronutrients on the Epigenetic Programming of Offspring." *Cell Mol Life Sci* 71(2) (Jan 2014):1427–9.

14. Stein, A.D., et al. "Anthropometric Measures in Middle Age after Exposure to Famine During Gestation: Evidence from the Dutch Famine." *Am J Clin Nutr* 85(3) (2007):869–876.

15. Gut, P., E. Verdin. "The Nexus of Chromatin Regulation and Intermediary Metabolism." *Nature* 502(7472) (2013):489–498.

16. Ibid.

17. Apostolou, E., K. Hochedlinger. "Chromatin Dynamics during Cellular Reprogramming." *Nature*. 502(7472) (2013):462–471.

18. Gut, P., E. Verdin. "The Nexus of Chromatin Regulation and Intermediary Metabolism." *Nature* 502(7472) (2013):489–498.

19. Kaati, G., et al. "Transgenerational Response to Nutrition, Early Life Circumstances and Longevity." *Eur J Hum Genet.* 15(7) (Jul 2007):784–90.

20. van Ommen B. "Personalized Nutrition from a Health Perspective: Luxury or Necessity?" *Genes Nutr* 2(1) (Oct 2007):3–4.

21. Nicholson, J.K., et al."Metabolic Phenotyping in Clinical and Surgical Environments." *Nature* 491 (2012):384–392.

22. Human Genome Project. http://web.ornl.gov/sci/techresources/Human_Genome/project/index.shtml. (accessed Apr 2014).

23. Parcell, S. "Sulfur in Human Nutrition and Applications in Medicine." *Altern Med Rev* 7(1) (Feb 2002):22–44.

24. Institute of Medicine (IOM). Panel on Dietary Reference Intakes for Electrolytes and Water. "Dietary Reference Intakes for Water, Potassium, Sodium, Chloride, and Sulfate." (2005): http://books.nap.edu/openbook.php?record_id=10925

25. Usha, P.R., M.U. Naidu."Randomised, Double-Blind, Parallel, Placebo-Controlled Study of Oral Glucosamine, Methylsulfonylmethane and their Combination in Osteoarthritis." *Clin Drug Investig* 24(6) (2004):353–63. Kim, L.S., et al. "Efficacy of Methylsulfonylmethane (MSM) in Osteoarthritis Pain of the Knee: A Pilot Clinical Trial." Osteoarthritis Cartilage. 14(3) . (Mar 2006):286–94. Debbi, E.M., et al. "Efficacy of Methylsulfonylmethane Supplementation on Osteoarthritis of the Knee: A Randomized Controlled Study." *BMC Complement Altern Med* 11 (Jun 27, 2011):50. Notarnicola, A., et al. "The "MESACA" Study: Methylsulfonylmethane and Boswellic Acids in the Treatment of Gonarthrosis." *Adv Ther* 28(10) (Oct 2011):894–906.

26. di Padova, C. "S-Adenosylmethionine in the Treatment of Osteoarthritis. Review of the Clinical Studies." *Am J Med* 83(5A) (Nov 20, 1987):60–5. Harmand, M.F., et al. "Effects of S-Adenosylmethionine on Human Articular Chondrocyte Differentiation. An In Vitro Study." *Am J Med* 83(5A) (Nov 20, 1987):48–54.

27. Gaby, A.R. *Nutritional Medicine.* Concord, NH: Fritz Perlberg Pub, 2011.

28. Wrenn, K.D., F. Murphy, C.M. Slovis. "A toxicity study of parenteral thiamine hydrochloride." *Ann Emerg Med* 18(8) (1980):867–870.

29. Nakada, T., R.T. Knight. "Alcohol and the Central Nervous System." *Med Clin North Am* 68(1) (Jan 1984):121–131. Lindberg, M,C,, R.A. Oyler. "Wernicke's Encephalopathy." *Am Fam Physician* 41(4) (Apr 1990):1205–9.

30. McCann, J.C., B.N. Ames. "Vitamin K, An Example of Triage Theory: Is Micronutrient Inadequacy Linked to Diseases of Aging?" *Am J Clin Nutr* 90(4) (Oct 2009):889–907.

31. McCann, J.C., B.N. Ames. "Vitamin K, An Example of Triage Theory: Is Micronutrient Inadequacy Linked to Diseases of Aging?" *Am J Clin Nutr* 90(4) (Oct 2009):889–907. Theuwissen, E., E. Smit, C. Vermeer. "The Role of Vitamin K in Soft-Tissue Calcification." *Adv Nutr* 3(2) (Mar 2012):166–173.

32. Ishii, Y., et al. "Distribution of Vitamin K2 in Subchondral Bone in Osteoarthritic Knee Joints." *Knee Surg Sports Traumatol Arthrosc* 21(8) (2013):1813–8.

33. Gropper, S.S., J.L. Smith. *Advanced Nutrition and Human Metabolism,* 6th edition. New York: Cengage Learning, 2013.

34. Nakagawa, K. "Biological Significance and Metabolic Activation of Vitamin K." *Yakugaku Zasshi* 133(12) (2013):1337–41.

35. Morishita, T., et al. "Production of Menaquinones by Lactic Acid Bacteria." *J Dairy Sci* 82(9) (Sep 1999):1897–903. Sato, T., et al. "Production of Menaquinone (Vitamin K2)-

7 by Bacillus subtilis." *J Biosci Bioeng* 91(1) (2001):16–20. McCann, J.C., B.N. Ames. "Vitamin K, An Example of Triage Theory: Is Micronutrient Inadequacy Linked to Diseases of Aging?" *Am J Clin Nutr* 90(4) (Oct 2009):889–907. Walther, B., et al. "Menaquinones, Bacteria, and the Food Supply: The Relevance of Dairy and Fermented Food Products to Vitamin K Requirements." *Adv Nutr* 4(4) (2013):463–473. LeBlanc, et al. "Bacteria as Vitamin Suppliers to Their Host: A Gut Microbiota Perspective." *Curr Opin Biotechnol* 24(2) (Apr 2013):160–8.

36. Hojo, K., et al. "Quantitative Measurement of Tetrahydromenaquinone-9 in Cheese Fermented by Propionibacteria." *J Dairy Sci* 90(9) (Sep 2007):4078–83. Manoury, E., et al. "Quantitative Measurement of Vitamin K2 (Menaquinones) in Various Fermented Dairy Products Using a Reliable High-Performance Liquid Chromatography Method." *J Dairy Sci* 96(3) (2013):1335–46.

37. Gropper, S.S., J.L. Smith. *Advanced Nutrition and Human Metabolism,* 6th edition. New York: Cengage Learning, 2013.

38. Ibid.

39. Ronden, J.E., H.H. Thijssen, C. Vermeer. "Tissue Distribution of K-Vitamers Under Different Nutritional Regimens in the Rat." Biochim Biophys Acta. 1379(1) (Jan 8, 1998):16–22.

40. Rheaume-Bleue, K. *Vitamin K2 and the Calcium Paradox: How a Little-Known Vitamin Could Save Your Life* New York: John Wiley & Sons, 2011.

41. Gast, G.C., et al. "A High Menaquinone Intake Reduces the Incidence of Coronary Heart Disease." *Nutr Metab Cardiovasc Dis* 19(7) (2008):504–510.

42. Ishii, Y., et al. "Distribution of Vitamin K2 in Subchondral Bone in Osteoarthritic Knee Joints." *Knee Surg Sports Traumatol Arthrosc* 21(8) (2013):1813–8.

43. Detrano, R., et al. "Coronary Calcium as a Predictor of Coronary Events in Four Racial or Ethnic Groups." *N Engl J Med* 358(13) (2008):1336–45.

44. Geleijnse, J.M., et al. "Dietary Intake of Menaquinone is Associated with a Reduced Risk of Coronary Heart Disease: The Rotterdam Study." *J Nutr* 134(11) (2004):3100–5.

45. Roberts, H., S. Hickey. *The Vitamin Cure for Heart Disease: How to Prevent and Treat Heart Disease Using Nutrition and Vitamin Supplementation.* Laguna Beach, CA: Basic Health Publications, 2011.

46. Neogi, T., et al. "Low Vitamin K Status is Associated with Osteoarthritis in the Hand and Knee." *Arthritis Rheum* 54(4) (2006):1255–61. Misra, D., et al. "Vitamin K Deficiency is Associated with Incident Knee Osteoarthritis." *Am J Med* 126(3) (Mar 2013):243–8.

47. Neogi, T., et al. "Vitamin K in Hand Osteoarthritis: Results from a Randomised Clinical Trial." *Ann Rheum Dis* 67(11) (Nov 2008):1570–73.

48. Okamoto, H., et al. "Anti-Arthritis Effects of Vitamin K(2) (Menaquinone-4)—A New Potential Therapeutic Strategy for Rheumatoid Arthritis." *FEBS J* 274(17) (Sep 2007):4588–94.

49. Okamoto, H. "Vitamin K and Rheumatoid Arthritis." *IUBMB Life* 60(6) (Jun 2008):355–61.

Chapter 5. Nutritional Treatments for Arthritis: The Evidence

1. Deschner, J., et al. "Signal Transduction by Mechanical Strain in Chondrocytes." *Curr Opin Clin Nutr Metab Care* 6(3) (May 2003):289–293.

2. Ward, B.W., J.S. Schiller. "Prevalence of Multiple Chronic Conditions Among US Adults:

Estimates from the National Health Interview Survey, 2010." *Prev Chronic Dis* 10 (Apr 25, 2013):E65.

3. Campbell, T.C., T.M. Campbell, II. *The China Study: The Most Comprehensive Study of Nutrition Ever Conducted and Startling Implications for Diet, Weight Loss, and Long-Term Health.* Dallas, TX: Ben-Bella Books, 2006. Ornish, D. *The Spectrum: How to Customize a Way of Eating and Living Just Right for You and Your Family.* New York: Ballantine Books, 2008. Campbell, T.C. *Whole: Rethinking the Science of Nutrition.* Dallas, TX: BenBella Books, 2013. Ruel, G., et al. "Association between Nutrition and the Evolution of Multimorbidity: The Importance of Fruits and Vegetables and Whole Grain Products." *Clin Nutr* (Jul 22, 2013): pii: S0261-5614(13)00200-8. [Epub ahead of print].

4. Deschner, J., et al. "Signal Transduction by Mechanical Strain in Chondrocytes." *Curr Opin Clin Nutr Metab Care* 6(3) (May 2003):289–93. Fransen, M., S. McConnell. "Exercise for Osteoarthritis of the Knee." *Cochrane Database Syst Rev* (4) (Oct 8, 2008): CD004376. doi: 10.1002/14651858.CD004376.pub2. Chen, H., K. Onishi. "Effect of Home Exercise Program Performance in Patients with Osteoarthritis of the Knee or the Spine on the Visual Analog Scale After Discharge from Physical Therapy." *Int J Rehabil Res* 35(3) (Sep 2012):275–277. Garrison, D. "Osteoarthritis, Osteoporosis, and Exercise." *Workplace Health Saf* 60(9) (Sep 2012):381–3. Musumeci, G., et al. "The Effects of Physical Activity on Apoptosis and Lubricin Expression in Articular Cartilage in Rats with Glucocorticoid-Induced Osteoporosis." *J Bone Miner Metab* 31(3) (May 2013):274–284. Bergman, J. *How to Reverse Arthritis Naturally.* CreateSpace Independent Publishing. ISBN-13: 978-1482701524.

5. Deschner, J., et al. "Signal Transduction by Mechanical Strain in Chondrocytes." *Curr Opin Clin Nutr Metab Care* 6(3) (May 2003):289–293.

6. Feldman, D.E., et al. "Effects of Adherence to Treatment on Short-Term Outcomes in Children with Juvenile Idiopathic Arthritis." *Arthritis Rheum* 57(6) (Aug 2007):905–12.

7. Hildebrand, J.S., et al. "Recreational Physical Activity and Leisure-Time Sitting in Relation to Postmenopausal Breast Cancer Risk." *Cancer Epidemiol Biomarkers Prev* 22(10) (2013):1906–12.

8. Miller, et al. "Why Don't Most Runners Get Knee Osteoarthritis? A Case for Per-Unit-Distance Loads." *Med Sci Sports Exerc* (Sep 12, 2013) [Epub ahead of print].

9. Molnar-Kimber, K.L. "No Matter the State of Your Bones, Joints and Muscles, Here are the Best Exercises to Get Muscle Tone, Boost Energy and Increase Flexibility for the Elderly, or Rheumatoid Arthritis Patients." (2013): www.rheumatoid-arthritis-decisions.com/bones-joints-and-muscles.html (accessed Apr 2014).

10. Theodosakis, J., S. Buff. *The Arthritis Cure.* Revised edition. St. Martin's Paperbacks, 2004. Arthritis Foundation (2013): www.arthritistoday.org/what-you-can-do (accessed Apr 2014). Molnar-Kimber, K.L. Rheumatoid-Arthritis-Decisions.com. www.rheumatoid-arthritis-decisions.com (2013) (accessed Jan 2014).

11. Theodosakis, J., S. Buff. *The Arthritis Cure.* Revised edition. St. Martin's Paperbacks, 2004.

12. Filaire, E., H. Toumi. "Reactive Oxygen Species and Exercise on Bone Metabolism: Friend or Enemy?" *Joint Bone Spine* 79(4) (Jul 2012):341–6.

13. Brody, J.E. The New York Times. Well. "Commuting's Hidden Cost." (Oct 26, 2013) http://well.blogs.nytimes.com/2013/10/28/commutings-hidden-cost.

14. Ibid.

15. Hoehner, C.M., et al. "Commuting Distance, Cardiorespiratory Fitness, and Metabolic Risk." *Am J Prev Med* 42(6) (Jun 2012):571–8.

16. Gossan, N., et al. "The Circadian Clock in Chondrocytes Regulates Genes Controlling Key Aspects of Cartilage Homeostasis." *Arthritis Rheum* 65(9) (2013):2334–45. Fisher, S.P., R.G. Foster, S.N. Peirson. "The Circadian Control of Sleep." *Handb Exp Pharmacol* 217 (2013):157–83.

17. Czeisler, C.A. "Perspective: Casting Light on Sleep Deficiency." *Nature* 497(7450) (May 23, 2013):S13. Münch, M., V. Bromundt. "Light and Chronobiology: Implications for Health and Disease." *Dialogues Clin Neurosci* 14(4) (Dec 2012):448–53. Münch, M., A. Kawasaki. "Intrinsically Photosensitive Retinal Ganglion Cells: Classification, Function and Clinical Implications." *Curr Opin Neurol* 26(1) (Feb 2013):45–51. Zee, P.C., H. Attarian, A. Videnovic. "Circadian Rhythm Abnormalities." *Continuum (Minneap Minn)*. 19(1 Sleep Disorders) (Feb 2013):132–47.

18. Czeisler, C.A. "Perspective: Casting Light on Sleep Deficiency." *Nature* 497(7450) (May 23, 2013):S13. Eisenstein, M. "Chronobiology: Stepping Out of Time." *Nature* 497(7450) (May 23, 2013):S10–2. Münch, M., A. Kawasaki. "Intrinsically Photosensitive Retinal Ganglion Cells: Classification, Function and Clinical Implications." *Curr Opin Neurol* 26(1) (Feb 2013):45–51. Fisher, S.P., R.G. Foster, S.N. Peirson. "The Circadian Control of Sleep." *Handb Exp Pharmacol* 217 (2013):157–83.

19. Pigeon, W.R., et al. "Effects of a Tart Cherry Juice Beverage on the Sleep of Older Adults with Insomnia: A Pilot Study." *J Med Food* 13(3) (Jun 2010):579–83. McCune, L.M., et al. "Cherries and Health: A Review." *Crit Rev Food Sci Nutr* 51(1) (Jan 2011):1–12. Zhao, Y., et al. "Melatonin and Its Potential Biological Functions in the Fruits of Sweet Cherry." *J Pineal Res* 55(1) (Aug 2013):79–88.

20. Huang, L.B., et al. The Effectiveness of Light/Dark Exposure to Treat Insomnia in Female Nurses Undertaking Shift Work during the Evening/Night Shift." *J Clin Sleep Med* 9(7) (Jul 15, 2013):641–6.

21. Burkhart, K., J.R. Phelps. "Amber Lenses to Block Blue Light and Improve Sleep: A Randomized Trial." *Chronobiol Int* 26(8) (Dec 2009):1602–12.

22. Huang, W., et al. "Improvement of Pain, Sleep, and Quality of Life in Chronic Pain Patients with Vitamin D Supplementation." *Clin J Pain* 29(4) (Apr 2013):341–7.

23. Price, P., et al. "The Use of a New Overlay Mattress in Patients with Chronic Pain: Impact on Sleep and Self-Reported Pain." *Clin Rehabil* 17(5) (Aug 2003):488–92.

24. Jenkins M. *What's Gotten into Us?: Staying Healthy in a Toxic World*. New York: Random House, 2011.

25. Molnar-Kimber KL. "24 Ways to Help Rheumatoid Arthritis Patients Neutralize Toxic Substances, Decrease Exposure and Reduce Your Flares." Rheumatoid-Arthritis-Decisions.com (2013) www.rheumatoid-arthritis-decisions.com/rheumatoid-arthritis-toxic-substances.html. (accessed Mar 2014).

26. Kwok, S.K., et al. "Retinoic Acid Attenuates Rheumatoid Inflammation in Mice." *J Immunol* 189(2) (Jul 15, 2012):1062–71.

27. Ames, B.N. "Optimal Micronutrients Delay Mitochondrial Decay and Age-Associated Diseases." *Mech Ageing Dev* 131(7–8) (Jul-Aug 2010):473–479. Ames, B.N. "Prevention of Mutation, Cancer, and Other Age-Associated Diseases by Optimizing Micronutrient Intake." *J Nucleic Acids* (Sep 22, 2010). pii:725071. Penberthy, W.T. "Niacin, Riboflavin, and Thiamine." In: *Biochemical, Physiological, and Molecular Aspects of Human Nutrition* M.H. Stipanuk and M.A. Caudill, eds. 3rd edition. St. Louis, MO: Saunders, 2012. p. 540–564.

28. Schuitemaker, G. "Restrictions on Food Supplements are Based on Misinformation." Orthomolecular News Service (OMNS). Oct 16, 2012. www.orthomolecular.org/resources/omns/v08n31.shtml (accessed Apr 2014). Alliance for Natural Health, Europe. "Codex Alimentarius. Codex—Government and Corporate Control of Our Food Supply." (2013): www.anh-europe.org/campaigns/codex. (accessed Apr 2014).

29. Alliance for Natural Health, Europe. "European Court Set to Judge Water Hydration Claim." (2013): http://anh-europe.org/news/european-court-set-to-judge-water-hydration-claim. www.anh-europe.org/news/more-alice-in-wonderland-decisions-on-health-claims (accessed Apr 2014).

30. Dean, C. *The Magnesium Miracle.* New York: Ballantine, 2007. Goodman, D. *Magnificent Magnesium.* Square One Publishers, 2013.

31. Ibid.

32. Dean, C. *The Magnesium Miracle.* New York: Ballantine, 2007.

33. Alliance for Natural Health, USA. Codex Committee: "You Can't Tell People that Food Prevents Disease!" (2103): www.anh-usa.org/codex-committee (accessed Apr 2014).

34. U.S. Food and Drug Administration (FDA). "Acetaminophen and Liver Injury: Q & A for Consumers." www.fda.gov/forconsumers/consumerupdates/ucm168830.htm (accessed Jan 2014).

35. Null, G., et al. "Death By Medicine", Independent review commissioned by the Nutrition Institute of America. (2005): *J Orthomol Med* 20(1) (2005): http://orthomolecular.org/library/jom/2005/pdf/2005-v20n01-p021.pdf (accessed Apr 2014). Meyer, T.V. "A Case for Natural Health Treatment." Orthomolecular News Service (OMNS) Oct 3, 2013. www.orthomolecular.org/resources/omns/v09n19.shtml (accessed Apr 2014). Centers for Disease Control (CDC). NCHS Fact Sheet. NCHS Data on Drug Poisoning Deaths. (Dec 2012): www.cdc.gov/nchs/data/factsheets/factsheet_drug_poisoning.htm www.cdc.gov/homeandrecreationalsafety/overdose/facts.html (accessed Apr 2014). U.S. Food and Drug Administration (FDA). "Acetaminophen and Liver Injury: Q & A for Consumers." www.fda.gov/forconsumers/consumerupdates/ucm168830.htm (accessed Jan 2014).

36. Centers for Disease Control (CDC). NCHS Fact Sheet. NCHS Data on Drug Poisoning Deaths. (Dec 2012): www.cdc.gov/nchs/data/factsheets/factsheet_drug_poisoning.htm www.cdc.gov/homeandrecreationalsafety/overdose/facts.html (accessed Apr 2014).

37. Lazarou, J., B. Pomeranz, P.N. Corey. "Incidence of Adverse Drug Reactions in Hospitalized Patients: A Meta-Analysis of Prospective Studies." *JAMA* 279(15) (Apr 15, 1998):1200–5. Null, G., et al. "Death By Medicine", Independent review commissioned by the Nutrition Institute of America. (2005): *J Orthomol Med* 20(1) (2005): http://orthomolecular.org/library/jom/2005/pdf/2005-v20n01-p021.pdf (accessed Apr 2014).

38. Centers for Disease Control (CDC). Injury Prevention and Control. "*Saving Lives and Protecting People:* Preventing Prescription Painkiller Overdoses." (2013): www.cdc.gov/injury/about/focus-rx.html (accessed Apr 2014).

39. Hefti, R. "Anti-Vitamin Publications: Misinformation Presented As Truth" Orthomolecular News Service (OMNS). Jul 18, 2013. http://orthomolecular.org/resources/omns/v09n14.shtml (accessed Apr 2014).

40. Orthomolecular News Service (OMNS). "Restrictions on Food Supplements are Based on Misinformation." Oct 16, 2012. www.orthomolecular.org/resources/omns/v08n31.shtml (accessed Apr 2014).

41. Saul, A.W. "NBC's Vitamin Ignorance: An Apology." Orthomolecular News Service

(OMNS). Nov 12, 2013. http://orthomolecular.org/resources/omns/v09n24.shtml (accessed Apr 2014).

42. Dean, C. *The Magnesium Miracle.* New York: Ballantine, 2007.

43. Shi, Y., et al. "Protective Effects of Nicotinamide Against Acetaminophen-Induced Acute Liver Injury." *Int Immunopharmacol* 14(4) (2012):530–7.

44. Penberthy, W.T. "Niacin, Riboflavin, and Thiamine." In: *Biochemical, Physiological, and Molecular Aspects of Human Nutrition* M.H. Stipanuk and M.A. Caudill, eds. 3rd edition. St. Louis, MO: Saunders, 2012. p. 540–564.

45. Gaby, A.R. "Natural Treatments for Osteoarthritis." *Altern Med Rev* 4(5) (Oct 1999):330–41. Kobayashi, T., et al. "Fursultiamine, A Vitamin B1 Derivative, Enhances Chondroprotective Effects of Glucosamine Hydrochloride and Chondroitin Sulfate in Rabbit Experimental Osteoarthritis." *Inflamm Res* 54(6) (Jun 2005):249–55.

46. White-O'Connor, B., J. Sobal. "Nutrient Intake and Obesity in a Multidisciplinary Assessment of Osteoarthritis." *Clin Ther* 9 Suppl B (1986):30–42.

47. Stanislavchuk, N.A., et al. "Influence of Enzyme Inducers and Inhibitors of the Metabolism of Xenobiotics and of the Coenzyme Forms of Vitamins B1 and B2 on the Anti-Inflammatory Effect of Voltaren." *Farmakol Toksikol* 51(2) (Mar-Apr 1988):69–71. Wang, Y., et al. "The Effect of Nutritional Supplements on Osteoarthritis." *Altern Med Rev* 9(3) (Sep 2004):275–96. Verdrengh, M., A. Tarkowski. "Riboflavin in Innate and Acquired Immune Responses." *Inflamm Res* 54(9) (Sep 2005):390–3.

48. Mulherin, D.M., D.I. Thurnham, R.D. Situnayake. "Glutathione Reductase Activity, Riboflavin Status, and Disease Activity in Rheumatoid Arthritis." *Ann Rheum Dis* 55(11) (Nov 1996):837–40.

49. Wang, Y., et al. "The Effect of Nutritional Supplements on Osteoarthritis." *Altern Med Rev* 9(3) (Sep 2004):275–96. Ng, T.P., et al. "Homocysteine, Folate, Vitamin B-12, and Physical Function in Older Adults: Cross-Sectional Findings from the Singapore Longitudinal Ageing Study." *Am J Clin Nutr* 96(6) (Dec 2012):1362–8.

50. Mock, D.M. "Biotin" Chapter 21 in *Modern Nutrition in Health and Disease,* editors A.C. Ross, et al., 11th ed. Baltimore: Lippincott Williams & Wilkins, 2012. Eng, W.K., et al. "Identification and Assessment of Markers of Biotin Status in Healthy Adults." *Br J Nutr* 110(2) (2013):321–9.

51. Al-Qudah, K.M., Z.B. Ismail. "The Relationship between Serum Biotin and Oxidant/Antioxidant Activities in Bovine Lameness." *Res Vet Sci.* 92(1) (Feb 2012):138–141.

52. Xue, J., J. Zempleni. "Epigenetic Synergies between Biotin and Folate in the Regulation of Pro-Inflammatory Cytokines and Repeats." *Scand J Immunol* 78(5) (Nov 2013):419–25.

53. Lanska, D.J. "The Discovery of Niacin, Biotin, and Pantothenic Acid." *Ann Nutr Metab* 61(3) (2012):246–253.

54. Eng, W.K., et al. "Identification and Assessment of Markers of Biotin Status in Healthy Adults." *Br J Nutr* 110(2) (2013):321–9.

55. Mock, D.M. "Biotin" Chapter 21 in *Modern Nutrition in Health and Disease,* editors A.C. Ross, et al., 11th ed. Baltimore: Lippincott Williams & Wilkins, 2012.

56. Kaufman, W. *The Common Form of Joint Dysfunction: Its Incidence and Treatment.* Brattleboro, VT: E.L. Hildreth, 1949. Wang, Y., et al. "The Effect of Nutritional Supplements on Osteoarthritis." *Altern Med Rev* 9(3) (Sep 2004):275–96.

57. Gaby, A.R. *Nutritional Medicine.* Concord, NH: Fritz Perlberg Pub, 2011.

58. Gaby, A.R. "Natural Treatments for Osteoarthritis." *Altern Med Rev* 4(5) (Oct 1999):330–41. Gaby, A.R. *Nutritional Medicine*. Concord, NH: Fritz Perlberg Pub, 2011.

59. Jonas, W.B., C.P. Rapoza, W.F. Blair. "The Effect of Niacinamide on Osteoarthritis: A Pilot Study." *Inflamm Res* 45(7) (Jul 1996):330–4.

60. Gaby, A.R. "Natural Treatments for Osteoarthritis." *Altern Med Rev* 4(5) (Oct 1999):330–41. Hoffer, A., A.W. Saul. *Orthomolecular Medicine for Everyone: Megavitamin Therapeutics for Families and Physicians*. Laguna Beach, CA: Basic Health Publications, 2008.

61. McCarty, M.F., A.L. Russell. "Niacinamide Therapy for Osteoarthritis—Does It Inhibit Nitric Oxide Synthase Induction by Interleukin 1 in Chondrocytes?" *Med Hypotheses*;53(4) (Oct 1999):350–60. Lopez, H.L. "Nutritional Interventions to Prevent and Treat Osteoarthritis. Part II: Focus on Micronutrients and Supportive Nutraceuticals." *PM R* 4(5 Suppl) (May 2012):S155–68.

62. Lotz, M. "The Role of Nitric Oxide in Articular Cartilage Damage." *Rheum Dis Clin North Am*;25(2) (May 1999):269–82.

63. de Guise Vaillancourt, G. "The Cutaneous Application of a Nicotinic Cream as a Diagnostic Aid in Various Rheumatic Diseases." *Can Med Assoc J*. 71(3) (1954):283–5.

64. Shi, Y., et al. "Protective Effects of Nicotinamide Against Acetaminophen-Induced Acute Liver Injury." *Int Immunopharmacol* 14(4) (2012):530–7.

65. Kaufman, W. *The Common Form of Joint Dysfunction: Its Incidence and Treatment*. Brattleboro, VT: E.L. Hildreth, 1949.

66. Kremer, J.M., J. Bigaouette. "Nutrient Intake of Patients with Rheumatoid Arthritis is Deficient in Pyridoxine, Zinc, Copper, and Magnesium." *J Rheumatol* 23(6) (1996):990–4. Friso, S., et al. "Low Circulating Vitamin B(6) is Associated with Elevation of the Inflammation Marker C-Reactive Protein Independently of Plasma Homocysteine Levels." *Circulation* 103(23) (2001):2788–91. Hoffer, A., A.W. Saul. *Orthomolecular Medicine for Everyone: Megavitamin Therapeutics for Families and Physicians*. Laguna Beach, CA: Basic Health Publications, 2008. Woolf, K., M.M. Manore. "Elevated Plasma Homocysteine and Low Vitamin B-6 Status in Nonsupplementing Older Women with Rheumatoid Arthritis." *J Am Diet Assoc* 108(3) (Mar 2008):443–53; discussion 454. Chiang, E.P., et al. "Pyridoxine Supplementation Corrects Vitamin B6 Deficiency but Does Not Improve Inflammation in Patients with Rheumatoid Arthritis." *Arthritis Res Ther* 7(6) (2005):R1404–11.

67. Rall, L.C., S.N. Meydani. "Vitamin B6 and Immune Competence." *Nutr Rev* 51(8) (1993):217–25. Sakakeeny, L., et al. "Plasma Pyridoxal-5-Phosphate is Inversely Associated with Systemic Markers of Inflammation in a Population of U.S. Adults. *J Nutr* 142(7) (2012):1280–5.

68. Huang, S.C., et al. "Vitamin B(6) Supplementation Improves Pro-Inflammatory Responses in Patients with Rheumatoid Arthritis." *Eur J Clin Nutr* 64(9) (2010):1007–13. Huang, S.C., et al. "Plasma Pyridoxal 5'-Phosphate Is Not Associated with Inflammatory and Immune Responses after Adjusting for Serum Albumin in Patients with Rheumatoid Arthritis: A Preliminary Study." *Ann Nutr Metab*. 60(2) (2012):83–9.

69. Lotto, V., S.W. Choi, S. Friso. "Vitamin B6: A Challenging Link Between Nutrition and Inflammation in CVD." *Br J Nutr* 106(2) (2011):183–95.

70. Vreugdenhil, G., et al. "Anaemia in Rheumatoid Arthritis: The Role of Iron, Vitamin B12, and Folic Acid Deficiency, and Erythropoietin Responsiveness." *Ann Rheum Dis* 49(2) (Feb 1990):93–8.

71. Masuko, K., S. Tohma, T. Matsui. "Potential Food-Drug Interactions in Patients with Rheumatoid Arthritis." *Int J Rheum Dis* 16(2) (Apr 2013):122–8.

72. Morgan, S.L., et al. "The Effect of Folic Acid and Folinic Acid Supplements on Purine Metabolism in Methotrexate-Treated Rheumatoid Arthritis." *Arthritis Rheum* 50(10) (Oct 2004):3104–3111.

73. Molnar-Kimber, K.L. Rheumatoid-Arthritis-Decisions.com. www.rheumatoid-arthritis-decisions.com (2013) (accessed Jan 2014).

74. Alban, C., D. Job, R. Douce. "Biotin Metabolism in Plants." *Annu Rev Plant Physiol Plant Mol Biol* 51(Jun 2000):17–47.

75. McGee, H. *On Food and Cooking: The Science and Lore of the Kitchen.* New York, NY: Scribner, Revised, updated edition, 2004. ISBN-13: 978–0684800011

76. Hertz, R. "Biotin and the Avidin-Biotin Complex." *Physiol Rev* 26(4) (1946):479–94. Green, N.M. "Avidin. 1. The Use of [14C]Biotin for Kinetic Studies and for Assay" *Biochem J.* 89(3) (1963):585–591. Laitinen, O.H., et al. "Genetically Engineered Avidins and Streptavidins." *Cell Mol Life Sci* 63(24) (2006):2992–3017. *but see* Holmberg, A., et al. "The Biotin-Streptavidin Interaction Can Be Reversibly Broken Using Water at Elevated Temperatures." *Electrophoresis* 26(3) (2005):501–10.

77. Eng, W.K., et al. "Identification and Assessment of Markers of Biotin Status in Healthy Adults." *Br J Nutr* 110(2) (2013):321–9.

78. Boas, M.A. "An Observation on the Value of Egg-White as the Sole Source of Nitrogen for Young Growing Rats." *Biochem J* 18(2) (1924):422–4.

79. Eakin, R.E., W.A. McKinley, R.J. Williams. "Egg-White Injury in Chicks and Its Relationship to a Deficiency of Vitamin H (Biotin)." *Science* 92(2384) (Sep 1940):224–5. György, P., et al. "Egg-White Injury as the Result of Nonabsorption or Inactivation of Biotin." *Science* 93(2420) (1941):477–8.

80. Holmberg, A., et al. "The Biotin-Streptavidin Interaction Can Be Reversibly Broken Using Water at Elevated Temperatures." *Electrophoresis* 26(3) (2005):501–10.

81. Pauling, L. *How to Live Longer and Feel Better.* Corvallis, OR: Oregon State University Press, 1986, 2006. György, P., et al. "Egg-White Injury as the Result of Nonabsorption or Inactivation of Biotin." *Science* 93(2420) (1941):477–8. Levine, M., S.J. Padayatty "Vitamin C." Chapter 29 in *Modern Nutrition in Health and Disease,* editors A.C. Ross, 11th ed. Baltimore: Lippincott Williams & Wilkins, 2012. Hickey, S, A.W. Saul. *Vitamin C: The Real Story, the Remarkable and Controversial Healing Factor.* Laguna Beach, CA: Basic Health Publications, 2008. Gropper, S.S., J.L. Smith. *Advanced Nutrition and Human Metabolism,* 6th edition. New York: Cengage Learning, 2013.

82. Frech, T.M., D.O. Clegg. "The Utility of Nutraceuticals in the Treatment of Osteoarthritis." *Curr Rheumatol Rep* 9(1) (Apr 2007):25–30. Lopez, H.L. "Nutritional Interventions to Prevent and Treat Osteoarthritis. Part II: Focus on Micronutrients and Supportive Nutraceuticals." *PM R* 4(5 Suppl) (May 2012):S155–68. Clark, A.G., et al. "The Effects of Ascorbic Acid on Cartilage Metabolism in Guinea Pig Articular Cartilage Explants." *Matrix Biol* 21 (Mar 2002): 175–84.

83. Schwartz, E.R., W.H. Oh, C.R. Leveille. "Experimentally Induced Osteoarthritis in Guinea Pigs: Metabolic Responses in Articular Cartilage to Developing Pathology." *Arthritis Rheum* 24(11) (1981):1345–55. Gerstenfeld, L.C., W.J. Landis. "Gene Expression and Extracellular Matrix Ultrastructure of a Mineralizing Chondrocyte Cell Culture System." *J Cell Biol* 112(3) (1991):501–13. Mobasheri, A. "Glucose: An Energy Currency and Structural Precursor in Articular Cartilage and Bone with Emerging Roles as an Extracellular

Signaling Molecule and Metabolic Regulator." *Front Endocrinol (Lausanne)* 3 (Dec 17, 2012):153.

84. Mobasheri, A., et al. "Glucose Transport and Metabolism in Chondrocytes: A Key to Understanding Chondrogenesis, Skeletal Development and Cartilage Degradation in Osteoarthritis." *Histol Histopathol* 17(4) (Oct 2002):1239–67. Clark, A.G., et al. "The Effects of Ascorbic Acid on Cartilage Metabolism in Guinea Pig Articular Cartilage Explants." *Matrix Biol* 21 (Mar 2002): 175–84.

85. Shargorodsky, M., et al. "Effect of Long-Term Treatment with Antioxidants (Vitamin C, Vitamin E, Coenzyme Q10 and Selenium) on Arterial Compliance, Humoral Factors and Inflammatory Markers in Patients with Multiple Cardiovascular Risk Factors." *Nutr Metab (Lond)* 7 (Jul 2010):55.

86. Dean, C. *The Magnesium Miracle.* New York: Ballantine, 2007. Shargorodsky, M., et al. "Effect of Long-Term Treatment with Antioxidants (Vitamin C, Vitamin E, Coenzyme Q10 and Selenium) on Arterial Compliance, Humoral Factors and Inflammatory Markers in Patients with Multiple Cardiovascular Risk Factors." *Nutr Metab (Lond)* 7 (Jul 2010):55.

87. McAlindon, T.E., et al. "Do Antioxidant Micronutrients Protect Against the Development and Progression of Knee Osteoarthritis?" *Arthritis Rheum* 39(4) (Apr 1996):648–56. McAlindon, T.E. "Nutraceuticals: Do They Work and When Should We Use Them?" *Best Pract Res Clin Rheumatol* 20(1) (Feb 2006):99–115.

88. Clark, A.G., et al. "The Effects of Ascorbic Acid on Cartilage Metabolism in Guinea Pig Articular Cartilage Explants." *Matrix Biol* 21 (Mar 2002): 175–84.

89. Kumar, V., P. Choudhury. "Scurvy—A Forgotten Disease with an Unusual Presentation." *Trop Doct* 39(3) (Jul 2009):190–2. Lau, H., D. Massasso, F. Joshua. "Skin,Muscle and Joint Disease from the 17th Century: Scurvy." *Int J Rheum Dis;* 12(4) (Dec 2009):361–5. Vitale, A., et al. "Arthritis and Gum Bleeding in Two Children." *J Paediatr Child Health* 45(3) (Mar 2009):158–60. Holley, A.D., et al. "Scurvy: Historically a Plague of the Sailor that Remains a Consideration in the Modern Intensive Care Unit." *Intern Med J* 41(3) (2011):283–5.

90. Lau, H., D. Massasso, F. Joshua. "Skin,Muscle and Joint Disease from the 17th Century: Scurvy." *Int J Rheum Dis;* 12(4) (Dec 2009):361–5.

91. Zollinger, P.E., et al. "Clinical Results of 40 Consecutive Basal Thumb Prostheses and No CRPS Type I After Vitamin C Prophylaxis." *Open Orthop J* 4 (Feb 17, 2010):62–6. Perez, R.S., et al. "Evidence Based Guidelines for Complex Regional Pain Syndrome Type 1." *BMC Neurol* 10 (Mar 2010):20.

92. Surapaneni, K.M., G. Venkataramana. "Status of Lipid Peroxidation, Glutathione, Ascorbic Acid, Vitamin E and Antioxidant Enzymes in Patients with Osteoarthritis." *Indian J Med Sci* 61 (2007):9–14

93. Regan, E.A., R.P. Bowler, J.D. Crapo. "Joint Fluid Antioxidants Are Decreased in Osteoarthritic Joints Compared to Joints with Macroscopically Intact Cartilage and Subacute Injury." *Osteoarthritis Cartilage* 16(4) (Apr 2008):515–521.

94. Traber, M.G., J.F. Stevens. "Vitamins C and E: Beneficial Effects from a Mechanistic Perspective." *Free Radic Biol Med* 51(5) (Sep 1, 2011):1,000–13.

95. Reppert, E., J. Donegan, L.E. Hines. "Ascorbic Acid and the Hyaluronidase. Hyaluronic Acid Reaction." *Proc Soc Exp Biol Med* 77 (1951):318–20. Spickenreither, M., et al. "Novel 6-O-Acylated Vitamin C Derivatives as Hyaluronidase Inhibitors with Selectivity for Bacterial Lyases." *Bioorg Med Chem Lett* 16 (2006):5313–6.

96. Massell, B.F., et al. "Antirheumatic Activity of Ascorbic Acid in Large Doses Preliminary Observations on Seven Patients with Rheumatic Fever." *N Engl J Med* 242(16) (1950):614–5. Baker, K., et al. "The Effects of Vitamin C Intake on Pain in Knee Osteoarthritis (OA)." *Arthritis Rheum* 48(9) (2003):S422. Jensen, N.H. "Reduced Pain from Osteoarthritis in Hip Joint or Knee Joint during Treatment with Calcium Ascorbate. A Randomized, Placebo-Controlled Cross-Over Trial in General Practice." *Ugeskr Laeger* 165 (2003):2563–6. Wang, Y., et al. "The Effect of Nutritional Supplements on Osteoarthritis." *Altern Med Rev* 9(3) (Sep 2004):275–96. Peregoy, J., F.V. Wilder. "The Effects of Vitamin C Supplementation on Incident and Progressive Knee Osteoarthritis: A Longitudinal Study." *Public Health Nutrition* 14(4) (Apr 2011):709–15.

97. Wang, Y., et al. "Effect of Antioxidants on Knee Cartilage and Bone in Healthy, Middle-Aged Participants: A Cross-Sectional Study." *Arthritis Res Ther* 9 (2007):R66.

98. Ibid.

99. McAlindon, T.E., et al. "Do Antioxidant Micronutrients Protect Against the Development and Progression of Knee Osteoarthritis?" *Arthritis Rheum* 39(4) (Apr 1996):648–56.

100. Zhu, L.L., et al. "Vitamin C Prevents Hypogonadal Bone Loss." *PLoS One* 7(10) (2012):e47058. doi: 10.1371/journal.pone.0047058.

101. Sakai, A., et al. "Large-Dose Ascorbic Acid Administration Suppresses the Development of Arthritis in Adjuvant-Injected Rats." *Arch Orthop Trauma Surg* 119 (1999):121–6

102. Yudoh, K., et al. "Potential Involvement of Oxidative Stress in Cartilage Senescence and Development of Osteoarthritis: Oxidative Stress Induces Chondrocyte Telomere Instability and Downregulation of Chondrocyte Function." *Arthritis Res Ther* 7(2) (2005):R380–91. McAlindon, T.E. "Nutraceuticals: Do They Work and When Should We Use Them?" *Best Pract Res Clin Rheumatol* 20(1) (Feb 2006):99–115.

103. Yudoh, K., et al. "Potential Involvement of Oxidative Stress in Cartilage Senescence and Development of Osteoarthritis: Oxidative Stress Induces Chondrocyte Telomere Instability and Downregulation of Chondrocyte Function." *Arthritis Res Ther* 7(2) (2005):R380–91.

104. Clark, A.G., et al. "The Effects of Ascorbic Acid on Cartilage Metabolism in Guinea Pig Articular Cartilage Explants." *Matrix Biol* 21 (Mar 2002): 175–84.

105. Cohen, M. "Rosehip—An Evidence Based Herbal Medicine for Inflammation and Arthritis." *Aust Fam Phys* 41 (2012):495–8.

106. Kawaguchi, K., et al. "Suppression of Collagen-Induced Arthritis by Oral Administration of the Citrus Flavonoid Hesperidin." *Planta Med* 72(5) (2006):477–9. Umar, S., et al. "Hesperidin Inhibits Collagen-Induced Arthritis Possibly through Suppression of Free Radical Load and Reduction in Neutrophil Activation and Infiltration." *Rheumatol Int* 33(3) (2013):657–63.

107. Traber, M.G., J.F. Stevens. "Vitamins C and E: Beneficial Effects from a Mechanistic Perspective." *Free Radic Biol Med* 51(5) (Sep 1, 2011):1,000–13.

108. Schectman, G., J.C. Byrd, H.W. Gruchow. "The Influence of Smoking on Vitamin C Status in Adults." *Am J Public Health* 79(2) (Feb 1989):158–62. Handelman, G.J., L. Packer, C.E. Cross. "Destruction of Tocopherols, Carotenoids, and Retinol in Human Plasma by Cigarette Smoke. *Am J Clin Nutr* 63(4) (Apr 1996):559–65. Frikke-Schmidt, et al. "High Dietary Fat and Cholesterol Exacerbates Chronic Vitamin C Deficiency in Guinea Pigs." *Br J Nutr* 105(1) (Jan 2011):54–61. Wilson, K.M., et al. "Micronutrient Levels in Children Exposed to Secondhand Tobacco Smoke." *Nicotine Tob Res* 13(9) (Sep 2011):800–8. Das, A., et al. "Molecular and Cellular Mechanisms of Cigarette Smoke-Induced Myocardial Injury: Prevention by Vitamin C." *PLoS One* 7(9) (2012):e44151.

Das, B., P.C. Maity, A.K. Sil. "Vitamin C Forestalls Cigarette Smoke Induced NF-kB activation in Alveolar Epithelial Cells." *Toxicol Lett* 220(1) (2013):76–81.

109. Wang, Y., et al. "Effects of Vitamin C and Vitamin D Administration on Mood and Distress in Acutely Hospitalized Patients?" *Am J Clin Nutr* 98(3) (Sep 2013):705–11.

110. Hickey, S., H. Roberts. *Tarnished Gold: The Sickness of Evidence-based Medicine.* CreateSpace Independent Publishing, 2011.

111. Holick M.F. *The Vitamin D Solution: A 3-Step Strategy to Cure Our Most Common Health Problems.* New York: Penguin Group USA, 2011.

112. Wang, Y., et al. "Effects of Vitamin C and Vitamin D Administration on Mood and Distress in Acutely Hospitalized Patients?" *Am J Clin Nutr* 98(3) (Sep 2013):705–11.

113. Pattison, D.J., P.G. Winyard. "Dietary Antioxidants in Inflammatory Arthritis: Do They Have Any Role in Etiology or Therapy?" *Nat Clin Pract Rheumatol* 4(11) (Nov 4, 2008):590–6.

114. Massell, B.F., et al. "Antirheumatic Activity of Ascorbic Acid in Large Doses Preliminary Observations on Seven Patients with Rheumatic Fever." *N Engl J Med* 242(16) (1950):614–5.

115. Darlington, L.G., T.W. Stone. "Antioxidants and Fatty Acids in the Amelioration of Rheumatoid Arthritis and Related Disorders." *Br J Nutr* 85(3) (Mar 2001):251–69.

116. Pattison, D.J., P.G. Winyard. "Dietary Antioxidants in Inflammatory Arthritis: Do They Have Any Role in Etiology or Therapy?" *Nat Clin Pract Rheumatol* 4(11) (Nov 4, 2008):590–6.

117. Winyard, P.G., et al. "Measurement and Meaning of Markers of Reactive Species of Oxygen, Nitrogen and Sulfur in Healthy Human Subjects and Patients with Inflammatory Joint Disease." *Biochem Soc Trans* 39(5) (Oct 2011):1226–1232.

118. Pattison, D.J., P.G. Winyard. "Dietary Antioxidants in Inflammatory Arthritis: Do They Have Any Role in Etiology or Therapy?" *Nat Clin Pract Rheumatol* 4(11) (Nov 4, 2008):590–6.

119. Levy, T.E. *Primal Panacea.* Henderson, NV: MedFox Publishing, 2011.

120. Ibid.

121. Hagfors, L., et al. "Antioxidant Intake, Plasma Antioxidants and Oxidative Stress in a Randomized, Controlled, Parallel, Mediterranean Dietary Intervention Study on Patients with Rheumatoid Arthritis." *Nutr J* 2 (Jul 30, 2003):5.

122. Molnar-Kimber, K.L., H.E. Buttram. "Evidence that Intravenous Administration of Glutathione and Vitamin C Relieved Acute Pain from Rheumatoid Arthritis Flare." *Townsend Letter* 304 (Nov 2008): 60–1. Molnar-Kimber, K.L. Rheumatoid-Arthritis-Decisions.com. www.rheumatoid-arthritis-decisions.com (2013) (accessed Jan 2014).

123. Mikirova, N., et al. "Effect of High Dose Intravenous Ascorbic Acid on the Level of Inflammation in Patients with Rheumatoid Arthritis." *Modern Res Inflamm* 1(2) (Nov 2012):26–32.

124. Hagel, A.F., et al. "Intravenous Infusion of Ascorbic Acid Decreases Serum Histamine Concentrations in Patients with Allergic and Non-Allergic Diseases." *Naunyn Schmiedebergs Arch Pharmacol* 386(9) (Sep 2013):789–93.

125. Khalsa, S. *The Vitamin D Revolution: How the Power of This Amazing Vitamin Can Change Your Life.* Hay House, 2009. Madrid, E. *Vitamin D Prescription: The Healing Power of the Sun & How It Can Save Your Life.* BookSurge Publishing, 2009. Holick M.F. *The Vitamin D Solution: A 3-Step Strategy to Cure Our Most Common Health Problems.*

New York: Penguin Group USA, 2011. Jones, G. "Vitamin D." Chapter 18 in *Modern Nutrition in Health and Disease,* editors A.C. Ross, et al., 11th ed. Baltimore: Lippincott Williams & Wilkins, 2012.

126. Earl, S., et al. "Session 2: Other Diseases: Dietary Management of Osteoporosis Throughout the Life Course." *Proc Nutr Soc;*69(1) (Feb 2010):25–33.

127. Holick M.F. *The Vitamin D Solution: A 3-Step Strategy to Cure Our Most Common Health Problems.* New York: Penguin Group USA, 2011.

128. McAlindon, T.E. "Nutraceuticals: Do They Work and When Should We Use Them?" *Best Pract Res Clin Rheumatol* 20(1) (Feb 2006):99–115.

129. Holick M.F. *The Vitamin D Solution: A 3-Step Strategy to Cure Our Most Common Health Problems.* New York: Penguin Group USA, 2011.

130. McAlindon, T.E. "Nutraceuticals: Do They Work and When Should We Use Them?" *Best Pract Res Clin Rheumatol* 20(1) (Feb 2006):99–115.

131. Castillo, E.C., et al. "Effects of Vitamin D Supplementation during the Induction and Progression of Osteoarthritis in a Rat Model." *Evid Based Complement Alternat Med* 2012 (2012):156563.

132. Chlebowski, R.T., et al. "25-hydroxyVitamin D Concentration, Vitamin D Intake and Joint Symptoms in Postmenopausal Women." *Maturitas;*68(1) (Jan 2011):73–8.

133. Huang, W., et al. "Improvement of Pain, Sleep, and Quality of Life in Chronic Pain Patients with Vitamin D Supplementation." *Clin J Pain* 29(4) (Apr 2013):341–7.

134. Bergink, A.P., et al. "Vitamin D Status, Bone Mineral Density, and the Development of Radiographic Osteoarthritis of the Knee: The Rotterdam Study." J Clin *Rheumatol* 15(5) (Aug 2009):230–7. doi: 10.1097/RHU.0b013e3181b08f20.

135. Heidari, B., P. Heidari, K. Hajian-Tilaki. "Association between Serum Vitamin D deficiency and Knee Osteoarthritis." *Int Orthop* 35(11) (2011):1627–31.

136. Wang, T.J., et al. "Common Genetic Determinants of Vitamin D Insufficiency: A Genome-Wide Association Study." *Lancet;*376(9736) (Jul 17, 2010):180–8.

137. Glover, T.L., et al. "Vitamin D, Race, and Experimental Pain Sensitivity in Older Adults with Knee Osteoarthritis." *Arthritis Rheum;*64(12) (Dec 2012):3926–35.

138. Abu El Maaty, M.A., et al. "Association of Suboptimal 25-HydroxyVitamin D Levels with Knee Osteoarthritis Incidence in Post-Menopausal Egyptian Women." *Rheumatol Int* 33(11) (Nov 2013):2903–7.

139. Yan, X., et al. "Vitamin D-Binding Protein (Group-Specific Component) Has Decreased Expression in Rheumatoid Arthritis." *Clin Exp Rheumatol* 30(4) (Jul-Aug 2012):525–533.

140. Yaron, I., et al. "Effect of 1,25-Dihydroxyvitamin D3 on Interleukin 1 Beta Actions and Cell Growth in Human Synovial Fibroblast Cultures." *J Rheumatol* 20(9) :1527–1532. Yan, X., et al. "Vitamin D-Binding Protein (Group-Specific Component) Has Decreased Expression in Rheumatoid Arthritis." *Clin Exp Rheumatol* 30(4) (Jul-Aug 2012):525–533.

141. Sen, D., P. Ranganathan. "Vitamin D in Rheumatoid Arthritis: Panacea or Placebo?" *Discov Med* 14(78) (Nov 2012):311–19. Sabbagh, Z., J. Markland, H. Vatanparast. "Vitamin D Status Is Associated with Disease Activity among Rheumatology Outpatients." *Nutrients* 5(7) (Jul 2013):2268–75. Zakeri, Z., et al. "Serum Vitamin D Level and Disease Activity in Patients with Recent Onset Rheumatoid Arthritis." *Int J Rheum Dis* (Oct 18, 2013): doi: 10.1111/1756–185X.12181. [Epub ahead of print]

142. Yan, X., et al. "Vitamin D-Binding Protein (Group-Specific Component) Has Decreased Expression in Rheumatoid Arthritis." *Clin Exp Rheumatol* 30(4) (Jul-Aug 2012):525–533.

143. Furuya, et al. "Prevalence of and Factors Associated with Vitamin D Deficiency in 4,793 Japanese Patients with Rheumatoid Arthritis." *Clin Rheumatol* 32(7) (Feb 20, 2013):1081–7.

144. Kostoglou-Athanassiou, I., et al. "Vitamin D and Rheumatoid Arthritis." *Ther Adv Endocrinol Metab* 3(6):181–7. Haga, H.J., et al. "Severe Deficiency of 25-Hydroxyvitamin D(3) (25-OH-D (3)) is Associated with High Disease Activity of Rheumatoid Arthritis." Clin Rheumatol 32(5) (May 2013):629–33. Yarwood, A., et al. "Enrichment of Vitamin D Response Elements in RA-Associated Loci Supports a Role for Vitamin D in the Pathogenesis of RA." *Genes Immun* 14(5) (Jul-Aug 2013): 325–9.

145. Sen, D., P. Ranganathan. "Vitamin D in Rheumatoid Arthritis: Panacea or Placebo?" *Discov Med* 14(78) (Nov 2012):311–19.

146. Villaggio, B., S. Soldano, M. Cutolo. "1,25-Dihydroxyvitamin D3 Downregulates Aromatase Expression and Inflammatory Cytokines in Human Macrophages." *Clin Exp Rheumatol* 30(6) (Nov-Dec 2012):934–938.

147. Neve, A., A. Corrado, F.P. Cantatore. "Immunomodulatory Effects of Vitamin D in Peripheral Blood Monocyte-Derived Macrophages from Patients with Rheumatoid Arthritis." *Clin Exp Med* (Jul 4, 2013). [Epub ahead of print]

148. Ranganathan, P., et al. "Vitamin D Deficiency, Interleukin 17, and Vascular Function in Rheumatoid Arthritis." *J Rheumatol* 2013 Jul 1. [Epub ahead of print]

149. Agmon-Levin, N., et al. "Vitamin D in Systemic and Organ-Specific Autoimmune Diseases." *Clin Rev Allergy Immunol* 45(2) (Oct 2013):256–66.

150. Jablonski, N.G. *Skin: A Natural History.* University of California Press, 2006. Jablonski, N.G. "Skin Color is an Illusion." Ted Talks. (2009) www.ted.com/talks/nina_jablonski_breaks_the_illusion_of_skin_color.html. (accessed Apr 2014) Jablonski, N.G.. "Human Skin Pigmentation as an Example of Adaptive Evolution." *Proc Am Philos Soc* 15691) (Mar 2012):45–57.

151. Jablonski, N.G. *Skin: A Natural History.* University of California Press, 2006.

152. McDougall, I., F.H. Brown, J.G. Fleagle. "Stratigraphic Placement and Age of Modern Humans from Kibish, Ethiopia." *Nature* 433 (7027) (2005):733–6. Liu, H., et al. "A Geographically Explicit Genetic Model of Worldwide Human-Settlement History." *Am J Hum Genet* 79(2) (Aug 2006):230–7. Day, M. "Fossil Reanalysis Pushes Back Origin of *Homo Sapiens*." *Sci Amer* Feb 17, 2005. www.scientificamerican.com/article.cfm?id=fossil-reanalysis-pushes (accessed Apr 2014).

153. Jablonski, N.G. *Skin: A Natural History.* University of California Press, 2006. Jablonski, N.G. "Skin Color is an Illusion." Ted Talks. (2009) www.ted.com/talks/nina_jablonski_breaks_the_illusion_of_skin_color.html. (accessed Apr 2014). Jablonski, N.G.. "Human Skin Pigmentation as an Example of Adaptive Evolution." *Proc Am Philos Soc* 15691) (Mar 2012):45–57.

154. Burbano, H.A., et al. "Analysis of Human Accelerated DNA Regions Using Archaic Hominin Genomes." *PLoS ONE* 7(3) (Mar 7.2012): e32877. doi:10.1371/journal.pone.0032877. Sankararaman, S., et al. "The Date of Interbreeding between Neandertals and Modern Humans." *PLoS Genet* 8(10) (Oct 2012): e1002947.

155. Jablonski, N.G. *Skin: A Natural History.* University of California Press, 2006.

156. Ibid.

157. Holick M.F. *The Vitamin D Solution: A 3-Step Strategy to Cure Our Most Common Health Problems.* New York: Penguin Group USA, 2011.

158. Godar, D.E., R.J. Landry, A.D. Lucas. "Increased UVA Exposures and Decreased Cutaneous Vitamin D(3) Levels May Be Responsible for the Increasing Incidence of Melanoma." *Med Hypotheses* 72(4) (Apr 2009):434–443.

159. Gaby, A.R. "Natural Treatments for Osteoarthritis." *Altern Med Rev* 4(5) (Oct 1999):330–41. Jacquet, A., et al. "Phytalgic, a Food Supplement, vs Placebo in Patients with Osteoarthritis of the Knee or Hip: A Double-Blind Placebo-Controlled Clinical Trial." *Arthritis Res Ther* 2009;11(6) (2009):R192.

160. Machtey, I., L. Ouaknine. "Tocopherol in Osteoarthritis: A Controlled Pilot Study." *J Am Geriatr Soc* 26(7) (1978):328–30.

161. Shuid, A.N., et al. "Vitamin E Exhibits Bone Anabolic Actions in Normal Male Rats." *J Bone Miner Metab* 28(2) (2010):149–56. Hamidi, M.S., P.N. Corey, A.M. Cheung. "Effects of Vitamin E on Bone Turnover Markers Among US Postmenopausal Women." *J Bone Miner Res* 27(6) (Jun 2012):1368–80.

162. Gaby, A.R. "Natural Treatments for Osteoarthritis." *Altern Med Rev* 4(5) (Oct 1999):330–41.

163. Hamidi, M.S., P.N. Corey, A.M. Cheung. "Effects of Vitamin E on Bone Turnover Markers Among US Postmenopausal Women." *J Bone Miner Res* 27(6) (Jun 2012):1368–80.

164. Papas, A. *The Vitamin E Factor: The Miraculous Antioxidant for the Prevention and Treatment of Heart Disease, Cancer, and Aging.* HarperCollins, 1999. Aggarwal, B.B., et al. "Tocotrienols, the Vitamin E of the 21st Century: Its Potential Against Cancer and Other Chronic Diseases." *Biochem Pharmacol.* 80(11) (Dec 1, 2010):1613–31.

165. McCann, J.C., B.N. Ames. "Vitamin K, An Example of Triage Theory: Is Micronutrient Inadequacy Linked to Diseases of Aging?" *Am J Clin Nutr* 90(4) (Oct 2009): 889–907.

166. McCann, J.C., B.N. Ames. "Vitamin K, An Example of Triage Theory: Is Micronutrient Inadequacy Linked to Diseases of Aging?" *Am J Clin Nutr* 90(4) (Oct 2009): 889–907. Misra, D., et al. "Vitamin K Deficiency is Associated with Incident Knee Osteoarthritis." *Am J Med* 126(3) (Mar 2013):243–8.

167. Neogi, T., et al. "Low Vitamin K Status is Associated with Osteoarthritis in the Hand and Knee." *Arthritis Rheum* 54(4) (2006):1255–61.

168. Heiss, C., et. "Diagnosis of Osteoporosis with Vitamin K as a New Biochemical Marker." *Vitam Horm* 78 (2008):417–34. doi: 10.1016/S0083-6729(07)00017-9.

169. Misra, D., et al. "Vitamin K Deficiency is Associated with Incident Knee Osteoarthritis." *Am J Med* 126(3) (Mar 2013):243–8.

170. Heiss, C., et. "Diagnosis of Osteoporosis with Vitamin K as a New Biochemical Marker." *Vitam Horm* 78 (2008):417–34. doi: 10.1016/S0083-6729(07)00017-9. McCann, J.C., B.N. Ames. "Vitamin K, An Example of Triage Theory: Is Micronutrient Inadequacy Linked to Diseases of Aging?" *Am J Clin Nutr* 90(4) (Oct 2009):889–907.

171. Bügel S. "Vitamin K and Bone Health in Adult Humans." *Vitam Horm* 78 (2008):393–416.

172. Walther, B., et al. "Menaquinones, Bacteria, and the Food Supply: The Relevance of Dairy and Fermented Food Products to Vitamin K Requirements." *Adv Nutr* 4(4) (2013):463–473.

173. McCann, J.C., B.N. Ames. "Vitamin K, An Example of Triage Theory: Is Micronu-

trient Inadequacy Linked to Diseases of Aging?" *Am J Clin Nutr* 90(4) (Oct 2009):889–907.

174. Ishii, Y., et al. "Distribution of Vitamin K2 in Subchondral Bone in Osteoarthritic Knee Joints." *Knee Surg Sports Traumatol Arthrosc* 21(8) (2013):1813–8.

175. Walther, B., et al. "Menaquinones, Bacteria, and the Food Supply: The Relevance of Dairy and Fermented Food Products to Vitamin K Requirements." *Adv Nutr* 4(4) (2013):463–473.

176. Ebina, K., et al. "Vitamin K2 Administration is Associated with Decreased Disease Activity in Patients with Rheumatoid Arthritis." *Mod Rheumatol* 23(5) (Sep 2013):1001–7.

177. Iwamoto, I., et al. "A Longitudinal Study of the Effect of Vitamin K2 on Bone Mineral Density in Postmenopausal Women a Comparative Study with Vitamin D3 and Estrogen-Progestin Therapy." Maturitas. 31(2) (Jan 4, 1999):161–4.

178. Rheaume-Bleue, K. *Vitamin K2 and the Calcium Paradox: How a Little-Known Vitamin Could Save Your Life* New York: John Wiley & Sons, 2011.

179. Ibid.

180. Fuerst, M., et al. "Articular Cartilage Mineralization in Osteoarthritis of the Hip." *BMC Musculoskelet Disord* 10 (2009):166. Fuerst, M., et al. "Calcification of Articular Cartilage in Human Osteoarthritis." *Arthritis Rheum* 60(9) (2009):2694–703.

181. Darlington, L.G., T.W. Stone. "Antioxidants and Fatty Acids in the Amelioration of Rheumatoid Arthritis and Related Disorders." *Br J Nutr* 85(3) (Mar 2001):251–69. Cleland, L.G., M.J. James. "Osteoarthritis. Omega-3 Fatty Acids and Synovitis in Osteoarthritic Knees." *Nat Rev Rheumatol* 8(6) (2012):314–5.

182. Harbige, L.S. "Fatty Acids, the Immune Response, and Autoimmunity: A Question of n-6 Essentiality and the Balance between n-6 and n-3. *Lipids;*38(4) (Apr 2003):323–41. Russo, G.L. "Dietary n-6 and n-3 Polyunsaturated Fatty Acids: from Biochemistry to Clinical Implications in Cardiovascular Prevention." *Biochem Pharmacol* 77(6) (Mar 15 2009):937–46. Lopez, H.L. "Nutritional Interventions to Prevent and Treat Osteoarthritis. Part I: Focus on Fatty Acids and Macronutrients." *PM R* 4(5 Suppl) (May 2012):S145–54. Gropper, S.S., J.L. Smith. *Advanced Nutrition and Human Metabolism,* 6th Edition. New York: Cengage Learning, 2013.

183. Cleland, L.G., M.J. James, S.M. Proudman. "The Role of Fish Oils in the Treatment of Rheumatoid Arthritis. *Drugs* 63(9) (2003):845–53. Galarraga, B., et al. "Cod Liver Oil (n-3 fatty acids) as an Non-Steroidal Anti-Inflammatory Drug Sparing Agent in Rheumatoid Arthritis." *Rheumatology (Oxford)* 47(5) (2008):665–9. Lopez, H.L. "Nutritional Interventions to Prevent and Treat Osteoarthritis. Part I: Focus on Fatty Acids and Macronutrients." *PM R* 4(5 Suppl) (May 2012):S145–54.

184. Hutchins-Wiese, H.L., et al. "The Impact of Supplemental n-3 Long Chain Polyunsaturated Fatty Acids and Dietary Antioxidants on Physical Performance in Postmenopausal Women." *J Nutr Health Aging* 17(1) (2013):76–80.

185. Cleland, L.G., et al. "Reduction of Cardiovascular Risk Factors with Longterm Fish Oil Treatment in Early Rheumatoid Arthritis." *J Rheumatol* 33(10) (2006):1973–9.

186. Knott, L., et al. Regulation of Osteoarthritis by Omega-3 (n-3) Polyunsaturated Fatty Acids in a Naturally Occurring Model of Disease." *Osteoarthritis Cartilage* 19(9) (Sep 2011):1150–7.

187. Kantor, E.D., et al. "Association between Use of Specialty Dietary Supplements and C-Reactive Protein Concentrations." *Am J Epidemiol* 176(11) (Dec 1, 2012):1002–13.

188. Jacquet, A., et al. "Phytalgic, a Food Supplement, vs Placebo in Patients with Osteoarthritis of the Knee or Hip: A Double-Blind Placebo-Controlled Clinical Trial." *Arthritis Res Ther* 2009;11(6) (2009):R192.

189. Papas, A. *The Vitamin E Factor: The Miraculous Antioxidant for the Prevention and Treatment of Heart Disease, Cancer, and Aging.* HarperCollins, 1999.

190. Darlington, L.G., T.W. Stone. "Antioxidants and Fatty Acids in the Amelioration of Rheumatoid Arthritis and Related Disorders." *Br J Nutr* 85(3) (Mar 2001):251–69.

191. Cleland, L.G., M.J. James, S.M. Proudman. "The Role of Fish Oils in the Treatment of Rheumatoid Arthritis. *Drugs* 63(9) (2003):845–53. Cleland, L.G., M.J. James. "Osteoarthritis. Omega-3 Fatty Acids and Synovitis in Osteoarthritic Knees." *Nat Rev Rheumatol* 8(6) (2012):314–5.

192. Miles, E.A., P.C. Calder. "Influence of Marine n-3 Polyunsaturated Fatty Acids on Immune Function and a Systematic Review of Their Effects on Clinical Outcomes in Rheumatoid Arthritis." *Br J Nutr* 107 (Suppl 2) (2012):S171–84. Vanden Heuvel, J.P. "Nutrigenomics and Nutrigenetics of Omega-3 Polyunsaturated Fatty Acids." *Prog Mol Biol Transl Sci* 108 (2012):75–112.

193. Kruger, M.C., D.F. Horrobin. "Calcium Metabolism, Osteoporosis and Essential Fatty Acids: A Review." *Prog Lipid Res* 36(2–3) (Sep 1997):131–151.

194. Vanhorn, J., et al. "Attenuation of Niacin-Induced Prostaglandin D(2) Generation by Omega-3 Fatty Acids in THP-1 Macrophages and Langerhans Dendritic Cells." *J Inflamm Res* 5 (2012):37–50.

195. Zafarullah, M., et al. "Molecular Mechanisms of N-Acetylcysteine Actions." *Cell Mol Life Sci* 60(1) (2003):6–20.

196. Roosendaal, G., et al. "Blood-Induced Joint Damage: A Human in Vitro Study." *Arthritis Rheum* 42(5) (1999):1025–32.

197. Kröger, H., et al. "Suppression of Type II Collagen-Induced Arthritis by N-Acetyl-L-Cysteine in Mice." *Gen Pharmacol* 29(4) (Oct 1997):671–4.

198. Zafarullah, M., et al. "Molecular Mechanisms of N-Acetylcysteine Actions." *Cell Mol Life Sci* 60(1) (2003):6–20. Nakagawa, S., et al. "N-Acetylcysteine Prevents Nitric Oxide-Induced Chondrocyte Apoptosis and Cartilage Degeneration in an Experimental Model of Osteoarthritis." *J Orthop Res* 28(2) (2010):156–63.

199. Beecher, B.R., et al. "Antioxidants Block Cyclic Loading Induced Chondrocyte Death." *Iowa Orthop J* 27 (2007):1–8.

200. Lai, Z.W., et al. "N-Acetylcysteine Reduces Disease Activity by Blocking Mammalian Target of Rapamycin in T Cells from Systemic Lupus Erythematosus Patients: A Randomized, Double-Blind, Placebo-Controlled Trial." *Arthritis Rheum* 64(9) (2012):2937–46.

201. Lee, H.G., J.H. Yang. "PCB126 Induces Apoptosis of Chondrocytes via ROS-Dependent Pathways." *Osteoarthritis Cartilage* 20(10) (2012):1179–85.

202. Biniecka, M., et al. "Hypoxia Induces Mitochondrial Mutagenesis and Dysfunction in Inflammatory Arthritis." *Arthritis Rheum* 63(8) (Aug 2011):2172–82.

203. Oliver, S.J., et al. "Vanadate, an Inhibitor of Stromelysin and Collagenase Expression, Suppresses Collagen Induced Arthritis." *J Rheumatol* 34(9) (2007):1802–9.

204. Lee, E.Y., et al. "Alpha-Lipoic Acid Suppresses the Development of Collagen-Induced Arthritis and Protects Against Bone Destruction in Mice." *Rheumatol Int* 27(3) (2007):225–33. Shay, K.P., et al. "Alpha-Lipoic Acid as a Dietary Supplement: Molecular Mechanisms and Therapeutic Potential." *Biochim Biophys Acta* 1790(10) (Oct 2009):

1149–60. Hah, Y.S., et al. "Dietary Alpha Lipoic Acid Supplementation Prevents Synovial Inflammation and Bone Destruction in Collagen-Induced Arthritic Mice." *Rheumatol Int* 31(12) (2011):1583–90.

205. Iwai, K., et al. "Identification of Food-Derived Collagen Peptides in Human Blood after Oral Ingestion of Gelatin Hydrolysates." *J Agric Food Chem* 53(16) (2005):6531–6. Ohara, H., et al. "Effects of Pro-Hyp, a Collagen Hydrolysate-Derived Peptide, on Hyaluronic Acid Synthesis Using In Vitro Cultured Synovium Cells and Oral Ingestion of Collagen Hydrolysates in a Guinea Pig Model of Osteoarthritis." *Biosci Biotechnol Biochem* 74(10) (2010):2096–9.

206. Schauss, A.G., et al. "Effect of the Novel Low Molecular Weight Hydrolyzed Chicken Sternal Cartilage Extract, BioCell Collagen, on Improving Osteoarthritis-Related Symptoms: A Randomized, Double-Blind, Placebo-Controlled Trial." *J Agric Food Chem.* 60(16) (2012):4096–101.

207. Lopez, H.L. "Nutritional Interventions to Prevent and Treat Osteoarthritis. Part II: Focus on Micronutrients and Supportive Nutraceuticals." *PM R* 4(5 Suppl) (May 2012):S155–68. Ragle, R.L., A.D. Sawitzke. "Nutraceuticals in the Management of Osteoarthritis : A Critical Review." *Drugs Aging* 29(9) (2012):717–31.

208. Gaby, A.R. "Natural Treatments for Osteoarthritis." *Altern Med Rev* 4(5) (Oct 1999):330–41.

209. Nagaoka, I., M. Igarashi, K. Sakamoto. "Biological Activities of Glucosamine and Its Related Substances." *Adv Food Nutr Res* 65(2012):337–52.

210. Theodosakis, J., S. Buff. *The Arthritis Cure.* Revised edition. St. Martin's Paperbacks, 2004.

211. Leffler, C.T., et al. "Glucosamine, Chondroitin, and Manganese Ascorbate for Degenerative Joint Disease of the Knee or Low Back: A Randomized, Double-Blind, Placebo-Controlled Pilot Study." *Mil Med.* 164(2) (1999):85–91.

212. Kantor, E.D., et al. "Association between Use of Specialty Dietary Supplements and C-Reactive Protein Concentrations." *Am J Epidemiol* 176(11) (Dec 1, 2012):1002–13.

213. Kobayashi, T., et al. "Fursultiamine, A Vitamin B1 Derivative, Enhances Chondroprotective Effects of Glucosamine Hydrochloride and Chondroitin Sulfate in Rabbit Experimental Osteoarthritis." *Inflamm Res* 54(6) (Jun 2005):249–55.

214. Theodosakis, J., S. Buff. *The Arthritis Cure.* Revised edition. St. Martin's Paperbacks, 2004. Frech, T.M., D.O. Clegg. "The Utility of Nutraceuticals in the Treatment of Osteoarthritis." *Curr Rheumatol Rep* 9(1) (Apr 2007):25–30.Ragle, R.L., A.D. Sawitzke. "Nutraceuticals in the Management of Osteoarthritis : A Critical Review." *Drugs Aging* 29(9) (2012):717–31.

215. Schauss, A.G., et al. "Effect of the Novel Low Molecular Weight Hydrolyzed Chicken Sternal Cartilage Extract, BioCell Collagen, on Improving Osteoarthritis-Related Symptoms: A Randomized, Double-Blind, Placebo-Controlled Trial." *J Agric Food Chem.* 60(16) (2012):4096–101.

216. Mobasheri, A., et al. "Glucose Transport and Metabolism in Chondrocytes: A Key to Understanding Chondrogenesis, Skeletal Development and Cartilage Degradation in Osteoarthritis." *Histol Histopathol* 17(4) (Oct 2002):1239–67. Gropper, S.S., J.L. Smith. *Advanced Nutrition and Human Metabolism*, 6th edition. New York: Cengage Learning, 2013.

217. Ohara, H., et al. "Effects of Pro-Hyp, a Collagen Hydrolysate-Derived Peptide, on Hyaluronic Acid Synthesis Using In Vitro Cultured Synovium Cells and Oral Ingestion of

Collagen Hydrolysates in a Guinea Pig Model of Osteoarthritis." *Biosci Biotechnol Biochem* 74(10) (2010):2096–9.

218. Lopez, H.L. "Nutritional Interventions to Prevent and Treat Osteoarthritis. Part II: Focus on Micronutrients and Supportive Nutraceuticals." *PM R* 4(5 Suppl) (May 2012): S155–68.

219. Ibid.

220. Crowley, D.C., et al. "Safety and Efficacy of Undenatured Type II Collagen in the Treatment of Osteoarthritis of the Knee: A Clinical Trial." *Int J Med Sci* 6(6) (2009): 312–21.

221. Lopez, H.L. "Nutritional Interventions to Prevent and Treat Osteoarthritis. Part II: Focus on Micronutrients and Supportive Nutraceuticals." *PM R* 4(5 Suppl) (May 2012):S155–68.

222. Ibid.

223. Ibid.

224. Lopez, H.L. "Nutritional Interventions to Prevent and Treat Osteoarthritis. Part II: Focus on Micronutrients and Supportive Nutraceuticals." *PM R* 4(5 Suppl) (May 2012):S155–68. Ragle, R.L., A.D. Sawitzke. "Nutraceuticals in the Management of Osteoarthritis : A Critical Review." *Drugs Aging* 29(9) (2012):717–31.

225. De Silva, V., et al. "Evidence for the Efficacy of Complementary and Alternative Medicines in the Management of Osteoarthritis: A Systematic Review." *Rheumatology (Oxford)* 50(5) (2011):911–20.

226. Yoshida, M., et al. "Expression Analysis of Three Isoforms of Hyaluronan Synthase and Hyaluronidase in the Synovium of Knees in Osteoarthritis and Rheumatoid Arthritis by Quantitative Real-Time Reverse Transcriptase Polymerase Chain Reaction." *Arthritis Res Ther* 6(6) (2004):R514–20.

227. Waller, K.A., et al. "Preventing Friction-Induced Chondrocyte Apoptosis: Comparison of Human Synovial Fluid and Hylan G-F 20." *J Rheumatol* 39(7) (2012):1473–80.

228. Khanasuk ,Y., T. Dechmaneenin, A. Tanavalee. "Prospective Randomized Trial Comparing the Efficacy of Single 6-ml Injection of Hylan G-F 20 and Hyaluronic Acid for Primary Knee Arthritis: A Preliminary Study." *J Med Assoc Thai* 95 Suppl 10 (2012):S92-S97. Cianflocco, A.J. "Viscosupplementation in Patients with Osteoarthritis of the Knee." *Postgrad Med* 125(1) (Jan 2013):97–105. Turajane, T., et al. "Combination of Intra-Articular Autologous Activated Peripheral Blood Stem Cells with Growth Factor Addition/ Preservation and Hyaluronic Acid in Conjunction with Arthroscopic Microdrilling Mesenchymal Cell Stimulation Improves Quality of Life and Regenerates Articular Cartilage in Early Osteoarthritic Knee Disease." *J Med Assoc Thai* 96(5) (2013):580–8.

229. Tsai, W.Y., et al. "Early Intraarticular Injection of Hyaluronic Acid Attenuates Osteoarthritis Progression in Anterior Cruciate Ligament-Transected Rats." *Connect Tissue Res* 54(1) (2013):49–54.

230. Civinini, R., et al. "Growth Factors in the Treatment of Early Osteoarthritis." *Clin Cases Miner Bone Metab* 10(1) (2013):26–9.

231. Shemesh, S., et al. "Septic Arthritis of the Knee Following Intraarticular Injections in Elderly Patients: Report of Six Patients." Isr Med Assoc J. 13(12) (Dec 13, 2011):757–60.

232. Powell, S.R. "The Antioxidant Properties of Zinc." *J Nutr* 130(5S Suppl) (2000):1447S-54S.

233. Powell, S.R. "The Antioxidant Properties of Zinc." *J Nutr* 130(5S Suppl)

(2000):1447S-54S. Gropper, S.S., J.L. Smith. *Advanced Nutrition and Human Metabolism*, 6th edition. New York: Cengage Learning, 2013.

234. Afridi, H.I., et al. "Interaction between Zinc, Cadmium, and Lead in Scalp Hair Samples of Pakistani and Irish Smokers Rheumatoid Arthritis Subjects in Relation to Controls." *Biol Trace Elem Res* 148(2) (Aug 2012):139–47. Afridi, H.I., et al. "Evaluation of Status of Arsenic, Cadmium, Lead and Zinc Levels in Biological Samples of Normal and Arthritis Patients of Age Groups (46–60) and (61–75) Years." *Clin Lab* 59(1–2) (2013):143–53.

235. Honkanen, V.E., et al. "Plasma Zinc and Copper Concentrations in Rheumatoid Arthritis: Influence of Dietary Factors and Disease Activity." *Am J Clin Nutr* 54(6) (Dec 1991):1082–6.

236. Afridi, H.I., et al. "Evaluation of Status of Arsenic, Cadmium, Lead and Zinc Levels in Biological Samples of Normal and Arthritis Patients of Age Groups (46–60) and (61–75) Years." *Clin Lab* 59(1–2) (2013):143–53.

237. Lopez, H.L. "Nutritional Interventions to Prevent and Treat Osteoarthritis. Part II: Focus on Micronutrients and Supportive Nutraceuticals." *PM R* 4(5 Suppl) (May 2012):S155–68. Gropper, S.S., J.L. Smith. *Advanced Nutrition and Human Metabolism*, 6th edition. New York: Cengage Learning, 2013.

238. Yazar, M., et al. "Synovial Fluid and Plasma Selenium, Copper, Zinc, and Iron Concentrations in Patients with Rheumatoid Arthritis and Osteoarthritis." *Biol Trace Elem Res* 106(2) (2005):123–132.

239. Lopez, H.L. "Nutritional Interventions to Prevent and Treat Osteoarthritis. Part II: Focus on Micronutrients and Supportive Nutraceuticals." *PM R* 4(5 Suppl) (May 2012):S155–68.

240. Cerhan, J.R., et al. "Antioxidant Micronutrients and Risk of Rheumatoid Arthritis in a Cohort of Older Women." *Am J Epidemiol* 57(4) (Feb 15, 2003):345–54. Sanmartin, C., et al. "Selenium and Clinical Trials: New Therapeutic Evidence for Multiple Diseases." *Curr Med Chem* 18(30) (2011):4635–50.

241. Yazar, M., et al. "Synovial Fluid and Plasma Selenium, Copper, Zinc, and Iron Concentrations in Patients with Rheumatoid Arthritis and Osteoarthritis." *Biol Trace Elem Res* 106(2) (2005):123–132.

242. Vieira, A.T., et al. "Treatment with Selemax®, a Selenium-Enriched Yeast, Ameliorates Experimental Arthritis in Rats and Mice." *Br J Nutr* 108(10) (Nov 28, 2012): 1829–38.

243. Kamanli, A., et al. "Plasma Lipid Peroxidation and Antioxidant Levels in Patients with Rheumatoid Arthritis." *Cell Biochem Funct* 22(1) (Jan-Feb 2004):53–57.

244. McCann, J.C., B.N. Ames. "Adaptive Dysfunction of Selenoproteins from the Perspective of the Triage Theory: Why Modest Selenium Deficiency May Increase Risk of Diseases of Aging." *FASEB J* 25(6) (Jun 2011):1793–814.

245. Cerhan, J.R., et al. "Antioxidant Micronutrients and Risk of Rheumatoid Arthritis in a Cohort of Older Women." *Am J Epidemiol* 57(4) (Feb 15, 2003):345–54. Merlino, L.A., et al. "Vitamin D Intake is Inversely Associated with Rheumatoid Arthritis: Results from the Iowa Women's Health Study." Arthritis Rheum. 50(1) (Jan 2004):72–7.

246. Lopez, H.L. "Nutritional Interventions to Prevent and Treat Osteoarthritis. Part II: Focus on Micronutrients and Supportive Nutraceuticals." *PM R* 4(5 Suppl) (May 2012):S155–68.

247. Newnham, R.E. "Essentiality of Boron for Healthy Bones and Joints." *Environ Health Perspect* 102(Suppl 7) (1994):83–5.

248. Guggenbuhl, P., P. Brissot, O. Loréal. "Haemochromatosis: The Bone and the Joint." *Best Pract Res Clin Rheumatol* 25(5) (2011):649–64.

249. Emery, T.F. *Iron and your Health: Facts and Fallacies.* Boca Raton, FL: CRC Press, 1991. Weinberg, E.D. "Is Addition of Iron to Processed Foods Safe for Iron Replete Consumers?" *Med Hypotheses* 73(6) (Dec 2009):948–9.

250. Emery, T.F. *Iron and your Health: Facts and Fallacies.* Boca Raton, FL: CRC Press, 1991. Knutson, M.D., et al. "Both Iron Deficiency and Daily Iron Supplements Increase Lipid Peroxidation in Rats." *J Nutr* 130(3) (2000):621–8.

251. Killilea, D.W., et al. "Iron Accumulation During Cellular Senescence." *Ann NY Acad Sci* 1019 (2004):365–7.

252. Guggenbuhl, P., P. Brissot, O. Loréal. "Haemochromatosis: The Bone and the Joint." *Best Pract Res Clin Rheumatol* 25(5) (2011):649–64.

253. Emery, T.F. *Iron and your Health: Facts and Fallacies.* Boca Raton, FL: CRC Press, 1991. Hurrell, R., I. Egli. "Iron Bioavailability and Dietary Reference Values." *Am J Clin Nutr* 91(5) (2010):1461S-1467S.

254. Hurrell, R., I. Egli. "Iron Bioavailability and Dietary Reference Values." *Am J Clin Nutr* 91(5) (2010):1461S-1467S.

255. Weinberg, E.D. "Iron Loading: A Risk Factor for Osteoporosis." *Biometals* 19(6) (2006):633–5.

256. Guggenbuhl, P., P. Brissot, O. Loréal. "Haemochromatosis: The Bone and the Joint." *Best Pract Res Clin Rheumatol* 25(5) (2011):649–64. Dallos, T., et al. "Idiopathic Hand Osteoarthritis vs Haemochromatosis Arthropathy—A Clinical, Functional and Radiographic Study." *Rheumatology (Oxford)* 52(5) (2013):910–5.

257. Guggenbuhl, P., P. Brissot, O. Loréal. "Haemochromatosis: The Bone and the Joint." *Best Pract Res Clin Rheumatol* 25(5) (2011):649–64.

258. Weinberg, E.D. "Role of Iron in Osteoporosis." *Pediatr Endocrinol Rev* 6(Suppl 1) (2009):81–5.

259. LeBlanc, et al. "Bacteria as Vitamin Suppliers to Their Host: A Gut Microbiota Perspective." *Curr Opin Biotechnol* 24(2) (Apr 2013):160–8.

260. Ibid.

261. Le Chatelier, E., et al. "Richness of Human Gut Microbiome Correlates with Metabolic Markers." *Nature* 500(7464) (2013):541–6.

262. Cotillard, A., et al, "Dietary Intervention Impact on Gut microbial Gene Richness." *Nature* 500(7464) (2013):585–8.

263. Kano, H., O. Mogami, M. Uchida. "Oral Administration of Milk Fermented with Lactobacillus Delbrueckii ssp. Bulgaricus OLL1073R-1 to DBA/1 Mice Inhibits Secretion of Proinflammatory Cytokines." *Cytotechnology* 40(1–3) (2002):67–73. Amdekar, S., et al. "Lactobacillus Casei and Lactobacillus Acidophilus Regulate Inflammatory Pathway and Improve Antioxidant Status in Collagen-Induced Arthritic Rats." *J Interferon Cytokine Res* 33(1) (Jan 2013):1–8.

264. So, J.S., et al. "Lactobacillus Casei Enhances Type II Collagen/Glucosamine-Mediated Suppression of Inflammatory Responses in Experimental Osteoarthritis." *Life Sci* 88(7–8) (2011):358–66.

265. Peltonen, R., et al. "Faecal Microbial Flora and Disease Activity in Rheumatoid Arthritis During a Vegan Diet." *Br J Rheumatol* 36(1) (Jan 1997):64–8.

266. Mandel, D.R., K. Eichas, J. Holmes. "Bacillus Coagulans: A Viable Adjunct Therapy for Relieving Symptoms of Rheumatoid Arthritis According to a Randomized, Controlled Trial." *BMC Complement Altern Med* 10 (Jan 12, 2010):1.

267. Schiffer, C., et al. "A Strain of Lactobacillus Casei Inhibits the Effector Phase of Immune Inflammation." *J Immunol* 187(5) (2011):2646–55.

268. Monachese, M., J.P. Burton, G. Reid. "Bioremediation and Tolerance of Humans to Heavy Metals through Microbial Processes: A Potential Role for Probiotics?" *Appl Environ Microbiol* 78(18) (2012):6397–404. Afridi, H.I., et al. "Interaction between Zinc, Cadmium, and Lead in Scalp Hair Samples of Pakistani and Irish Smokers Rheumatoid Arthritis Subjects in Relation to Controls." *Biol Trace Elem Res* 148(2) (Aug 2012):139–47. Afridi, H.I., et al. "Evaluation of Status of Arsenic, Cadmium, Lead and Zinc Levels in Biological Samples of Normal and Arthritis Patients of Age Groups (46–60) and (61–75) Years." *Clin Lab* 59(1–2) (2013):143–53.

269. Weinberg, E.D. "Iron Availability and Infection." *Biochim Biophys Acta* 1790(7) (2009):600–5.

270. Emery, T.F. *Iron and your Health: Facts and Fallacies.* Boca Raton, FL: CRC Press, 1991. Weinberg, E.D. "The Lactobacillus Anomaly: Total Iron Abstinence. Perspectives in Biology and Medicine." 40(4) (1997):578–83.

271. Archibald, F. "Manganese: Its Acquisition by and Function in the Lactic Acid Bacteria." *Crit Rev Microbiol* 13(1) (1986):63–109. Weinberg, E.D. "Iron Availability and Infection." *Biochim Biophys Acta* 1790(7) (2009):600–5.

272. Troxell, B., H. Xu, X.F. Yang. "Borrelia Burgdorferi, a Pathogen That Lacks Iron, Encodes Manganese-Dependent Superoxide Dismutase Essential for Resistance to Streptonigrin." *J Biol Chem* 287(23) (2012):19284–93. Aguirre, J.D., et al. "A Manganese-Rich Environment Supports Superoxide Dismutase Activity in a Lyme Disease Pathogen, *Borrelia burgdorferi*." *J Biol Chem* 288(12) (2013):8468–78.

273. Wang, P., et al. "A Novel Iron- and Copper-Binding Protein in the Lyme Disease Spirochaete." *Mol Microbiol* 86(6) (2012):1441–51.

274. Jacob, R.A., et al. "Consumption of Cherries Lowers Plasma Urate in Healthy Women. *J Nutr* 133 (2003):1826–9. Kelley, D.S., et al. "Consumption of Bing Sweet Cherries Lowers Circulating Concentrations of Inflammation Markers in Healthy Men and Women." *J Nutr* 136 (2006):981–6. Recio, M.C., I. Andujar, J.L. Rios. "Anti-Inflammatory Agents from Plants: Progress and Potential." *Curr Med Chem* 19(14) (2012):2088–103. Bell, P.G., et al. "The Role of Cherries in Exercise and Health." *Scand J Med Sci Sports* (May 27, 2013). doi: 10.1111/sms.12085. [Epub ahead of print] Glehr, M., A. Leithner, R. Windhager. "Influence of Resveratrol on Rheumatoid Fibroblast-Like Synoviocytes Analysed with Gene Chip Transcription. *Phytomedicine* 20 (2013):310–8. Kelley, D.S., et al. "Sweet Bing Cherries Lower Circulating Concentrations of Markers for Chronic Inflammatory Diseases in Healthy Humans." *J Nutr* 143(3) (Mar 2013):340–4.

275. Ferretti, G., et al. "Cherry Antioxidants: From Farm to Table." *Molecules* 15(10) (Oct 12, 2010):6993–7005. Kuehl, K.S. "Cherry Juice Targets Antioxidant Potential and Pain Relief." *Med Sport Sci* 59 (2012):86–93.

276. Shen, C.L., et al. "Dietary Polyphenols and Mechanisms of Osteoarthritis." *J Nutr Biochem* 23 (2012):1367–77. Bell, P.G., et al. "The Role of Cherries in Exercise and Health." *Scand J Med Sci Sports* (May 27, 2013). doi: 10.1111/sms.12085. [Epub ahead of print]. Jean-Gilles, D., et al. "Inhibitory Effects of Polyphenol Punicalagin on Type-II

Collagen Degradation in Vitro and Inflammation in Vivo." *Chem Biol Interact* 205(2) (Sep 25, 2013):90–9.

277. Bråkenhielm, E., R. Cao, Y. Cao. "Suppression of Angiogenesis, Tumor Growth, and Wound Healing by Resveratrol, a Natural Compound in Red Wine and Grapes." *FASEB J* 15 (2001):1798–800. Lee, A.S., et al. "A Current Review of Molecular Mechanisms Regarding Osteoarthritis and Pain." *Gene* 527(2) (Sep 25, 2013): 440–7. Tian, J., et al. "Resveratrol Inhibits TNF-Alpha-Induced IL-1-beta, MMP-3 Production in Human Rheumatoid Arthritis Fibroblast-Like Synoviocytes via Modulation of PI3kinase/Akt Pathway." *Rheumatol Int* 33 (2013):1829–35.

278. McCormack, D., D. McFadden. "A Review of Pterostilbene Antioxidant Activity and Disease Modification." *Oxid Med Cell Longev* (2013):575482.

279. Im, H.J., et al. "Biological Effects of the Plant-Derived Polyphenol Resveratrol in Human Articular Cartilage and Chondrosarcoma Cells." *J Cell Physiol* 227 (2012):3488–97. Mobasheri, A, et al. "Scientific Evidence and Rationale for the Development of Curcumin and Resveratrol as Nutraceutricals for Joint Health." *Int J Mol Sci* 13(4) (2012):4202–32. Glehr, M., A. Leithner, R. Windhager. "Influence of Resveratrol on Rheumatoid Fibroblast-Like Synoviocytes Analysed with Gene Chip Transcription. *Phytomedicine* 20 (2013):310–8. Lee, A.S., et al. "A Current Review of Molecular Mechanisms Regarding Osteoarthritis and Pain." *Gene* 527(2) (Sep 25, 2013): 440–7.

280. Shen, C.L., et al. "Dietary Polyphenols and Mechanisms of Osteoarthritis." *J Nutr Biochem* 23 (2012):1367–77. Jean-Gilles, D., et al. "Inhibitory Effects of Polyphenol Punicalagin on Type-II Collagen Degradation in Vitro and Inflammation in Vivo." *Chem Biol Interact* 205(2) (Sep 25, 2013):90–9.

281. Jacob, R.A., et al. "Consumption of Cherries Lowers Plasma Urate in Healthy Women. *J Nutr* 133 (2003):1826–9.

282. Kelley, D.S., et al. "Consumption of Bing Sweet Cherries Lowers Circulating Concentrations of Inflammation Markers in Healthy Men and Women." *J Nutr* 136 (2006):981–6. Kelley, D.S., et al. "Sweet Bing Cherries Lower Circulating Concentrations of Markers for Chronic Inflammatory Diseases in Healthy Humans." *J Nutr* 143(3) (Mar 2013):340–4.

283. McCune, L.M., et al. "Cherries and Health: A Review." *Crit Rev Food Sci Nutr* 51(1) (Jan 2011):1–12. Zhao, Y., et al. "Melatonin and Its Potential Biological Functions in the Fruits of Sweet Cherry." *J Pineal Res* 55(1) (Aug 2012):79–88.

284. Zhao, Y., et al. "Melatonin and Its Potential Biological Functions in the Fruits of Sweet Cherry." *J Pineal Res* 55(1) (Aug 2012):79–88.

285. Pigeon, W.R., et al. "Effects of a Tart Cherry Juice Beverage on the Sleep of Older Adults with Insomnia: A Pilot Study." *J Med Food* 13(3) (Jun 2010):579–83.

286. Bell, P.G., et al. "The Role of Cherries in Exercise and Health." *Scand J Med Sci Sports* (May 27, 2013). doi: 10.1111/sms.12085. [Epub ahead of print]

287. van Leeuwen, W.M., et al. "Sleep Restriction Increases the Risk of Developing Cardiovascular Diseases by Augmenting Proinflammatory Responses through IL-17 and CRP." *PLoS One* 4(2) (2009):e4589.

288. Bell, P.G., et al. "The Role of Cherries in Exercise and Health." *Scand J Med Sci Sports* (May 27, 2013). doi: 10.1111/sms.12085. [Epub ahead of print]

289. Ferretti, G., et al. "Cherry Antioxidants: From Farm to Table." *Molecules* 15(10) (Oct 12, 2010):6993–7005. Kuehl, K.S. "Cherry Juice Targets Antioxidant Potential and Pain Relief." *Med Sport Sci* 59 (2012):86–93. Tian, J., et al. "Resveratrol Inhibits TNF-

Alpha-Induced IL-1-beta, MMP-3 Production in Human Rheumatoid Arthritis Fibroblast-Like Synoviocytes via Modulation of PI3kinase/Akt Pathway." *Rheumatol Int* 33 (2013):1829–35.

290. Ferretti, G., et al. "Cherry Antioxidants: From Farm to Table." *Molecules* 15(10) (Oct 12, 2010):6993–7005. Kuehl, K.S. "Cherry Juice Targets Antioxidant Potential and Pain Relief." *Med Sport Sci* 59 (2012):86–93.

291. Kuehl, K.S. "Cherry Juice Targets Antioxidant Potential and Pain Relief." *Med Sport Sci* 59 (2012):86–93. Bell, P.G., et al. "The Role of Cherries in Exercise and Health." *Scand J Med Sci Sports* (May 27, 2013). doi: 10.1111/sms.12085. [Epub ahead of print]

292. Kuehl, K.S. "Cherry Juice Targets Antioxidant Potential and Pain Relief." *Med Sport Sci* 59 (2012):86–93.

293. Lopez, H.L. "Nutritional Interventions to Prevent and Treat Osteoarthritis. Part II: Focus on Micronutrients and Supportive Nutraceuticals." *PM R* 4(5 Suppl) (May 2012):S155–68.

294. Wahls, T.L. *Minding My Mitochondria 2nd Edition: How I Overcame Secondary Progressive Multiple Sclerosis (MS) and got out of my wheelchair.* 2nd edition. Iowa City, IA: TZ Press; 2010. Wahls, T.L. (2013) The Wahls Protocol: How I Beat Progressive MS Using Paleo Principles and Functional Medicine. New York: Avery, 2014. www.terry-wahls.com.

295. Davidson, R.K., et al. "Sulforaphane Represses Matrix-Degrading Proteases and Protects Cartilage from Destruction In Vitro and In Vivo." *Arthritis & Rheumatism* 65(12) (Dec 2013):31330–40.

296. Ammon, H.P. "Modulation of the Immune System by Boswellia Serrata Extracts and Boswellic Acids." *Phytomedicine* 17(11) (Sep 2010):862–7.

297. Aggarwal, B.B., et al. "Curcumin: The Indian Solid Gold." *Adv Exp Med Biol* 595 (2007):1–75. Aggarwal, B.B., B. Sung. "Pharmacological Basis for the Role of Curcumin in Chronic Diseases: An Age-Old Spice with Modern Targets." *Trends Pharmacol Sci* 30(2) (Feb 2009):85–94.

298. Jackson, J.K., et al. "The Antioxidants Curcumin and Quercetin Inhibit Inflammatory Processes Associated with Arthritis." *Inflamm Res* 55(4) (Apr 2006):168–75. Aggarwal, B.B., B. Sung. "Pharmacological Basis for the Role of Curcumin in Chronic Diseases: An Age-Old Spice with Modern Targets." *Trends Pharmacol Sci* 30(2) (Feb 2009):85–94. Mobasheri, A, et al. "Scientific Evidence and Rationale for the Development of Curcumin and Resveratrol as Nutraceutricals for Joint Health." *Int J Mol Sci* 13(4) (2012):4202–32. Lopez, H.L. "Nutritional Interventions to Prevent and Treat Osteoarthritis. Part II: Focus on Micronutrients and Supportive Nutraceuticals." *PM R* 4(5 Suppl) (May 2012):S155–68. Shen, C.L., et al. "Dietary Polyphenols and Mechanisms of Osteoarthritis." *J Nutr Biochem* 23 (2012):1367–77.

299. Mobasheri, A, et al. "Scientific Evidence and Rationale for the Development of Curcumin and Resveratrol as Nutraceutricals for Joint Health." *Int J Mol Sci* 13(4) (2012):4202–32.

300. Altenburg, J.D., et al. "A Synergistic Antiproliferation Effect of Curcumin and Docosahexaenoic Acid in SK-BR-3 Breast Cancer Cells: Unique Signaling Not Explained by the Effects of Either Compound Alone." *BMC Cancer* 11 (2011):149.

301. Lopez, H.L. "Nutritional Interventions to Prevent and Treat Osteoarthritis. Part II: Focus on Micronutrients and Supportive Nutraceuticals." *PM R* 4(5 Suppl) (May 2012):S155–68.

302. Mobasheri, A, et al. "Scientific Evidence and Rationale for the Development of Curcumin and Resveratrol as Nutraceuticals for Joint Health." *Int J Mol Sci* 13(4) (2012):4202–32.

303. Mobasheri, A, et al. "Scientific Evidence and Rationale for the Development of Curcumin and Resveratrol as Nutraceuticals for Joint Health." *Int J Mol Sci* 13(4) (2012):4202–32.

304. Chalasani, N., et al. "Acute Liver Injury Due to Flavocoxid (Limbrel), A medical Food for Osteoarthritis: A Case Series." *Ann Intern Med* 156(12) (Jun 19, 2012):857–60. Panduranga, V., et al. "Hypersensitivity Pneumonitis Due to Flavocoxid: Are Corticosteroids Necessary?" *Conn Med* 77(2) (Feb 2013):87–90.

305. Mobasheri, A, et al. "Scientific Evidence and Rationale for the Development of Curcumin and Resveratrol as Nutraceuticals for Joint Health." *Int J Mol Sci* 13(4) (2012):4202–32.

306. De Silva, V., et al. "Evidence for the Efficacy of Complementary and Alternative Medicines in the Management of Osteoarthritis: A Systematic Review." *Rheumatology (Oxford)* 50(5) (2011):911–920.

307. Bode, A.M., Z. Dong. "The Amazing and Mighty Ginger." Chapter 7 in: *Herbal Medicine: Biomolecular and Clinical Aspects.* editors I.F.F. Benzie, S. Wachtel-Galor, 2nd edition. Boca Raton, FL: CRC Press, 2011.. Online at: www.ncbi.nlm.nih.gov/books/NBK92775

308. Drozdov, V.N., et al. "Influence of a Specific Ginger Combination on Gastropathy Conditions in Patients with Osteoarthritis of the Knee or Hip." *J Altern Complement Med* 18(6) (Jun 2012):583–8. Niempoog, S., P. Siriarchavatana, T. Kajsongkram. "The Efficacy of Plygersic Gel for Use in the Treatment of Osteoarthritis of the Knee." *J Med Assoc Thai* 95 Suppl 10 (2012):S113–9. Ribel-Madsen, S., et al. "A Synoviocyte Model for Osteoarthritis and Rheumatoid Arthritis: Response to Ibuprofen, Betamethasone, and Ginger Extract-A Cross-Sectional In Vitro Study." *Arthritis* 2012 (2012):505842.

309. Drozdov, V.N., et al. "Influence of a Specific Ginger Combination on Gastropathy Conditions in Patients with Osteoarthritis of the Knee or Hip." *J Altern Complement Med* 18(6) (Jun 2012):583–8. 890.

310. Altman, R.D., K.C. Marcussen. "Effects of a Ginger Extract on Knee Pain in Patients with Osteoarthritis." *Arthritis Rheum* 44(11) (Nov 2001):2531–8. Funk, J.L., et al. "Comparative Effects of Two Gingerol-Containing Zingiber Officinale Extracts on Experimental Rheumatoid Arthritis" *J Nat Prod* 72(3) (Mar 27, 2009):403–7. Bode, A.M., Z. Dong. "The Amazing and Mighty Ginger." Chapter 7 in: *Herbal Medicine: Biomolecular and Clinical Aspects.* editors I.F.F. Benzie, S. Wachtel-Galor, 2nd edition. Boca Raton, FL: CRC Press, 2011.. Online at: www.ncbi.nlm.nih.gov/books/NBK92775.

311. Srivastava, K.C., T. Mustafa. "Ginger (Zingiber Officinale) in Rheumatism and Musculoskeletal Disorders." Med Hypotheses. 39(4) (1992):342–348. Bode, A.M., Z. Dong. "The Amazing and Mighty Ginger." Chapter 7 in: *Herbal Medicine: Biomolecular and Clinical Aspects.* editors I.F.F. Benzie, S. Wachtel-Galor, 2nd edition. Boca Raton, FL: CRC Press, 2011.. Online at: www.ncbi.nlm.nih.gov/books/NBK92775

312. Srivastava, K.C., T. Mustafa. "Ginger (Zingiber Officinale) in Rheumatism and Musculoskeletal Disorders." Med Hypotheses. 39(4) (1992):342–348. Bode, A.M., Z. Dong. "The Amazing and Mighty Ginger." Chapter 7 in: *Herbal Medicine: Biomolecular and Clinical Aspects.* editors I.F.F. Benzie, S. Wachtel-Galor, 2nd edition. Boca Raton, FL: CRC Press, 2011.. Online at: www.ncbi.nlm.nih.gov/books/NBK92775

313. Bode, A.M., Z. Dong. "The Amazing and Mighty Ginger." Chapter 7 in: *Herbal Med-*

icine: Biomolecular and Clinical Aspects. editors I.F.F. Benzie, S. Wachtel-Galor, 2nd edition. Boca Raton, FL: CRC Press, 2011.. Online at: www.ncbi.nlm.nih.gov/books/NBK92775.

314. Bhadoriya, S.S., et al. "Tamarindus Indica: Extent of Explored Potential." *Pharmacogn Rev* 5(9) (Jan 2011):73–81.

315. Chen, X.Y., et al. "Effect of Total Flavonoids of Chrysanthemum Indicum on the Apoptosis of Synoviocytes in Joint of Adjuvant Arthritis Rats." *Am J Chin Med* 36(4) (2008):695–704. Man, M.Q., et al. "Topical Apigenin Alleviates Cutaneous Inflammation in Murine Models." *Evid Based Complement Alternat Med.* 2012 (2012):912028.

316. Akhtar, N., T.M. Haqqi. "Epigallocatechin-3-Gallate Suppresses the Global Interleukin-1beta-Induced Inflammatory Response in Human Chondrocytes." *Arthritis Res Ther* 13(3) (Jun 2011):R93. Recio, M.C., I. Andujar, J.L. Rios. "Anti-Inflammatory Agents from Plants: Progress and Potential." *Curr Med Chem* 19(14) (2012):2088–103. Shen, C.L., et al. "Dietary Polyphenols and Mechanisms of Osteoarthritis." *J Nutr Biochem* 23 (2012):1367–77.

317. Chandra, L., et al. "White Button and Shiitake Mushrooms Reduce the Incidence and Severity of Collagen-Induced Arthritis in Dilute Brown Non-Agouti Mice." *J Nutr* 141(1) (Jan 2011):131–6. Yayeh, T., et al. "Phellinus Baumii Ethyl Acetate Extract Alleviated Collagen Type II Induced Arthritis in DBA/1 Mice." *J Nat Med* 2013 (Oct 2013):807–13.

318. Cerhan, J.R., et al. "Antioxidant Micronutrients and Risk of Rheumatoid Arthritis in a Cohort of Older Women." *Am J Epidemiol* 57(4) (Feb 15, 2003):345–54.

319. Shaik, Y.B., et al. "Role of Quercetin (A Natural Herbal Compound) in Allergy and Inflammation." *J Biol Regul Homeost Agents* 20(3–4) (Jul-Dec 2006):47–52.

320. Boyer, J., R.H. Liu. "Apple Phytochemicals and Their Health Benefits." *Nutr J* 3 (May 2004):5.

321. Pennathur, S., et al. "Potent Antioxidative Activity of Lycopene: A Potential Role in Scavenging Hypochlorous Acid." *Free Radic Biol Med* 49(2) (2010):205–13.

322. Al-Okbi, S.Y. "Nutraceuticals of Anti-inflammatory Activity as Complementary Therapy for Rheumatoid Arthritis." *Toxicol Ind Health* (Oct 26, 2012).

323. Yang, L., et al. "Herbal Hepatoxicity from Chinese Skullcap: A Case Report." *World J Hepatol* 4(7) (2012):231–3.

324. Richette, P., T. Bardin. "Gout." *Lancet* 375(9711) (Jan 23, 2010):318–28. Crittenden, D..B., M.H. Pillinger. "New Therapies for Gout." *Annu Rev Med* 64 (2013):325–37. Harrold, L. "New Developments in Gout." *Curr Opin Rheumatol* 25(3) (May 2013):304–9.

325. Zhang, Y., et al. "Alcohol Consumption as a Trigger of Recurrent Gout Attacks." *Am J Med* 119(9) (Sep 2006):800.e13–8. Richette, P., T. Bardin. "Gout." *Lancet* 375(9711) (Jan 23, 2010):318–28.

326. Choi, H.K. "A Prescription for Lifestyle Change in Patients with Hyperuricemia and Gout." *Curr Opin Rheumatol* 22(2) (Mar 2010):165–72. Richette, P., T. Bardin. "Gout." *Lancet* 375(9711) (Jan 23, 2010):318–28. Juraschek, S.P., E.R. Miller 3rd, A.C. Gelber. "Effect of Oral Vitamin C Supplementation on Serum Uric Acid: A Meta-Analysis of Randomized Controlled Trials." *Arthritis Care Res (Hoboken)* 63(9) (2011):1295–306. Crittenden, D..B., M.H. Pillinger. "New Therapies for Gout." *Annu Rev Med* 64 (2013):325–37.

327. Choi, W.J., et al. "Independent Association of Serum Retinol and Beta-Carotene Lev-

els with Hyperuricemia: A National Population Study." *Arthritis Care Res (Hoboken)* 64(3) (2012):389–96.

328. Choi, H.K. "A Prescription for Lifestyle Change in Patients with Hyperuricemia and Gout." *Curr Opin Rheumatol* 22(2) (Mar 2010):165–72. Shen, L., H.F. Ji. "Potential of Vitamin C in the Prevention and Treatment of Gout." *Nature Reviews Rheumatology* 7(368) (June 2011):doi:10.1038/nrrheum.2010.222-c1 Saul, A. *Doctor Yourself: Natural Healing That Works.* 2nd edition. Laguna Beach, CA: Basic Health Publications, 2012. www.doctoryourself.com.

329. Saul, A. *Doctor Yourself: Natural Healing That Works.* 2nd edition. Laguna Beach, CA: Basic Health Publications, 2012. www.doctoryourself.com.

330. Jacob, R.A., et al. "Consumption of Cherries Lowers Plasma Urate in Healthy Women. *J Nutr* 133 (2003):1826–9. Kelley, D.S., et al. "Sweet Bing Cherries Lower Circulating Concentrations of Markers for Chronic Inflammatory Diseases in Healthy Humans." *J Nutr* 143(3) (Mar 2013):340–4.

331. Saul, A. *Doctor Yourself: Natural Healing That Works.* 2nd edition. Laguna Beach, CA: Basic Health Publications, 2012. www.doctoryourself.com.

332. Zhang, Y., et al. "Cherry Consumption and Decreased Risk of Recurrent Gout Attacks." *Arthritis Rheum* 64(12) (Dec 2012):4004–11.

Chapter 6. Restoring Cartilage after Complete Loss

1. Han, M., et al. "Limb Regeneration in Higher Vertebrates: Developing a Roadmap." *Anat Rec B New Anat* 287(1) (2005):14–24.

2. Rinkevich, Y., et al. "Germ-Layer and Lineage-Restricted Stem/Progenitors Regenerate the Mouse Digit Tip." *Nature* 476 (Aug 25, 2011):409–413.

3. Gangji, V., J.P. Hauzeur. "Treatment of Osteonecrosis of the Femoral Head with Implantation of Autologous Bone-Marrow Cells. Surgical Technique." *J Bone Joint Surg Am* 87 Suppl 1(Pt 1) (Mar 2005):106–12.

4. Gangji, V., J.P. Hauzeur. "Treatment of Osteonecrosis of the Femoral Head with Implantation of Autologous Bone-Marrow Cells. Surgical Technique." *J Bone Joint Surg Am* 87 Suppl 1(Pt 1) (Mar 2005):106–12. Gangji, V., V. De Maertelaer, J.P. Hauzeur. "Autologous Bone Marrow Cell Implantation in the Treatment of Non-Traumatic Osteonecrosis of the Femoral head: Five Year Follow-Up of a Prospective Controlled Study." *Bone* 49(5) Nov (2011):1005–9.

5. Chen, J., et al. "Niaspan Treatment Increases Tumor Necrosis Factor-Alpha-Converting Enzyme and Promotes Arteriogenesis after Stroke." *J Cereb Blood Flow Metab* 29(5) (2009):911–920. Chen, J., et al. "Niaspan Increases Angiogenesis and Improves Functional Recovery after Stroke." *Ann Neurol* 62(1) (2007):49–58.

6. Ying, W., et al. "Intranasal Administration with NAD+ Profoundly Decreases Brain Injury in a Rat Model of Transient Focal Ischemia." *Front Biosci.* 12 (Jan 2007):2728–34.

7. Gadau, S., et al. "Benfotiamine Accelerates the Healing of Ischaemic Diabetic Limbs in Mice through Protein Kinase B/Akt-Mediated Potentiation of Angiogenesis and Inhibition of Apoptosis." *Diabetologia* 49(2) (Feb 2006):405–20.

8. Daghini, E., et al. "Antioxidant Vitamins Induce Angiogenesis in the Normal Pig Kidney." *Am J Physiol Renal Physiol* 293(1) (2007):F371–81.

9. Omeroglu, S., et al. "High-Dose Vitamin C Supplementation Accelerates the Achilles Tendon Healing in Healthy Rats." *Arch Orthop Trauma Surg* 129(2) 2009: 281–6.

10. Lee, C.S., et al. "Tailoring Adipose Stem Cell Trophic Factor Production with Differentiation Medium Components to Regenerate Chondral Defects." *Tissue Eng Part A* 19(11–12) (Jun 19, 2013): 1451–64. Stumpf, U., et al. "Selection of Proangiogenic Ascorbate Derivatives and Their Exploitation in a Novel Drug-Releasing System for Wound Healing." *Wound Repair Regen.* 19(5) (2011):597–607.

11. Wang, Y., et al. "Vitamin K Epoxide Reductase: A Protein Involved in Angiogenesis." *Mol Cancer Res* 3(6) (2005): 317–23.

12. Rocamonde, B., et al. "Neuroprotection of Lipoic Acid Treatment Promotes Angiogenesis and Reduces the Glial Scar Formation after Brain Injury." *Neuroscience.* 224 (Nov 8, 2012):102–15.

13. Daghini, E., et al. "Antioxidant Vitamins Induce Angiogenesis in the Normal Pig Kidney." *Am J Physiol Renal Physiol* 293(1) (2007):F371–81.

14. Sheffield, F.J. "Adaptation of Tilt Table for Lumbar Traction." *Arch Phys Med Rehabil* 45 (1964):469–72. Nosse, L.J. "Inverted Spinal Traction." *Arch Phys Med Rehabil* 59(8) 1978:367–70.

15. Haaz, S., S.J. Bartlett. "Yoga for Arthritis: A Scoping Review." *Rheum Dis Clin North Am* 37(1) (2011):33–46.

16. Mokbel, A.N., et al. " Homing and Reparative Effect of Intra-Articular Injection of Autologus Mesenchymal Stem Cells in Osteoarthritic Animal Model." *BMC Musculoskelet Disord* 12 (2011):259.

17. Melief, S.M., et al.. "Adipose Tissue-Derived Multipotent Stromal Cells Have a Higher Immunomodulatory Capacity than Their Bone Marrow-Derived Counterparts." *Stem Cells Transl Med* 2(6) (Jun 2013):455–63.

18. Pak, J. "Regeneration of Human Bones in Hip Osteonecrosis and Human Cartilage in Knee Osteoarthritis with Autologous Adipose-Tissue-Derived Stem Cells: A Case Series." *J Med Case Rep* 5 (Jul 7, 2011):296.

19. Emadedin, M., et al. "Intra-Articular Injection of Autologous Mesenchymal Stem Cells in Six Patients with Knee Osteoarthritis." *Arch Iran Med* 15(7) (Jul 2012):422–8.

20. Stem Cell Doctors (2013): Dr. Nathan Wei (1-301-694-5800; Maryland), Dr. Ross Hauser (1-708-848-7789; Illinois), Dr. Marc Darrow (1-800-734-2210), Dr. Wellington Chen (1-941-330-8553; Florida), Dr. Kenneth Mautner (1-404-778-3350; Georgia), or Dr. Donna Alderman (1-661-295-1110; California).

21. Toh, W.S., et al. "Cartilage Repair Using Hyaluronan Hydrogel-Encapsulated Human Embryonic Stem Cell-Derived Chondrogenic Cells." *Biomaterials* 31(27) (2010):6968–80. Ogawa, R., et al. "Osteogenic and Chondrogenic Differentiation by Adipose-Derived Stem Cells Harvested from GFP Transgenic Mice." *Biochem Biophys Res Commun* 313(4) (2004):871–7.

22. Esteban, M.A., et al. "Vitamin C Enhances the Generation of Mouse and Human Induced Pluripotent Stem Cells." *Cell Stem Cell* 6(1) 2010:71–9.

23. Chen, J., et al. "Vitamin C Modulates TET1 Function During Somatic Cell Reprogramming." *Nat Genet* 45(12) (2013):1504–9. Monfort, A., A. Wutz. "Breathing-in Epigenetic Change with Vitamin C." *EMBO Rep* 14(4) (2013):337–46. Pera, M.F. "Epigenetics, Vitamin Supplements and Cellular Reprogramming." *Nat Genet* 45(12) (Dec 2013): 1412–3.

24. Esteban, M.A., D. Pei. "Vitamin C Improves the Quality of Somatic Cell Reprogramming." *Nat Genet* 44(4) 2012:366–7.

25. Fong, E.L., C.K. Chan, S.B.Goodman. "Stem Cell Homing in Musculoskeletal Injury." *Biomaterials* 32(2) (2011):395–409. Mitkari, B., et al. "Intra-Arterial Infusion of Human Bone Marrow-Derived Mesenchymal Stem Cells Results in Transient Localization in the Brain after Cerebral Ischemia in Rats." *Exp Neurol* 239 (2013):158–62.

26. Zubair, A.C., et al. "Evaluation of Mobilized Peripheral Blood CD34(+) Cells from Patients with Severe Coronary Artery Disease as a Source of Endothelial Progenitor Cells." *Cytotherapy* 12(2) (2010):178–89. Kong, X.D., et al. "Endothelial Progenitor Cells with Alzheimer's Disease." *Chin Med J (Engl)* 124(6) (2011):901–6. Batycka-Baran, A., et al. "Reduced Number of Circulating Endothelial Progenitor Cells (CD133+/KDR+) in Patients with Plaque Psoriasis." *Dermatology* 225(1) (2012):88–92.

27. Orthomolecular News Service (OMNS). "Restrictions on Food Supplements are Based on Misinformation." Oct 16, 2012. www.orthomolecular.org/resources/omns/v08n31 .shtml (accessed Apr 2014).

28. González M.J., et al. "Orthomolecular Oncology: A Mechanistic View of Intravenous Ascorbate's Chemotherapeutic Activity." *PR Health Sci J* 21(1) (2002):39–41.

29. Batycka-Baran, A., et al. "Reduced Number of Circulating Endothelial Progenitor Cells (CD133+/KDR+) in Patients with Plaque Psoriasis." *Dermatology* 225(1) (2012):88–92.

30. Mikirova, N.A., et al. "Circulating Endothelial Progenitor Cells: A New Approach to Anti-Aging Medicine?" *J Transl Med* 7 (2009):106. Mikirova, N.A., et al. "Nutraceutical Augmentation of Circulating Endothelial Progenitor Cells and Hematopoietic Stem Cells in Human Subjects." *J Transl Med.* 8 (2010):34.

31. Patchen, M.L., T.J. MacVittie. "Dose-Dependent Responses of Murine Pluripotent Stem Cells and Myeloid and Erythroid Progenitor Cells Following Administration of the Immunomodulating Agent Glucan." *Immunopharmacology* 5(4) (1983):303–13.

32. Vetvicka, V., Z. Vancikova. "Anti-Stress Action of Several Orally-Given ß-Glucans." *Biomed Pap Med Fac Univ Palacky Olomouc Czech Repub* 154(3) (Sep 2010):235–8.

33. Wong, C.Y., et al. "Daily Intake of Thiamine Correlates with the Circulating Level of Endothelial Progenitor Cells and the Endothelial Function in Patients with Type II Diabetes." *Mol Nutr Food Res* 52(12) (2008):1421–7. Katare, R., et al. "Boosting the Pentose Phosphate Pathway Restores Cardiac Progenitor Cell Availability in Diabetes. *Cardiovasc Res* 97(1) (2013):55–65.

34. Wong, C.Y., et al. "Daily Intake of Thiamine Correlates with the Circulating Level of Endothelial Progenitor Cells and the Endothelial Function in Patients with Type II Diabetes." *Mol Nutr Food Res* 52(12) (2008):1421–7.

35. Huang, P.H., et al. "Niacin Improves Ischemia-Induced Neovascularization in Diabetic Mice by Enhancement of Endothelial Progenitor Cell Functions Independent of Changes in Plasma Lipids." *Angiogenesis* 15(3) (2012):377–89.

36. Sorrentino, S.A., et al. "Endothelial-Vasoprotective Effects of High-Density Lipoprotein are Impaired in Patients with Type 2 Diabetes Mellitus But are Improved after Extended-Release Niacin Therapy." *Circulation* 121(1) (Jan 5,2010):110–22.

37. North, T.E., et al. "Prostaglandin E2 Regulates Vertebrate Haematopoietic Stem Cell Homeostasis." *Nature* 447(7147) (Jun 21, 2007):1007–111.

38. Khanna-Gupta, A., N. Berliner. "Vitamin B3 Boosts Neutrophil Counts." *Nat Med* 15(2) (2009):139–41. Kyme, P., et al. "C/EBPe Mediates Nicotinamide-Enhanced Clearance of Staphylococcus Aureus in Mice." *J Clin Invest;*122(9) (Sep 4, 2012):3316–29.

Chapter 7. Prevent and Reverse Arthritis through Lifestyle and Food

1. Bittman, M. "Not All Industrial Food Is Evil." *The New York Times*. (Aug 17, 2013) http://opinionator.blogs.nytimes.com/2013/08/17/not-all-industrial-food-is-evil (accessed Apr 2014).

2. Dean, C. *The Magnesium Miracle*. New York: Ballantine, 2007. Thomas, D. "The Mineral Depletion of Foods Available to Us as a Nation (1940–2002). A Review of the 6th Edition of McCance and Widdowson." *Nutr Health* 19(1–2) (2007):21–55. Bittman, M. "Everyone Eats There." *The New York Times Magazine* (Oct 10, 2012) www.nytimes.com/2012/10/14/magazine/californias-central-valley-land-of-a-billion-vegetables.html (accessed Apr 2014).

3. Montgomery, D.R. "Soil Erosion and Agricultural Sustainability." *Proc Natl Acad Sci USA* 104(33) (Aug 14, 2007):13268–13272.

4. Thomas, D. "The Mineral Depletion of Foods Available to Us as a Nation (1940–2002). A Review of the 6th Edition of McCance and Widdowson." *Nutr Health* 19(1–2) (2007):21–55. Fan, M.S., et al. "Evidence of Decreasing Mineral Density in Wheat Grain Over the Last 160 Years." *J Trace Elem Med Biol* 22(4) (2008):315–324.

5. Thomas, D. "The Mineral Depletion of Foods Available to Us as a Nation (1940–2002). A Review of the 6th Edition of McCance and Widdowson." *Nutr Health* 19(1–2) (2007):21–55.

6. Davis, D.R., M.D. Epp, H.D. Riordan. "Changes in USDA Food Composition Data for 43 Garden Crops, 1950 to 1999." *J Am Coll Nutr* 23 (Dec 2004):669–82. Fan, M.S., et al. "Evidence of Decreasing Mineral Density in Wheat Grain Over the Last 160 Years." *J Trace Elem Med Biol* 22(4) (2008):315–324.

7. Mollison, B. *Introduction to Permaculture*. Rev. edition. New York: Ten Speed Press, 1997. Fukuoka, M. *The One-Straw Revolution: An Introduction to Natural Farming*. New York: NYRB Classics, 2009. Jackson, W. *Consulting the Genius of the Place: An Ecological Approach to a New Agriculture*. Berkeley, CA: Counterpoint Press, 2011. Bittman, M. "Now This is Natural Food." *The New York Times* (Oct 22, 2013) www.nytimes.com/2013/10/23/opinion/bittman-now-this-is-natural-food.html (accessed Apr 2014). Shein, C. *The Vegetable Gardener's Guide to Permaculture: Creating an Edible Ecosystem*. Portland, OR: Timber Press, 2013.

8. Fukuoka, M. *Sowing Seeds in the Desert: Natural Farming, Global Restoration, and Ultimate Food Security*. White River Junction, VT: Chelsea Green Publishing, 2012.

9. Berry, W. *The Unsettling of America: Culture & Agriculture*. San Francisco: Sierra Club Books, 1996. Jackson, W. *Consulting the Genius of the Place: An Ecological Approach to a New Agriculture*. Berkeley, CA: Counterpoint Press, 2011. Jackson, W. *Nature as Measure: The Selected Essays of Wes Jackson*. Berkeley, CA: Counterpoint Press, 2011. Lappé, F.M. *EcoMind: Changing the Way We Think, to Create the World We Want*. New York: Nation Books, 2013. Bittman, M. "Now This is Natural Food." *The New York Times* (Oct 22, 2013) www.nytimes.com/2013/10/23/opinion/bittman-now-this-is-natural-food.html (accessed Apr 2014).

10. Lappé, F.M. *Diet for a Small Planet*. 20th anniv edition. New York: Ballantine Books, 1971, 1985.

11. Campbell, T.C. *Whole: Rethinking the Science of Nutrition*. Dallas, TX: BenBella Books, 2013. Morrell, A. "Can This Man Feed the World? Billionaire Harry Stine's Quest to Reinvent Agriculture—Again." *Forbes* (Apr 14, 2014) www.forbes.com/sites/alexmorrell/2014/03/26/can-this-man-feed-the-world-billionaire-harry-stines-quest-to-reinvent-agriculture-again (accessed Apr 2014).

12. Hauter, W. *Foodopoly: the Battle Over the Future of Food and Farming in America.* New York: The New Press, 2012. Campbell, T.C. *Whole: Rethinking the Science of Nutrition.* Dallas, TX: BenBella Books, 2013.

13. Bradley, F.M., B.W. Ellis, editors. *Rodale's All-New Encyclopedia of Organic Gardening: The Indispensable Resource for Every Gardener.* Rodale Books, 1993. ISBN-13: 978-0875965994

14. Crinnion WJ. "Organic Foods Contain Higher Levels of Certain Nutrients, Lower Levels of Pesticides, and May Provide Health Benefits for the Consumer." *Altern Med Rev* 15(1) (Apr 2010):4–12.

15. Molnar-Kimber, K.L. Rheumatoid-Arthritis-Decisions.com. www.rheumatoid-arthritis-decisions.com (2013) (accessed Jan 2014).

16. Jenkins M. *What's Gotten into Us?: Staying Healthy in a Toxic World.* New York: Random House, 2011.

17. Dean, C. *The Magnesium Miracle.* New York: Ballantine, 2007.

18. Ibid.

19. Consolazio, D.F., et al. "Excretion of Sodium, Potassium, Magnesium and Iron in Human Sweat and the Relation of Each to Balance and Requirements." *J Nutr* 79 (Apr 1963):407–15.

20. Levy, T.E. *Optimal Nutrition for Optimal Health.* New York, McGraw-Hill, 2001.

21. Scales, C.D. Jr, et al. "Prevalence of Kidney Stones in the United States." *Eur Urol* 62(1):160–5.

22. Gaby, A.R. *Nutritional Medicine.* Concord, NH: Fritz Perlberg Pub, 2011. Orthomolecular News Service (OMNS). "What Really Causes Kidney Stones (And Why Vitamin C Does Not)." Feb 11, 2013. www.orthomolecular.org/resources/omns/v09n05.shtml (accessed Jan 2014).

23. Orthomolecular News Service (OMNS). "What Really Causes Kidney Stones (And Why Vitamin C Does Not)." Feb 11, 2013. www.orthomolecular.org/resources/omns/v09n05.shtml (accessed Jan 2014).

24. Gaby, A.R. *Nutritional Medicine.* Concord, NH: Fritz Perlberg Pub, 2011.

25. Abratt, V.R., S.J. Reid. "Oxalate-Degrading Bacteria of the Human Gut as Probiotics in the Management of Kidney Stone Disease." *Adv Appl Microbiol* 72 (2010):63–87.

26. Gaby, A.R. *Nutritional Medicine.* Concord, NH: Fritz Perlberg Pub, 2011. Chutipongtanate, S., S. Chaiyarit, V. Thongboonkerd. "Citrate, Not Phosphate, Can Dissolve Calcium Oxalate Monohydrate Crystals and Detach These crystals from Renal Tubular Cells." *Eur J Pharmacol* 689(1–3) (Aug 15, 2012):219–25.

27. Ettinger, B., et al. "Potassium-Magnesium Citrate is an Effective Prophylaxis against Recurrent Calcium Oxalate Nephrolithiasis." *J Urol* 158(6) (1997):2069–73.

28. Dean, C. *The Magnesium Miracle.* New York: Ballantine, 2007. Gaby, A.R. *Nutritional Medicine.* Concord, NH: Fritz Perlberg Pub, 2011. Orthomolecular News Service (OMNS). "What Really Causes Kidney Stones (And Why Vitamin C Does Not)." Feb 11, 2013. www.orthomolecular.org/resources/omns/v09n05.shtml (accessed Jan 2014).

29. Molnar-Kimber, K.L. Rheumatoid-Arthritis-Decisions.com. www.rheumatoid-arthritis-decisions.com (2013) (accessed Jan 2014).

30. Dean, C. *The Magnesium Miracle.* New York: Ballantine, 2007.

31. Consolazio, D.F., et al. "Excretion of Sodium, Potassium, Magnesium and Iron in Human Sweat and the Relation of Each to Balance and Requirements." *J Nutr* 79 (Apr 1963):407–15.

32. Levy, T.E. *Primal Panacea*. Henderson, NV: MedFox Publishing, 2011.

33. Gaby, A.R. *Nutritional Medicine*. Concord, NH: Fritz Perlberg Pub, 2011.

34. Bertram, K.M., et al. "Molecular Regulation of Cigarette Smoke Induced-Oxidative Stress in Human Retinal Pigment Epithelial Cells: Implications for Age-Related Macular Degeneration." *Am J Physiol Cell Physiol* 297(5) (2009):C1200–10.

35. International Agency for Research on Cancer. IARC Monographs on the Evaluation of Carcinogenic Risks to Humans: *Tobacco Smoke and Involuntary Smoking*. Volume 83. 2004. http://monographs.iarc.fr/ENG/Monographs/vol83/ (accessed Apr 2014). Oliver, J.E., A.J. Silman. "What Epidemiology Has Told Us about Risk Factors and Aetiopathogenesis in Rheumatic Diseases." *Arthritis Res Ther* 11(3) (2009):223. Mnatzaganian, G., et al. "Smoking, Body Weight, Physical Exercise, and Risk of Lower Limb Total Joint Replacement in a Population-Based Cohort of Men." *Arthritis Rheum* 63(8) (Aug 2011):2523–30.

36. Jenkins M. *What's Gotten into Us?: Staying Healthy in a Toxic World*. New York: Random House, 2011.

37. Davis, M.L., et al. "Associations of Alcohol Use with Radiographic Disease Progression in African Americans with Recent-onset Rheumatoid Arthritis." *J Rheumatol.* 40(9) (Sep 2013):1498–504.

38. Torralba, K.D., E. De Jesus, S. Rachabattula. "The Interplay Between Diet, Urate Transporters and the Risk for Gout and Hyperuricemia: Current and Future Directions." *Int J Rheum Dis* 15(6) (2012):499–506. Wang, et al. "A Meta-Analysis of Alcohol Consumption and the Risk of Gout." *Clin Rheumatol* 32(11) (Nov 2013):1641–8.

39. Scott, I.C., et al. "The Protective Effect of Alcohol on Developing Rheumatoid Arthritis: A Systematic Review and Meta-Analysis." *Rheumatology (Oxford)* 52(5) (2013):856–67.

40. Hoffer, A., A.W. Saul. *The Vitamin Cure for Alcoholism: How to Protect Against and Fight Alcoholism Using Nutrition and Vitamin Supplementation*. Laguna Beach, CA: Basic Health Publications, 2009.

41. Dean, C. *The Magnesium Miracle*. New York: Ballantine, 2007.

42. Lustig, R.H., L.A. Schmidt, C.D. Brindis. "The Toxic Truth about Sugar." *Nature* 482(7383) (Feb 1, 2012):27–9. Orthomolecular News Service (OMNS). "Toxic Sugar." Editorial. Apr 24, 2012. www.orthomolecular.org/resources/omns/v08n14.shtml (accessed Jan 2014). Torralba, K.D., E. De Jesus, S. Rachabattula. "The Interplay Between Diet, Urate Transporters and the Risk for Gout and Hyperuricemia: Current and Future Directions." *Int J Rheum Dis* 15(6) (2012):499–506. Vos, M.B., J.E. Lavine. "Dietary Fructose in Nonalcoholic Fatty Liver Disease." *Hepatology* 57(6) (2013):2525–31.

43. Lustig, R.H., L.A. Schmidt, C.D. Brindis. "The Toxic Truth about Sugar." *Nature* 482(7383) (Feb 1, 2012):27–9. Vos, M.B., J.E. Lavine. "Dietary Fructose in Nonalcoholic Fatty Liver Disease." *Hepatology* 57(6) (2013):2525–31.

44. Lottenberg, A.M., et al. "The Role of Dietary Fatty Acids in the Pathology of Metabolic Syndrome." *J Nutr Biochem* 23(9) (Sep 2012):1027–40. Simopoulos, A.P. "Dietary Omega-3 Fatty Acid Deficiency and High Fructose Intake in the Development of Metabolic Syndrome, Brain Metabolic Abnormalities, and Non-Alcoholic Fatty Liver Disease." *Nutrients* 5(8) (2013):2901–23.

45. Lyssiotis, C.A., Cantley, L.C. (2013) Metabolic Syndrome: F Stands for Fructose and Fat." *Nature* 502(7470) (Oct 10, 2013):181–2.

46. Agricultural Research Service, United States Department of Agriculture (USDA). "Nutrient Database for Standard Reference," National Nutrient Database for Standard Reference. Release 26 v.1.3.1, 2011. http://ndb.nal.usda.gov/ndb/nutrients/index (accessed Apr 2014).

47. Ibid.

48. Bremer, A.A., M. Mietus-Snyder, R.H. Lustig. "Toward a Unifying Hypothesis of Metabolic Syndrome." *Pediatrics* 129(3) (Mar 2012):557–70. Lustig, R.H., L.A. Schmidt, C.D. Brindis. "The Toxic Truth about Sugar." *Nature* 482(7383) (Feb 1, 2012):27–9. Lyssiotis CA, Cantley LC. (2013) Metabolic Syndrome: F Stands for Fructose and Fat." *Nature* 502(7470) (Oct 10, 2013):181–2. Vos, M.B., J.E. Lavine. "Dietary Fructose in Nonalcoholic Fatty Liver Disease." *Hepatology* 57(6) (2013):2525–31.

49. Simopoulos, A.P. "Dietary Omega-3 Fatty Acid Deficiency and High Fructose Intake in the Development of Metabolic Syndrome, Brain Metabolic Abnormalities, and Non-Alcoholic Fatty Liver Disease." *Nutrients* 5(8) (2013):2901–23.

50. Boyer, J., R.H. Liu. "Apple Phytochemicals and Their Health Benefits." *Nutr J* 3 (May 2004):5.

51. Agricultural Research Service, United States Department of Agriculture (USDA). "Nutrient Database for Standard Reference," National Nutrient Database for Standard Reference. Release 26 v.1.3.1, 2011. http://ndb.nal.usda.gov/ndb/nutrients/index (accessed Apr 2014).

52. Lustig, R.H., L.A. Schmidt, C.D. Brindis. "The Toxic Truth about Sugar." *Nature* 482(7383) (Feb 1, 2012):27–9.

53. Hu, Y., et al. "Relations of Glycemic Index and Glycemic Load with Plasma Oxidative Stress Markers." *Am J Clin Nutr* 84(1) (2006):70–6.

54. Lopez, H.L. "Nutritional Interventions to Prevent and Treat Osteoarthritis. Part I: Focus on Fatty Acids and Macronutrients." *PM R* 4(5 Suppl) (May 2012):S145–54.

55. Strom, S. "Social Media as a Megaphone to Pressure the Food Industry." *The New York Times* (Dec 30, 2013) www.nytimes.com/2013/12/31/business/media/social-media-as-a-megaphone-to-push-food-makers-to-change.html (accessed Apr 2014).

56. Alshatwi, A.A., et al. "Al2O3 Nanoparticles Induce Mitochondria-Mediated Cell Death and Upregulate the Expression of Signaling Genes in Human Mesenchymal Stem Cells." J Biochem Mol Toxicol. 2012 Nov;26(11) (Nov 2012):469–76. Ding, Y., et al. "[Effects of Maternal Exposure to Nano-Alumina during Pregnancy on Neurodevelopment in Offspring Mice.]" *Zhonghua Lao Dong Wei Sheng Zhi Ye Bing Za Zhi.* 31(10) (Oct 2013):744–8. [article in Chinese]. Pakrashi, S., et al. "Ceriodaphnia Dubia as a Potential Bio-Indicator for Assessing Acute Aluminum Oxide Nanoparticle Toxicity in Fresh Water Environment." *PLoS One* 8(9) (Sep 5, 2013):e74003. Zhang, Q., et al. "Lysosomes Involved in the Cellular Toxicity of Nano-Alumina: Combined Effects of Particle Size and Chemical Composition." *J Biol Regul Homeost Agents* 27(2) (Apr-Jun 2013):365–75.

57. U.S. EPA. TEACH Chemical Summary. "Nitrates and Nitrites. Toxicity and Exposure Assessment for Children's Health." www.epa.gov/teach/chem_summ/Nitrates_summary.pdf (accessed Apr 2014).

58. Dean, C. *The Magnesium Miracle.* New York: Ballantine, 2007. Schiffman, S.S. "Rationale for Further Medical and Health Research on High-Potency Sweeteners." *Chem Sens-*

es 37(8) (2012):671–9. Sanders, F. *Sweet Poisons~The Toxic Truth About Artificial Sweeteners.* Pro @ctive Media, 2013.

59. Peterson, M.E. "Xylitol" *Top Companion Anim Med* 28(1) (Feb 2013):18–20.

60. Brown, R.J., K.I. Rother. "Non-Nutritive Sweeteners and Their Role in the Gastrointestinal Tract." *J Clin Endocrinol Metab* 97(8) (2012):2597–605. Schiffman, S.S. "Rationale for Further Medical and Health Research on High-Potency Sweeteners." *Chem Senses* 37(8) (2012):671–9. Wauson, E.M., Lorente-Rodríguez, A., M.H. Cobb. Minireview: Nutrient sensing by G protein-coupled receptors. *Mol Endocrinol.* 27(8) (Aug 2013):1188–97.

61. Brown, R.J., M. Walter, K.I. Rother. "Ingestion of Diet soda before a Glucose Load Augments Glucagon-Like Peptide-1 Secretion." *Diabetes Care* 32(12) (2009):2184–6. Brown, R.J., K.I. Rother. "Non-Nutritive Sweeteners and Their Role in the Gastrointestinal Tract." *J Clin Endocrinol Metab* 97(8) (2012):2597–605. Pepino, M.Y., C.Bourne. "Non-Nutritive Sweeteners, Energy Balance, and Glucose Homeostasis." *Curr Opin Clin Nutr Metab Care* 14(4) (Jul 2011):391–5. Pepino, M.Y., et al. "Sucralose Affects Glycemic and Hormonal Responses to an Oral Glucose Load." *Diabetes Care* 36(9) (Sep 2013):2530–5.

62. Abou-Donia, M.B., et al. "Splenda Alters Gut Microflora and Increases Intestinal P-Glycoprotein and Cytochrome P-450 in Male Rats." *J Toxicol Environ Health A* 71(21) (2008):1415–29. Schiffman, S.S., M.B. Abou-Donia. "Sucralose Revisited: Rebuttal of Two Papers about Splenda Safety." Regul Toxicol Pharmacol. 63(3) (Aug 2012):505–8. Schiffman, S.S. "Rationale for Further Medical and Health Research on High-Potency Sweeteners." *Chem Senses* 37(8) (2012):671–9. Cong, W.N., et al. "Long-Term Artificial Sweetener Acesulfame Potassium Treatment Alters Neurometabolic Functions in C57BL/6J Mice." *PLoS One* 8(8) (2013):e70257.

63. Campbell, T.C. *Whole: Rethinking the Science of Nutrition.* Dallas, TX: BenBella Books, 2013.

64. Agricultural Research Service, United States Department of Agriculture (USDA). "Nutrient Database for Standard Reference," National Nutrient Database for Standard Reference. Release 26 v.1.3.1, 2011. http://ndb.nal.usda.gov/ndb/nutrients/index (accessed Apr 2014).

65. Ibid.

66. Ibid.

67. Menaa, F., et al. "Technological Approaches to Minimize Industrial Trans Fatty Acids in Foods. *J Food Sci* 78(3) (2013):R377–86.

68. Roach, C., et al. "Comparison of Cis and Trans Fatty Acid Containing Phosphatidylcholines on Membrane Properties." *Biochemistry* 43(20) (May 25, 2004):6344–51.

69. Gropper, S.S., J.L. Smith. *Advanced Nutrition and Human Metabolism,* 6th edition. New York: Cengage Learning, 2013.

70. Cascio, G., G. Schiera, I. Di Liegro. "Dietary Fatty Acids in Metabolic Syndrome, Diabetes and Cardiovascular Diseases." *Curr Diabetes Rev* 8(1) (Jan 2012):2–17.

71. Ibid.

72. Bremer, A.A., M. Mietus-Snyder, R.H. Lustig. "Toward a Unifying Hypothesis of Metabolic Syndrome." *Pediatrics* 129(3) (Mar 2012):557–70.

73. Bremer, A.A., M. Mietus-Snyder, R.H. Lustig. "Toward a Unifying Hypothesis of Metabolic Syndrome." *Pediatrics* 129(3) (Mar 2012):557–70. Cascio, G., G. Schiera, I. Di

Liegro. "Dietary Fatty Acids in Metabolic Syndrome, Diabetes and Cardiovascular Diseases." *Curr Diabetes Rev* 8(1) (Jan 2012):2–17. Lottenberg, A.M., et al. "The Role of Dietary Fatty Acids in the Pathology of Metabolic Syndrome." *J Nutr Biochem* 23(9) (Sep 2012):1027–40. Menaa, F., et al. "Technological Approaches to Minimize Industrial Trans Fatty Acids in Foods. *J Food Sci* 78(3) (2013):R377–86.

74. Saul, A. *Doctor Yourself: Natural Healing That Works.* 2nd edition. Laguna Beach, CA: Basic Health Publications, 2012. www.doctoryourself.com.

75. Dean, C. *The Magnesium Miracle.* New York: Ballantine, 2007. Hagel, A.F., et al. "Intravenous Infusion of Ascorbic Acid Decreases Serum Histamine Concentrations in Patients with Allergic and Non-Allergic Diseases." *Naunyn Schmiedebergs Arch Pharmacol* 386(9) (Sep 2013):789–93. Hemilä, H. "Vitamin C and Common Cold-Induced Asthma: A Systematic Review and Statistical Analysis." *Allergy Asthma Clin Immunol* 9(1) (Nov 26, 2013):9–46.

76. Dean, C. *The Magnesium Miracle.* New York: Ballantine, 2007.

77. Vogt, R., et al. "Cancer and Non-Cancer Health Effects from Food Contaminant Exposures for Children and Adults in California: A Risk Assessment." *Environ Health* 11 (Nov 9, 2012):83.

78. Bell, R.R., C.A. Heller. "Nutrition Studies: An Appraisal of the Modern Northern Alaskan Eskimo Diet." in: Jamison, P.L., S.L. Zegura, F.A. Milan, eds. *Eskimos of Northwestern Alaska: A Biological Perspective.* Stroudsburg, PA: Dowden, Hutchinson and Ross, 1978:145–56. Draper, H.H. "Nutrition of Alaskan Natives." *Am J Clin Nutr* 57(5) (May 1993):698–699. Gadsby, P. "The Inuit Paradox: How Can People Who Gorge on Fat and Rarely See a Vegetable Be Healthier Than We Are?" *Discover Mag* (Oct 1, 2004). Bersamin, A., et al. "Nutrient Intakes Are Associated with Adherence to a Traditional Diet among Yup'ik Eskimos Living in Remote Alaska Native Communities: The CANHR Study." *Int J Circumpolar Health* 66(1) (2007):62–70.

79. Gadsby, P. "The Inuit Paradox: How Can People Who Gorge on Fat and Rarely See a Vegetable Be Healthier Than We Are?" *Discover Mag* (Oct 1, 2004).

80. Aesoph, L.M. *How to Eat Away Arthritis: Gain Relief from the Pain and Discomfort of Arthritis Through Nature's Remedies.* New York: Prentice Hall Press, 1996. Martin, R., K.J. Romano. J. Robbins. *Preventing and Reversing Arthritis Naturally: The Untold Story.* Rochester, NY: Healing Arts Press, 2000. Allan, B. *Conquering Arthritis: What Doctors Don't Tell You Because They Don't Know (9 Secrets I Learned the Hard Way).* 2nd ed. Phoenix: Shining Prairie Flower Productions, 2009. Gerson, C. *Defeating Arthritis, Bone and Joint Diseases.* Carmel, CA: Gerson Health Media, 2011.

81. Esselstyn, C.B. *Prevent and Reverse Heart Disease: The Revolutionary, Scientifically Proven, Nutrition-Based Cure.* New York: Avery, 2008.

82. Brighthope, I.E. *The Vitamin Cure for Diabetes: Prevent and Treat Diabetes Using Nutrition and Vitamin Supplementation.* Laguna Beach, CA: Basic Health Publications, 2012. Attia, P. "Is the Obesity Crisis Hiding a Bigger Problem?" TED Talks: TED Partner Series video. 2013 www.ted.com/talks/peter_attia_what_if_we_re_wrong_about_diabetes.html (accessed Jan 2014).

83. Campbell, T.C., T.M. Campbell, II. *The China Study: The Most Comprehensive Study of Nutrition Ever Conducted and Startling Implications for Diet, Weight Loss, and Long-Term Health.* Dallas, TX: BenBella Books, 2006. Ornish, D. *The Spectrum: How to Customize a Way of Eating and Living Just Right for You and Your Family.* New York: Ballantine Books, 2008. Campbell, T.C. *Whole: Rethinking the Science of Nutrition.* Dallas, TX: BenBella Books, 2013.

84. McGee, H. *On Food and Cooking: The Science and Lore of the Kitchen.* Revised, updated edition. New York, NY: Scribner, 2004. Miglio, C., et al. "Effects of Different Cooking Methods on Nutritional and Physicochemical Characteristics of Selected Vegetables." *J Agric Food Chem* 56(1) (Jan 9, 2008):139–47.

85. Boutenko, V. *Green Smoothie Revolution: The Radical Leap Towards Natural Health.* Berkeley, CA: North Atlantic Books, 2009. Wells, J. *The Green Smoothie: A Quick Start Guide about Vegetable Smoothies for Good Health.* CreateSpace Independent Publishing, 2013.

86. Crocker, P. *The Juicing Bible.* 2nd edition. Toronto, ON: Robert Rose, 2008. Saul, A. *Doctor Yourself: Natural Healing That Works.* 2nd edition. Laguna Beach, CA: Basic Health Publications, 2012. www.doctoryourself.com.

87. Gerson, C. *Defeating Arthritis, Bone and Joint Diseases.* Carmel, CA: Gerson Health Media, 2011.

88. Crocker, P. *The Juicing Bible.* 2nd edition. Toronto, ON: Robert Rose, 2008. Saul, A. *Doctor Yourself: Natural Healing That Works.* 2nd edition. Laguna Beach, CA: Basic Health Publications, 2012. www.doctoryourself.com. Saul, A.W., H.S. Case. *Vegetable Juicing for Everyone: How to Get Your Family Healthier and Happier, Faster*! Laguna Beach, CA: Basic Health Publications, 2013.

89. Boutenko, V. *Green Smoothie Revolution: The Radical Leap Towards Natural Health.* Berkeley, CA: North Atlantic Books, 2009. Wells, J. *The Green Smoothie: A Quick Start Guide about Vegetable Smoothies for Good Health.* CreateSpace Independent Publishing, 2013.

90. Boutenko, V. *Green Smoothie Revolution: The Radical Leap Towards Natural Health.* Berkeley, CA: North Atlantic Books, 2009. Wells, J. *The Green Smoothie: A Quick Start Guide about Vegetable Smoothies for Good Health.* CreateSpace Independent Publishing, 2013.

91. Saul, A. *Doctor Yourself: Natural Healing That Works.* 2nd edition. Laguna Beach, CA: Basic Health Publications, 2012. www.doctoryourself.com.

92. Ibid.

93. Ibid.

94. Arbour, G. "Are Buckwheat Greens Toxic?" *Townsend Letter* (Dec 2004) www.townsendletter.com/Dec2004/buckwheat1204.htm (accessed Apr 2014).

95. Bartholomew, M. *All New Square Foot Gardening: The Revolutionary Way to Grow More In Less Space.* 2nd edition. Minneapolis, MN: Cool Springs Press, 2013. Flores, H.C. *Food Not Lawns: How to Turn Your Yard into a Garden and Your Neighborhood into a Community.* White River Junction, VT: Chelsea Green Publishing, 2006. Jeavons, J. How to Grow More Vegetables: And Fruits, Nuts, Berries, Grains, and Other Crops Than You Ever Thought Possible on Less Land Than You Can Imagine. 8th edition. New York: Ten Speed Press, 2012.

96. Berry, W. *The Unsettling of America: Culture & Agriculture.* San Francisco: Sierra Club Books, 1996. Seymour, J. *The New Self-Sufficient Gardener.* New York: DK Publishing, 2008. Markham, B.L. *Mini Farming: Self-Sufficiency on 1/4 Acre.* New York: Skyhorse Publishing, 2010. Flores, H.C. *Food Not Lawns: How to Turn Your Yard into a Garden and Your Neighborhood into a Community.* White River Junction, VT: Chelsea Green Publishing, 2006. Hemenway, T. *Gaia's Garden: A Guide to Home-Scale Permaculture,* 2nd edition. White River Junction, VT: Chelsea Green Publishing, 2009. Jackson, W. *Consulting the Genius of the Place: An Ecological Approach to a New Agriculture.* Berkeley, CA:

Counterpoint Press, 2011. Jackson, W. *Nature as Measure: The Selected Essays of Wes Jackson*. Berkeley, CA: Counterpoint Press, 2011. Henderson, E., R. Van En. *Sharing the Harvest: A Citizen's Guide to Community Supported Agriculture*, 2nd edition. White River Junction, VT: Chelsea Green Publishing, 2007.

97. Farm To City. Uniting Communities, Families, and Farmers Year Round Through Good Local Food. 2013. www.farmtocity.org (accessed Apr 2014). California Federation of Certified Farmers' Markets. (2013) www.cafarmersmarkets.com (accessed Apr 2014).

98. United States Department of Agriculture. National Agricultural Library. Alternative Farming Systems Information System. Community Supported Agriculture. (2014) www.nal.usda.gov/afsic/pubs/csa/csa.shtml (accessed Apr 2014).

99. Van En, R. "Eating for Your Community. A Report from the Founder of Community Supported Agriculture." *A Good Harvest* Context Institute (1995):29. www.context.org/iclib/ic42/vanen (accessed Apr 2014). Wilson College. Robyn Van En Center (2013) www.wilson.edu/about-wilson-college/fulton/robyn-van-en-center/index.aspx (accessed Apr 2014).

100. Ladd, C. "Giant Greenhouses Mean Flavorful Tomatoes All Year." *The New York Times* (Mar 30, 2010) www.nytimes.com/2010/03/31/dining/31tomato.html (accessed Apr 2014).

101. Wijsman, A.J.T.M., G.A.M. van Meurs. "The Seasonal Heat Store in Groningen." In *First E.C. Conference on Solar Heating*.. Springer, 1984: 886–893. http://link.springer.com/chapter/10.1007%2F978-94-009-6508-9_161. (accessed Apr 2014). YouTube. "Renewable Energy Home Tour – Seasonal Heat Store, Solar PV, and Masonry Heater." (2012). www.youtube.com/watch?v=xJz4cKwddBs (accessed Apr 2014). Drake Landing Solar Community. (2013): www.dlsc.ca (accessed Apr 2014).

102. Weavers Way Co-Op. Community-owned Food Markets Open to Everyone. (2014) www.weaversway.coop (accessed Apr 2014).

103. Agricultural Research Service, United States Department of Agriculture (USDA). "Nutrient Database for Standard Reference," National Nutrient Database for Standard Reference. Release 26 v.1.3.1, 2011. http://ndb.nal.usda.gov/ndb/nutrients/index (accessed Apr 2014).

104. Boyer, J., R.H. Liu. "Apple Phytochemicals and Their Health Benefits." *Nutr J* 3 (May 2004):5.

105. Agricultural Research Service, United States Department of Agriculture (USDA). "Nutrient Database for Standard Reference," National Nutrient Database for Standard Reference. Release 26 v.1.3.1, 2011. http://ndb.nal.usda.gov/ndb/nutrients/index (accessed Apr 2014).

106. Lappé, F.M. *Diet for a Small Planet*. 20th anniv edition. New York: Ballantine Books, 1971, 1985.

107. Sun, G.X., et al. "Inorganic Arsenic in Rice Bran and Its Products Are an Order of Magnitude Higher Than in Bulk Grain." *Environ Sci Technol* 42(19) (Oct 1, 2008):7542–6. Lombi, E., et al. "Speciation and Distribution of Arsenic and Localization of Nutrients in Rice Grains." New Phytol. 184(1) (2009):193–201. Williams, P.N., et al., "Occurrence and Partitioning of Cadmium, Arsenic and Lead in Mine Impacted Paddy Rice: Hunan, China." *Environ Sci Technol* 43(3) (Feb 1,2009):637–42. Ruangwises, S., et al. "Total and Inorganic Arsenic in Rice and Rice Bran Purchased in Thailand." *J Food Prot* 75(4) (Apr 2012):771–4.

108. Lappé, F.M. *Diet for a Small Planet*. 20th anniv edition. New York: Ballantine Books,

1971, 1985. Campbell, T.C. *Whole: Rethinking the Science of Nutrition.* Dallas, TX: BenBella Books, 2013.

109. Agricultural Research Service, United States Department of Agriculture (USDA). "Nutrient Database for Standard Reference," National Nutrient Database for Standard Reference. Release 26 v.1.3.1, 2011. http://ndb.nal.usda.gov/ndb/nutrients/index (accessed Apr 2014).

110. Roberts, H., S. Hickey. *The Vitamin Cure for Heart Disease: How to Prevent and Treat Heart Disease Using Nutrition and Vitamin Supplementation.* Laguna Beach, CA: Basic Health Publications, 2011.

111. Hoffer, A., A.W. Saul. *Orthomolecular Medicine for Everyone: Megavitamin Therapeutics for Families and Physicians.* Laguna Beach, CA: Basic Health Publications, 2008.

112. Pauling, L. *How to Live Longer and Feel Better.* Corvallis, OR: Oregon State University Press, 1986, 2006. Saul, A. *Doctor Yourself: Natural Healing That Works.* 2nd edition. Laguna Beach, CA: Basic Health Publications, 2012. www.doctoryourself.com.

113. Ames, B.N. "Low Micronutrient Intake May Accelerate the Degenerative Diseases of Aging through Allocation of Scarce Micronutrients by Triage." *Proc Natl Acad Sci USA.* 103(47) (Nov 21, 2006):17589–94. Ames, B.N. "Optimal Micronutrients Delay Mitochondrial Decay and Age-Associated Diseases." *Mech Ageing Dev* 131(7–8) (Jul-Aug 2010):473–479. Ames, B.N. "Prevention of Mutation, Cancer, and Other Age-Associated Diseases by Optimizing Micronutrient Intake." *J Nucleic Acids* (Sep 22, 2010). pii:725071. McCann, J.C., B.N. Ames. "Vitamin K, An Example of Triage Theory: Is Micronutrient Inadequacy Linked to Diseases of Aging?" *Am J Clin Nutr* 90(4) (Oct 2009):889–907.

114. Williams, R.J. *Biochemical Individuality.* New Canaan, CT: Keats Publishing, 1998.

115. Hoffer, A., A.W. Saul. *Orthomolecular Medicine for Everyone: Megavitamin Therapeutics for Families and Physicians.* Laguna Beach, CA: Basic Health Publications, 2008.

116. Mietus-Snyder, M.L., et al. "A Nutrient-Dense, High-Fiber, Fruit-Based Supplement Bar Increases HDL Cholesterol, Particularly Large HDL, Lowers Homocysteine, and Raises Glutathione in a 2-Wk Trial." *FASEB J* 26(8) (Aug 2012):3515–27.

117. Rodahl, K., T. Moore. "The Vitamin A Content and Toxicity of Bear and Seal Liver." Biochem J. 37(2) (Jul 1943):166–8.

118. Hoffer, A., A.W. Saul. *Orthomolecular Medicine for Everyone: Megavitamin Therapeutics for Families and Physicians.* Laguna Beach, CA: Basic Health Publications, 2008.

119. Goralczyk, R. "Beta-Carotene and Lung Cancer in Smokers: Review of Hypotheses and Status of Research." *Nutr Cancer* 61(6) (2009):767–74.

120. Choi, W.J., et al. "Independent Association of Serum Retinol and Beta-Carotene Levels with Hyperuricemia: A National Population Study." *Arthritis Care Res (Hoboken)* 64(3) (2012):389–96.

121. Ross, A.C. "Vitamin A." Chapter 17 in *Modern Nutrition in Health and Disease,* editors A.C. Ross, et al., 11th ed. Baltimore: Lippincott Williams & Wilkins, 2012.

122. Ibid.

123. Agricultural Research Service, United States Department of Agriculture (USDA). "Nutrient Database for Standard Reference," National Nutrient Database for Standard Reference. Release 26 v.1.3.1, 2011. http://ndb.nal.usda.gov/ndb/nutrients/index (accessed Apr 2014).

124. Kaufman, W. *The Common Form of Joint Dysfunction: Its Incidence and Treatment.* Brattleboro, VT: E.L. Hildreth, 1949. Kaufman, W. *Common Form of Niacin Amide Defi-*

ciency Disease: Aniacinamidosis. Yale University Press, 1943. Kaufman, W. "Niacinamide as a Therapeutic Agent: A Memoir." 2001. www.doctoryourself.com/kaufman12.html.

125. Gaby, A.R. "Natural Treatments for Osteoarthritis." *Altern Med Rev* 4(5) (Oct 1999):330–41. Gaby, A.R. *Nutritional Medicine.* Concord, NH: Fritz Perlberg Pub, 2011. Hoffer, A., A.W. Saul, H.D. Foster. *Niacin: The Real Story: Learn about the Wonderful Healing Properties of Niacin.* Laguna Beach, CA: Basic Health Publications, 2012. Saul, A. *Doctor Yourself: Natural Healing That Works.* 2nd edition. Laguna Beach, CA: Basic Health Publications, 2012. www.doctoryourself.com. Penberthy, W.T., J.B. Kirkland. "Niacin." In: *Present Knowledge in Nutrition.* Erdman, J.W. et al. 10th edition. Ames, IA: International Life Sciences Institute, 2012. p 293–306. Penberthy, W.T. "Niacin, Riboflavin, and Thiamine." In: *Biochemical, Physiological, and Molecular Aspects of Human Nutrition* M.H. Stipanuk and M.A. Caudill, eds. 3rd edition. St. Louis, MO: Saunders, 2012. p. 540–564.

126. Hoffer, A., A.W. Saul. *The Vitamin Cure for Alcoholism: How to Protect Against and Fight Alcoholism Using Nutrition and Vitamin Supplementation.* Laguna Beach, CA: Basic Health Publications, 2009. Hoffer, A., A.W. Saul, H.D. Foster. *Niacin: The Real Story: Learn about the Wonderful Healing Properties of Niacin.* Laguna Beach, CA: Basic Health Publications, 2012. Jonsson, B.H. *The Vitamin Cure for Depression: How to Prevent and Treat Depression Using Nutrition and Vitamin Supplementation.* Laguna Beach, CA: Basic Health Publications, 2012.

127. Hoffer, A., A.W. Saul, H.D. Foster. *Niacin: The Real Story: Learn about the Wonderful Healing Properties of Niacin.* Laguna Beach, CA: Basic Health Publications, 2012. Saul, A. *Doctor Yourself: Natural Healing That Works.* 2nd edition. Laguna Beach, CA: Basic Health Publications, 2012. www.doctoryourself.com.

128. Hoffer, A., A.W. Saul, H.D. Foster. *Niacin: The Real Story: Learn about the Wonderful Healing Properties of Niacin.* Laguna Beach, CA: Basic Health Publications, 2012.

129. Hoffer, A., A.W. Saul. *Orthomolecular Medicine for Everyone: Megavitamin Therapeutics for Families and Physicians.* Laguna Beach, CA: Basic Health Publications, 2008. Penberthy, W.T., J.B. Kirkland. "Niacin." In: *Present Knowledge in Nutrition.* Erdman, J.W. et al. 10th edition. Ames, IA: International Life Sciences Institute, 2012. p 293–306. Hoffer, A., A.W. Saul, H.D. Foster. *Niacin: The Real Story: Learn about the Wonderful Healing Properties of Niacin.* Laguna Beach, CA: Basic Health Publications, 2012. Penberthy, W.T. "Niacin, Riboflavin, and Thiamine." In: *Biochemical, Physiological, and Molecular Aspects of Human Nutrition* M.H. Stipanuk and M.A. Caudill, eds. 3rd edition. St. Louis, MO: Saunders, 2012. p. 540–564.

130. Bajaj, S., A. Khan. "Antioxidants and Diabetes." *Indian J Endocrinol Metab* 16(8) (2012):267–71. Brighthope, I.E. *The Vitamin Cure for Diabetes: Prevent and Treat Diabetes Using Nutrition and Vitamin Supplementation.* Laguna Beach, CA: Basic Health Publications, 2012. Ceriello, A., et al. "Vitamin C Further Improves the Protective Effect of GLP-1 on the Ischemia-Reperfusion-Like Effect Induced by Hyperglycemia Post-Hypoglycemia in Type 1 Diabetes." *Cardiovasc Diabetol* 12(1) (Jun 27, 2013):97. Ceriello, A., et al. "Hyperglycemia Following Recovery from Hypoglycemia Worsens Endothelial Damage and Thrombosis Activation in Type 1 Diabetes and in Healthy Controls." *Nutr Metab Cardiovasc Dis* 24(2) (Feb 2014):116–23. Franke, S.I., et al. "Vitamin C Intake Reduces the Cytotoxicity Associated with Hyperglycemia in Prediabetes and Type 2 Diabetes." *Biomed Res Int* 2013 (2013):896536.

131. Hoffer, A., A.W. Saul, H.D. Foster. *Niacin: The Real Story: Learn about the Wonderful Healing Properties of Niacin.* Laguna Beach, CA: Basic Health Publications, 2012.

132. Hoffer, A., A.W. Saul, H.D. Foster. *Niacin: The Real Story: Learn about the Won-*

derful Healing Properties of Niacin. Laguna Beach, CA: Basic Health Publications, 2012. Penberthy, W.T. "Niacin, Riboflavin, and Thiamine." In: *Biochemical, Physiological, and Molecular Aspects of Human Nutrition* M.H. Stipanuk and M.A. Caudill, eds. 3rd edition. St. Louis, MO: Saunders, 2012. p. 540–564.

133. Barakat, M.R., et al. "Effect of Niacin on Retinal Vascular Diameter in Patients with Age-Related Macular Degeneration." *Curr Eye Res* 31(6–7) (2006):629–34. Dajani, H.M., A.K. Lauer. "Optical Coherence Tomography Findings in Niacin Maculopathy." *Can J Ophthalmol* 41(2) (2006):197–200. Millay, R.H., M.L. Klein, D.R. Illingworth. "Niacin Maculopathy." *Ophthalmology* 95(7) (1988):930–6. Freisberg, L., et al. "Diffuse Macular Edema in Niacin-Induced Maculopathy May Resolve With Dosage Decrease." *Retinal Cases Brief Rep* 5(3) (2011):227–8. Smith, R.G. *The Vitamin Cure for Eye Disease.* Laguna Beach, CA: Basic Health Publications, 2012.

134. Hoffer, A., A.W. Saul, H.D. Foster. *Niacin: The Real Story: Learn about the Wonderful Healing Properties of Niacin.* Laguna Beach, CA: Basic Health Publications, 2012. Orthomolecular News Service (OMNS). "Niacin is the Safest and Most Effective Way to Control Cholesterol." Mar 21, 2013." http://orthomolecular.org/resources/omns/v09n07.shtml (accessed Apr 2014).

135. Roberts, H., S. Hickey. *The Vitamin Cure for Heart Disease: How to Prevent and Treat Heart Disease Using Nutrition and Vitamin Supplementation.* Laguna Beach, CA: Basic Health Publications, 2011. Hoffer, A., A.W. Saul, H.D. Foster. *Niacin: The Real Story: Learn about the Wonderful Healing Properties of Niacin.* Laguna Beach, CA: Basic Health Publications, 2012.

136. Saul, A.W. "NBC's Vitamin Ignorance: An Apology." Orthomolecular News Service (OMNS). Nov 12, 2013. http://orthomolecular.org/resources/omns/v09n24.shtml (accessed Apr 2014).

137. Kaufman, W. *The Common Form of Joint Dysfunction: Its Incidence and Treatment.* Brattleboro, VT: E.L. Hildreth, 1949. Kaufman, W. *Common Form of Niacin Amide Deficiency Disease: Aniacinamidosis.* Yale University Press, 1943. Kaufman, W. "Niacinamide as a Therapeutic Agent: A Memoir." 2001. www.doctoryourself.com/kaufman12.html.

138. Hoffer, A., A.W. Saul, H.D. Foster. *Niacin: The Real Story: Learn about the Wonderful Healing Properties of Niacin.* Laguna Beach, CA: Basic Health Publications, 2012.

139. Pacholok, S.M., J.J. Stuart. *Could It Be B12?: An Epidemic of Misdiagnoses.* Fresno, CA: Quill Driver Books, 2011.

140. Ibid.

141. Ibid.

142. Agricultural Research Service, United States Department of Agriculture (USDA). "Nutrient Database for Standard Reference," National Nutrient Database for Standard Reference. Release 26 v.1.3.1, 2011. http://ndb.nal.usda.gov/ndb/nutrients/index (accessed Apr 2014).

143. Kwak, C.S., et al. "Dietary Source of Vitamin B(12) Intake and Vitamin B(12) Status in Female Elderly Koreans Aged 85 and Older Living in Rural Area." Nutr Res Pract. 4(3) (Jun 2010):229–34.

144. Jablonski, N.G. *Skin: A Natural History.* University of California Press, 2006. Jablonski, N.G. "Skin Color is an Illusion." Ted Talks. (2009) www.ted.com/talks/nina_jablonski_breaks_the_illusion_of_skin_color.html. (accessed Apr 2014) Jablonski, N.G.. "Human Skin Pigmentation as an Example of Adaptive Evolution." *Proc Am Philos Soc* 15691) (Mar 2012):45–57.

145. Hoffer, A., A.W. Saul. *Orthomolecular Medicine for Everyone: Megavitamin Therapeutics for Families and Physicians.* Laguna Beach, CA: Basic Health Publications, 2008.

146. Agricultural Research Service, United States Department of Agriculture (USDA). "Nutrient Database for Standard Reference," National Nutrient Database for Standard Reference. Release 26 v.1.3.1, 2011. http://ndb.nal.usda.gov/ndb/nutrients/index (accessed Apr 2014).

147. Quinlivan, E.P., J.F. Gregory 3rd. "Effect of Food Fortification on Folic Acid Intake in the United States." *Am J Clin Nutr* 77(1) (Jan 2003):221–5. Shane, B. "Folate Fortification: Enough Already?" *Am J Clin Nutr* 77(1) (Jan 2003):8–9.

148. Saul, A.W. "Folic acid does not cause cancer. So who made the mistake?" Orthomolecular News Service (OMNS). May 6, 2010. http://orthomolecular.org/resources/omns/v06n17.shtml (accessed Apr 2014).

149. Johansson, M., et al. "Serum B Vitamin Levels and Risk of Lung Cancer." *JAMA.* 303(23) (Jun 16, 2010):2377–85.Smith, R.G. "Vitamins Decrease Lung Cancer Risk by 50%." Orthomolecular News Service (OMNS). Nov 18, 2011. www.orthomolecular.org/resources/omns/v07n13.shtml (accessed Apr 2014).

150. Saul, A.W. "Folic acid does not cause cancer. So who made the mistake?" Orthomolecular News Service (OMNS). May 6, 2010. http://orthomolecular.org/resources/omns/v06n17.shtml (accessed Apr 2014). Rycyna, K.J., D.J. Bacich, D.S. O'Keefe. "Opposing Roles of Folate in Prostate Cancer." *Urology* 2013 82(6) (Dec 2013):1197–203.

151. Hoffer, A., A.W. Saul. *Orthomolecular Medicine for Everyone: Megavitamin Therapeutics for Families and Physicians.* Laguna Beach, CA: Basic Health Publications, 2008. Levy, T.E. *Primal Panacea.* Henderson, NV: MedFox Publishing, 2011.

152. Lopez, H.L. "Nutritional Interventions to Prevent and Treat Osteoarthritis. Part II: Focus on Micronutrients and Supportive Nutraceuticals." *PM R* 4(5 Suppl) (May 2012):S155–68.

153. Levy, T.E. *Primal Panacea.* Henderson, NV: MedFox Publishing, 2011.

154. Kurl, S., et al. "Plasma Vitamin C Modifies the Association between Hypertension and Risk of Stroke." *Stroke* 33(6) (Jun 2002):1568–73. Shargorodsky, M., et al. "Effect of Long-Term Treatment with Antioxidants (Vitamin C, Vitamin E, Coenzyme Q10 and Selenium) on Arterial Compliance, Humoral Factors and Inflammatory Markers in Patients with Multiple Cardiovascular Risk Factors." *Nutr Metab (Lond)* 7 (Jul 2010):55. Levy, T.E. *Primal Panacea.* Henderson, NV: MedFox Publishing, 2011.

155. Hoffer, A., A.W. Saul. *Orthomolecular Medicine for Everyone: Megavitamin Therapeutics for Families and Physicians.* Laguna Beach, CA: Basic Health Publications, 2008.

156. Montel-Hagen, A., M. Sitbon, N. Taylor. "Erythroid Glucose Transporters." *Curr Opin Hematol* 16(3) (May 2009):165–72.

157. Agricultural Research Service, United States Department of Agriculture (USDA). "Nutrient Database for Standard Reference," National Nutrient Database for Standard Reference. Release 26 v.1.3.1, 2011. http://ndb.nal.usda.gov/ndb/nutrients/index (accessed Apr 2014).

158. Carpenter, K.J. *The History of Scurvy and Vitamin C.* Cambridge: Cambridge Univ. Press, 1988. Crawford, E.M. "Scurvy in Ireland during the Great Famine." *Soc Hist Med* 1(3) (1988):281–300.

159. Pauling, L. *How to Live Longer and Feel Better.* Corvallis, OR: Oregon State Uni-

versity Press, 1986, 2006. Levy, T.E. *Primal Panacea.* Henderson, NV: MedFox Publishing, 2011.

160. Hagel, A.F., et al. "Intravenous Infusion of Ascorbic Acid Decreases Serum Histamine Concentrations in Patients with Allergic and Non-Allergic Diseases." *Naunyn Schmiedebergs Arch Pharmacol* 386(9) (Sep 2013):789–93. Hemilä, H. "Vitamin C and Common Cold-Induced Asthma: A Systematic Review and Statistical Analysis." *Allergy Asthma Clin Immunol* 9(1) (Nov 26, 2013):9–46.

161. Pauling, L. *How to Live Longer and Feel Better.* Corvallis, OR: Oregon State University Press, 1986, 2006. Levine, M., S.J. Padayatty "Vitamin C." Chapter 29 in *Modern Nutrition in Health and Disease,* editors A.C. Ross, 11th ed. Baltimore: Lippincott Williams & Wilkins, 2012. Hickey, S, A.W. Saul. *Vitamin C: The Real Story, the Remarkable and Controversial Healing Factor.* Laguna Beach, CA: Basic Health Publications, 2008.

162. Hickey, S, A.W. Saul. *Vitamin C: The Real Story, the Remarkable and Controversial Healing Factor.* Laguna Beach, CA: Basic Health Publications, 2008.

163. Handelman, G.J., L. Packer, C.E. Cross. "Destruction of Tocopherols, Carotenoids, and Retinol in Human Plasma by Cigarette Smoke. *Am J Clin Nutr* 63(4) (Apr 1996):559–65. Frikke-Schmidt, et al. "High Dietary Fat and Cholesterol Exacerbates Chronic Vitamin C Deficiency in Guinea Pigs." *Br J Nutr* 105(1) (Jan 2011):54–61.

164. Goodwin, J.S., M.R. Tangum. "Battling Quackery: Attitudes about Micronutrient Supplements in American Academic Medicine." *Arch Intern Med* 158(20) (Nov 9, 1998):2187–2191. Robitaille, L., et al. "Oxalic Acid Excretion after Intravenous Ascorbic Acid Administration. Metabolism." 58(2) (Feb 2009):263–9. Gaby, A.R. *Nutritional Medicine.* Concord, NH: Fritz Perlberg Pub, 2011. Levy, T.E. *Primal Panacea.* Henderson, NV: MedFox Publishing, 2011. Levy, T.E. *Death by Calcium.* Henderson, NV: MedFox Publishing, 2013. Levine, M., S.J. Padayatty "Vitamin C." Chapter 29 in *Modern Nutrition in Health and Disease,* editors A.C. Ross, 11th ed. Baltimore: Lippincott Williams & Wilkins, 2012. Orthomolecular News Service (OMNS). "What Really Causes Kidney Stones (And Why Vitamin C Does Not)." Feb 11, 2013. www.orthomolecular.org/resources/omns/ v09n05.shtml (accessed Jan 2014).

165. Orthomolecular News Service (OMNS). "What Really Causes Kidney Stones (And Why Vitamin C Does Not)." Feb 11, 2013. www.orthomolecular.org/resources/omns/v09n05.shtml (accessed Jan 2014).

166. Cheraskin, E., M. Ringsdorf Jr, E. Sisley. *The Vitamin C Connection.* New York: Bantam Books, 1983. Hickey, S, A.W. Saul. *Vitamin C: The Real Story, the Remarkable and Controversial Healing Factor.* Laguna Beach, CA: Basic Health Publications, 2008. Orthomolecular News Service (OMNS). "What Really Causes Kidney Stones (And Why Vitamin C Does Not)." Feb 11, 2013. www.orthomolecular.org/resources/omns/v09n05.shtml (accessed Jan 2014). Levy, T.E. *Death by Calcium.* Henderson, NV: MedFox Publishing, 2013.

167. Heilberg, I.P., D.S. Goldfarb. "Optimum Nutrition for Kidney Stone Disease." *Adv Chronic Kidney Dis* 20(2) . (Mar 2013):165–74.

168. Dean, C. *The Magnesium Miracle.* New York: Ballantine, 2007.

169. Dean, C. *The Magnesium Miracle.* New York: Ballantine, 2007. Orthomolecular News Service (OMNS). "What Really Causes Kidney Stones (And Why Vitamin C Does Not)." Feb 11, 2013. www.orthomolecular.org/resources/omns/v09n05.shtml (accessed Jan 2014). Riley, J.M., et al. "Effect of Magnesium on Calcium and Oxalate Ion Binding." *J Endourol* (Sep 2, 2013) [Epub ahead of print] doi:10.1089/end.2013-0173.ECB13.

170. Taylor, E.N., T.T. Fung, G.C. Curhan. "DASH-Style Diet Associates with Reduced Risk for Kidney Stones." *J Am Soc Nephrol* 20(10) (2009):2253–9.

171. Bailey JL, Sands JM, Franch HA (2012) "Electrolytes and acid-base metabolism" Chapter 6 in *Modern Nutrition in Health and Disease,* editors A.C. Ross, B Caballero, R.J.Cousins, et al., 11th ed. Baltimore, MD: Lippincott Williams & Wilkins, 2013.

172. Emery, T.F. *Iron and your Health: Facts and Fallacies.* Boca Raton, FL: CRC Press, 1991. Hurrell, R., I. Egli. "Iron Bioavailability and Dietary Reference Values." *Am J Clin Nutr* 91(5) (2010):1461S-1467S.

173. Emery, T.F. *Iron and your Health: Facts and Fallacies.* Boca Raton, FL: CRC Press, 1991.

174. Conrad, M.E., J.N. Umbreit. "Iron Absorption and Transport-An Update." *Am Hematol* 64(4) (Aug 2000):287–98.

175. Gaby, A.R. *Nutritional Medicine.* Concord, NH: Fritz Perlberg Pub, 2011.

176. Hickey, S, A.W. Saul. *Vitamin C: The Real Story, the Remarkable and Controversial Healing Factor.* Laguna Beach, CA: Basic Health Publications, 2008. Mikirova, N., et al. "Effect of High Dose Intravenous Ascorbic Acid on the Level of Inflammation in Patients with Rheumatoid Arthritis." *Modern Res Inflamm* 1(2) (Nov 2012):26–32.

177. Council for Responsible Nutrition (CRN). "Fact Sheet: Are Vitamins and Minerals Safe for Persons with G6PD deficiency?" Washington, DC: Council for Responsible Nutrition, 2005. www.crnusa.org/pdfs/CRN_G6PDDeficiency_0305.pdf. (accessed Apr 2014).

178. Ibid.

179. Williams, R.J. *Biochemical Individuality.* New Canaan, CT: Keats Publishing, 1998.

180. Hickey, S, A.W. Saul. *Vitamin C: The Real Story, the Remarkable and Controversial Healing Factor.* Laguna Beach, CA: Basic Health Publications, 2008. Gropper, S.S., J.L. Smith. *Advanced Nutrition and Human Metabolism,* 6th edition. New York: Cengage Learning, 2013.

181. Hickey, S, A.W. Saul. *Vitamin C: The Real Story, the Remarkable and Controversial Healing Factor.* Laguna Beach, CA: Basic Health Publications, 2008.

182. Bürzle, M., M.A. Hediger. "Functional and Physiological Role of Vitamin C Transporters." *Curr Top Membr* 70 (2012):357–75.

183. Hickey, S, A.W. Saul. *Vitamin C: The Real Story, the Remarkable and Controversial Healing Factor.* Laguna Beach, CA: Basic Health Publications, 2008. Bürzle, M., M.A. Hediger. "Functional and Physiological Role of Vitamin C Transporters." *Curr Top Membr* 70 (2012):357–75.

184. Cousins, N. *Anatomy of an Illness: As Perceived by the Patient.* Reprint ed. New York: W W Norton & Company; 1967, 2005.

185. Saul, A. *Doctor Yourself: Natural Healing That Works.* 2nd edition. Laguna Beach, CA: Basic Health Publications, 2012. www.doctoryourself.com.

186. Dalgård, C., et al. "Variation in the Sodium-Dependent Vitamin C Transporter 2 Gene Is Associated with Risk of Acute Coronary Syndrome among Women." *PLoS One* 8(8) (2013):e70421.

187. Pauling, L. *How to Live Longer and Feel Better.* Corvallis, OR: Oregon State University Press, 1986, 2006.

188. Levy, T.E. *Death by Calcium.* Henderson, NV: MedFox Publishing, 2013.

189. Ibid.

190. Hickey, S, A.W. Saul. *Vitamin C: The Real Story, the Remarkable and Controversial Healing Factor.* Laguna Beach, CA: Basic Health Publications, 2008.

191. Hickey, S, A.W. Saul. *Vitamin C: The Real Story, the Remarkable and Controversial Healing Factor.* Laguna Beach, CA: Basic Health Publications, 2008. Padayatty, S.J., et al. "Vitamin C: Intravenous Use by Complementary and Alternative Medicine Practitioners and Adverse Effects." *PLoS One* 5(7) (Jul 7, 2010):e11414.

192. Molnar-Kimber, K.L., H.E. Buttram. "Evidence that Intravenous Administration of Glutathione and Vitamin C Relieved Acute Pain from Rheumatoid Arthritis Flare." *Townsend Letter* 304 (Nov 2008): 60–1.

193. Mikirova, N., et al. "Effect of High Dose Intravenous Ascorbic Acid on the Level of Inflammation in Patients with Rheumatoid Arthritis." *Modern Res Inflamm* 1(2) (Nov 2012):26–32.

194. Khalsa, S. *The Vitamin D Revolution: How the Power of This Amazing Vitamin Can Change Your Life.* Hay House, 2009. Madrid, E. *Vitamin D Prescription: The Healing Power of the Sun & How It Can Save Your Life.* BookSurge Publishing, 2009. Holick M.F. *The Vitamin D Solution: A 3-Step Strategy to Cure Our Most Common Health Problems.* New York: Penguin Group USA, 2011. Jones, G. "Vitamin D." Chapter 18 in *Modern Nutrition in Health and Disease,* editors A.C. Ross, et al., 11th ed. Baltimore: Lippincott Williams & Wilkins, 2012.

195. Holick M.F. *The Vitamin D Solution: A 3-Step Strategy to Cure Our Most Common Health Problems.* New York: Penguin Group USA, 2011.

196. Ibid.

197. Khalsa, S. *The Vitamin D Revolution: How the Power of This Amazing Vitamin Can Change Your Life.* Hay House, 2009.

198. Holick M.F. *The Vitamin D Solution: A 3-Step Strategy to Cure Our Most Common Health Problems.* New York: Penguin Group USA, 2011.

199. Ibid.

200. Ibid.

201. Institute of Medicine (IOM). Food and Nutrition Board. "Dietary Reference Intake for Calcium and Vitamin D." (2010) www.iom.edu/~/media/Files/Report%20Files/2010/Dietary-Reference-Intakes-for-Calcium-and-Vitamin-D/Vitamin%20D%20and%20Calcium%202010%20Report%20Brief.pdf (accessed Apr 2014).

202. Heaney, R.P., M.F. Holick. "Why the IOM Recommendations for Vitamin D are Deficient." *J Bone Miner Res* 26(3) (Mar 2011):455–7.

203 Khalsa, S. *The Vitamin D Revolution: How the Power of This Amazing Vitamin Can Change Your Life.* Hay House, 2009.

204. Holick M.F. *The Vitamin D Solution: A 3-Step Strategy to Cure Our Most Common Health Problems.* New York: Penguin Group USA, 2011.

205. Papas, A. *The Vitamin E Factor: The Miraculous Antioxidant for the Prevention and Treatment of Heart Disease, Cancer, and Aging.* HarperCollins, 1999. Hoffer, A., A.W. Saul. *Orthomolecular Medicine for Everyone: Megavitamin Therapeutics for Families and Physicians.* Laguna Beach, CA: Basic Health Publications, 2008.

206. Hoffer, A., A.W. Saul. *Orthomolecular Medicine for Everyone: Megavitamin Therapeutics for Families and Physicians.* Laguna Beach, CA: Basic Health Publications, 2008.

Schürks, M., et al. "Effects of Vitamin E on Stroke Subtypes: Meta-Analysis of Randomised Controlled Trials." *BMJ* 341(Nov 4, 2010):c5702.

207. Papas, A. *The Vitamin E Factor: The Miraculous Antioxidant for the Prevention and Treatment of Heart Disease, Cancer, and Aging*. HarperCollins, 1999. Sen, C.K., S. Khanna, S. Roy. "Tocotrienols: Vitamin E Beyond Tocopherols." *Life Sci* 78(18) (Mar 27, 2006):2088–98. Traber, M.G. "Vitamin E." Chapter 19 in *Modern Nutrition in Health and Disease*, editors A.C. Ross, et al., 11th ed. Baltimore: Lippincott Williams & Wilkins, 2012.

208. Shuid, A.N., et al. "Vitamin E Exhibits Bone Anabolic Actions in Normal Male Rats." *J Bone Miner Metab* 28(2) (2010):149–56. Hamidi, M.S., P.N. Corey, A.M. Cheung. "Effects of Vitamin E on Bone Turnover Markers Among US Postmenopausal Women." *J Bone Miner Res* 27(6) (Jun 2012):1368–80.

209. Sen, C.K., S. Khanna, S. Roy. "Tocotrienols: Vitamin E Beyond Tocopherols." *Life Sci* 78(18) (Mar 27, 2006):2088–98. Sen, C.K., C. Rink, S. Khanna. "Palm Oil-Derived Natural Vitamin E alpha-Tocotrienol in Brain Health and Disease." *J Am Coll Nutr* 29(3 Suppl) (Jun 2010):314S-323S.

210. Hamidi, M.S., P.N. Corey, A.M. Cheung. "Effects of Vitamin E on Bone Turnover Markers Among US Postmenopausal Women." *J Bone Miner Res* 27(6) (Jun 2012):1368–80.

211. Klein, E.A., et al. "Vitamin E and the Risk of Prostate Cancer: The Selenium and Vitamin E Cancer Prevention Trial (SELECT)." *JAMA.*;306(14) (Oct 12, 2011):1549–56.

212. Papas, A. *The Vitamin E Factor: The Miraculous Antioxidant for the Prevention and Treatment of Heart Disease, Cancer, and Aging*. HarperCollins, 1999.

213. Thapa, D., R. Ghosh. "Antioxidants for Prostate Cancer Chemoprevention: Challenges and Opportunities." *Biochem Pharmacol* 83(10) (May 15, 2012):1319–30.

214. [No Authors Listed]. "The Effect of Vitamin E and Beta Carotene on the Incidence of Lung Cancer and Other Cancers in Male Smokers. The Alpha-Tocopherol, Beta Carotene Cancer Prevention Study Group." *N Engl J Med* 330(15) (Apr 14, 1994):1029–35. Lonn, E., "Effects of Long-Term Vitamin E Supplementation on Cardiovascular Events and Cancer: A Randomized Controlled Trial." *JAMA* 293(11) (Mar 16, 2005):1338–47. Miller, E.R. 3rd, et al. "Meta-Analysis: High-Dosage Vitamin E Supplementation May Increase All-Cause Mortality", *Ann Intern Med* 142(1) (2005):37–46.

215. Thapa, D., R. Ghosh. "Antioxidants for Prostate Cancer Chemoprevention: Challenges and Opportunities." *Biochem Pharmacol* 83(10) (May 15, 2012):1319–30.

216. Chew, E.Y., T. Clemons. "Vitamin E and Prostate Cancer." *Ophthalmology* 119(9) (Sep 2012):1938–9.

217. Orthomolecular News Service (OMNS). "Vitamin E: Safe, Effective, and Heart-Healthy." Mar 23, 2005. www.orthomolecular.org/resources/omns/v01n01.shtml (accessed Apr 2014). Orthomolecular News Service (OMNS). "Vitamin E Prevents Lung Cancer. News Media Virtually Silent on Positive Vitamin Research." Oct 28, 2008. www.orthomolecular .org/resources/omns/v04n18.shtml (accessed Apr 2014). Orthomolecular News Service (OMNS). "Vitamin E Research Ignored by Major News Media. Coast-to Coast Censorship." Oct 25, 2010. www.orthomolecular.org/resources/omns/v06n19.shtml (accessed Apr 2014). Orthomolecular News Service (OMNS). "Two Vitamin C Tablets Every Day Could Save 200,000 Lives Every Year: Ascorbate Supplementation Reduces Heart Failure." Nov 22, 2011. www.orthomolecular.org/resources/omns/v06n24.shtml (accessed Jan 2014). Saul, A.W. "Vitamin E Attacked Again. Of Course. Because It Works." Orthomolecular News Service (OMNS). Oct 14, 2011. www.orthomolecular.org/resources/omns/ v07n11.shtml

218. Hoffer, A., A.W. Saul. *Orthomolecular Medicine for Everyone: Megavitamin Therapeutics for Families and Physicians*. Laguna Beach, CA: Basic Health Publications, 2008.

219. Schürks, M., et al. "Effects of Vitamin E on Stroke Subtypes: Meta-Analysis of Randomised Controlled Trials." *BMJ* 341(Nov 4, 2010):c5702.

220. Hoffer, A., A.W. Saul. *Orthomolecular Medicine for Everyone: Megavitamin Therapeutics for Families and Physicians*. Laguna Beach, CA: Basic Health Publications, 2008.

221. Kurl, S., et al. "Plasma Vitamin C Modifies the Association between Hypertension and Risk of Stroke." *Stroke* 33(6) (Jun 2002):1568–73.

222. Schürks, M., et al. "Effects of Vitamin E on Stroke Subtypes: Meta-Analysis of Randomised Controlled Trials." *BMJ* 341(Nov 4, 2010):c5702.

223. Kurl, S., et al. "Plasma Vitamin C Modifies the Association between Hypertension and Risk of Stroke." *Stroke* 33(6) (Jun 2002):1568–73. Centers for Disease Control and Prevention. (CDC), "Types of Stroke." Dec 6, 2013. www.cdc.gov/stroke/types_of_stroke .htm (accessed Apr 2014). Lloyd-Jones, D., et al. "Heart Disease and Stroke Statistics—2009 Update: A Report from the American Heart Association Statistics Committee and Stroke Statistics Subcommittee." *Circulation* 119(3) (Jan 27, 2009):e21–161. http://circ.ahajournals.org/content/early/2008/ 12/15/CIRCULATIONAHA.108.191261

224. Kurl, S., et al. "Plasma Vitamin C Modifies the Association between Hypertension and Risk of Stroke." *Stroke* 33(6) (Jun 2002):1568–73. (accessed Apr 2014). Levy, T.E. *Stop America's #1 Killer: Reversible Vitamin Deficiency Found to be Origin of All Coronary Heart Disease*. Henderson, NV: Livon Books, 2006. Levy, T.E. *Primal Panacea*. Henderson, NV: MedFox Publishing, 2011.

225. Nathens, A.B,, et al. "Randomized, Prospective Trial of Antioxidant Supplementation in Critically Ill Surgical Patients." *Ann Surg* 236(6) (Dec 2002):814–22.

226. Levy, T.E. *Stop America's #1 Killer: Reversible Vitamin Deficiency Found to be Origin of All Coronary Heart Disease*. Henderson, NV: Livon Books, 2006. Shargorodsky, M., et al. "Effect of Long-Term Treatment with Antioxidants (Vitamin C, Vitamin E, Coenzyme Q10 and Selenium) on Arterial Compliance, Humoral Factors and Inflammatory Markers in Patients with Multiple Cardiovascular Risk Factors." *Nutr Metab (Lond)* 7 (Jul 2010):55.

227. Levy, T.E. *Death by Calcium*. Henderson, NV: MedFox Publishing, 2013. Misra, D., et al. "Vitamin K Deficiency is Associated with Incident Knee Osteoarthritis." *Am J Med* 126(3) (Mar 2013):243–8.

228. Agricultural Research Service, United States Department of Agriculture (USDA). "Nutrient Database for Standard Reference," National Nutrient Database for Standard Reference. Release 26 v.1.3.1, 2011. http://ndb.nal.usda.gov/ndb/nutrients/index (accessed Apr 2014).

229. Gropper, S.S., J.L. Smith. *Advanced Nutrition and Human Metabolism*, 6th edition. New York: Cengage Learning, 2013.

230. Adams, J., J. Pepping. "Vitamin K in the Treatment and Prevention of Osteoporosis and Arterial Calcification." *Am J Health Syst Pharm* 62(15) (Aug 1, 2005):1574–81.

231. Cranenburg, E.C., L.J. Schurgers, C. Vermeer. "Vitamin K: The Coagulation Vitamin That Became Omnipotent." *Thromb Haemost* 98(1) (Jul 2007):120–5.

232. Adams, J., J. Pepping. "Vitamin K in the Treatment and Prevention of Osteoporosis and Arterial Calcification." *Am J Health Syst Pharm* 62(15) (Aug 1, 2005):1574–81.

233. McCann, J.C., B.N. Ames. "Vitamin K, An Example of Triage Theory: Is Micronu-

trient Inadequacy Linked to Diseases of Aging?" *Am J Clin Nutr* 90(4) (Oct 2009):889–907.

234. Schurgers, L.J., et al. "Vitamin K-Containing Dietary Supplements: Comparison of Synthetic Vitamin K1 and Natto-Derived Menaquinone-7." *Blood* 109(8) (2007):3279–83.

235. Ibid.

236. Traber, M.G. "Vitamin E and K Interactions—A 50-Year-Old Problem." *Nutr Rev* 66(11) (2008):624–9.

237. Gomes, T., et al. "Rates of Hemorrhage During Warfarin Therapy for Atrial Fibrillation." *CMAJ* 185(2) (Feb 5, 2013):E121-E127.

238. McCann, J.C., B.N. Ames. "Vitamin K, An Example of Triage Theory: Is Micronutrient Inadequacy Linked to Diseases of Aging?" *Am J Clin Nutr* 90(4) (Oct 2009):889–907. Levy, T.E. *Death by Calcium*. Henderson, NV: MedFox Publishing, 2013.

239. Hoffer, A., A.W. Saul. *Orthomolecular Medicine for Everyone: Megavitamin Therapeutics for Families and Physicians*. Laguna Beach, CA: Basic Health Publications, 2008.

240. Morishita, T., et al. "Production of Menaquinones by Lactic Acid Bacteria." *J Dairy Sci* 82(9) (Sep 1999):1897–903. Sato, T., et al. "Production of Menaquinone (Vitamin K2)-7 by Bacillus subtilis." *J Biosci Bioeng* 91(1) (2001):16–20. McCann, J.C., B.N. Ames. "Vitamin K, An Example of Triage Theory: Is Micronutrient Inadequacy Linked to Diseases of Aging?" *Am J Clin Nutr* 90(4) (Oct 2009):889–907.

241. Gropper, S.S., J.L. Smith. *Advanced Nutrition and Human Metabolism*, 6th edition. New York: Cengage Learning, 2013.

242. Simopoulos, A.P. "Dietary Omega-3 Fatty Acid Deficiency and High Fructose Intake in the Development of Metabolic Syndrome, Brain Metabolic Abnormalities, and Non-Alcoholic Fatty Liver Disease." *Nutrients* 5(8) (2013):2901–23.

243. Russo, G.L. "Dietary n-6 and n-3 Polyunsaturated Fatty Acids: from Biochemistry to Clinical Implications in Cardiovascular Prevention." *Biochem Pharmacol* 77(6) (Mar 15 2009):937–46.

244. Lopez, H.L. "Nutritional Interventions to Prevent and Treat Osteoarthritis. Part I: Focus on Fatty Acids and Macronutrients." *PM R* 4(5 Suppl) (May 2012):S145–54.

245. Agricultural Research Service, United States Department of Agriculture (USDA). "Nutrient Database for Standard Reference," National Nutrient Database for Standard Reference. Release 26 v.1.3.1, 2011. http://ndb.nal.usda.gov/ndb/nutrients/index (accessed Apr 2014).

246. Lopez, H.L. "Nutritional Interventions to Prevent and Treat Osteoarthritis. Part I: Focus on Fatty Acids and Macronutrients." *PM R* 4(5 Suppl) (May 2012):S145–54.

247. Ibid.

248. Agricultural Research Service, United States Department of Agriculture (USDA). "Nutrient Database for Standard Reference," National Nutrient Database for Standard Reference. Release 26 v.1.3.1, 2011. http://ndb.nal.usda.gov/ndb/nutrients/index (accessed Apr 2014).

249. Silva, L., et al. "Oxidative Stability of Olive Oil after Food Processing and Comparison with Other Vegetable Oils." Food Chem. 121(4) (Aug 15, 2010):1177–87.

250. Seppanen, C.M., Q. Song, A.S. Csallany. "The Antioxidant Functions of Tocopherol and Tocotrienol Homologues in Oils, Fats, and Food Systems." *J Amer Oil Chem Soc* 87(5) (2010):469–81.

251. Agricultural Research Service, United States Department of Agriculture (USDA). "Nutrient Database for Standard Reference," National Nutrient Database for Standard Reference. Release 26 v.1.3.1, 2011. http://ndb.nal.usda.gov/ndb/nutrients/index (accessed Apr 2014).

252. Ibid.

253. Dean, C. *The Magnesium Miracle.* New York: Ballantine, 2007.

254. Ibid.

255. Ibid.

256. Ibid.

257. Ibid.

258. Ibid.

259. Ibid.

260. Levy, T.E. *Death by Calcium.* Henderson, NV: MedFox Publishing, 2013.

261. Ibid.

262. Dean, C. *The Magnesium Miracle.* New York: Ballantine, 2007. Levy, T.E. *Death by Calcium.* Henderson, NV: MedFox Publishing, 2013.

263. Dean, C. *The Magnesium Miracle.* New York: Ballantine, 2007.

264. Ibid.

265. Ibid.

266. Ibid.

267. Dean, C. *The Magnesium Miracle.* New York: Ballantine, 2007. Levy, T.E. *Death by Calcium.* Henderson, NV: MedFox Publishing, 2013.

268. Dean, C. *The Magnesium Miracle.* New York: Ballantine, 2007.

269. Lim, K.H., et al. "Iron and Zinc Nutrition in the Economically-Developed World: A Review." *Nutrients* 5(8) (2013):3184–211.

270. Shamsuddin, A.M. *IP6 + Inositol: Nature's Medicine For The Millennium!: Discover How A Cocktail of Simple Molecules Can Prevent And Fight Cancer And Other Diseases.* Baltimore, MD: IP-6 Research, Inc., 2011. Wawszczyk, J., et al. "The Effect of Phytic Acid on the Expression of NF-kappaB, IL-6 and IL-8 in IL-1beta-Stimulated Human Colonic Epithelial Cells." *Acta Pol Pharm* 69(6) (Nov-Dec 2012):1313–9.

271. Dean, C. *The Magnesium Miracle.* New York: Ballantine, 2007.

272. Ibid.

273. Weinberg, E.D. "Iron Toxicity: New Conditions Continue to Emerge." *Oxid Med Cell Longev* 2(2) (Apr-Jun 2009):107–9. Weinberg, E.D. "Is Addition of Iron to Processed Foods Safe for Iron Replete Consumers?" *Med Hypotheses* 73(6) (Dec 2009):948–9. Weinberg, E.D. "Role of Iron in Osteoporosis." Pediatr Endocrinol Rev. 6(Suppl 1) (Oct 2008):81–5.

274. Agricultural Research Service, United States Department of Agriculture (USDA). "Nutrient Database for Standard Reference," National Nutrient Database for Standard Reference. Release 26 v.1.3.1, 2011. http://ndb.nal.usda.gov/ndb/nutrients/index (accessed Apr 2014).

275. Emery, T.F. *Iron and your Health: Facts and Fallacies.* Boca Raton, FL: CRC Press,

1991. Saul, A. *Doctor Yourself: Natural Healing That Works.* 2nd edition. Laguna Beach, CA: Basic Health Publications, 2012. www.doctoryourself.com.

276. Geerligs, P.D., B.J. Brabin, A.A. Omari. "Food Prepared in Iron Cooking Pots as an Intervention for Reducing Iron Deficiency Anaemia in Developing Countries: A Systematic Review." *J Hum Nutr Diet* 16(4) (Aug 2003):275–81. Charles, C.V., A.J. Summerlee, C.E. Dewey. "Iron Content of Cambodian Foods When Prepared in Cooking Pots Containing an Iron Ingot." *Trop Med Int Health* 16(12) (2011):1518–24. Kulkarni, S.A., et al. "Beneficial Effect of Iron Pot Cooking on Iron Status." *Indian J Pediatr* 80(12) (2013):985–9.

277. Klevay, L.M. "Iron Overload Can Induce Mild Copper Deficiency." *J Trace Elem Med Biol* 14(4) (Apr 2001):237–40.

278. Hoffer, A., A.W. Saul. *Orthomolecular Medicine for Everyone: Megavitamin Therapeutics for Families and Physicians.* Laguna Beach, CA: Basic Health Publications, 2008. King, J.C., R.J. Cousins. "Zinc." Chapter 11 in *Modern Nutrition in Health and Disease,* editors A.C. Ross, et al., 11th ed. Baltimore: Lippincott Williams & Wilkins, 2012.

279. Collins, J.F. "Copper" Chapter 12 in *Modern Nutrition in Health and Disease.* editors A.C. Ross, et al., 11th ed. Baltimore: Lippincott Williams & Wilkins, 2012.

280. Hoffer, A., A.W. Saul. *Orthomolecular Medicine for Everyone: Megavitamin Therapeutics for Families and Physicians.* Laguna Beach, CA: Basic Health Publications, 2008.

281. Agricultural Research Service, United States Department of Agriculture (USDA). "Nutrient Database for Standard Reference," National Nutrient Database for Standard Reference. Release 26 v.1.3.1, 2011. http://ndb.nal.usda.gov/ndb/nutrients/index (accessed Apr 2014).

282. Eckhert, C.D. "Trace Elements." Chapter 16 in *Modern Nutrition in Health and Disease.* editors A.C. Ross, et al., 11th ed. Baltimore: Lippincott Williams & Wilkins, 2012. Gropper, S.S., J.L. Smith. *Advanced Nutrition and Human Metabolism,* 6th edition. New York: Cengage Learning, 2013.

283. Gropper, S.S., J.L. Smith. *Advanced Nutrition and Human Metabolism,* 6th edition. New York: Cengage Learning, 2013.

284. Kröger, H., et al. "Suppression of Type II Collagen-Induced Arthritis by N-Acetyl-L-Cysteine in Mice." *Gen Pharmacol* 29(4) (Oct 1997):671–4.

285. Epsom Salt Council. "Report on Sulfate absorption and benefits." www.epsomsaltcouncil.org/articles/report_on_absorption_of_magnesium_sulfate.pdf (2011) www.epsomsaltcouncil.org/articles/sulfation_benefits.pdf (accessed Apr 2014).

286. Dean, C. *The Magnesium Miracle.* New York: Ballantine, 2007.

287. Saul, A. *Doctor Yourself: Natural Healing That Works.* 2nd edition. Laguna Beach, CA: Basic Health Publications, 2012. www.doctoryourself.com. Hagel, A.F., et al. "Intravenous Infusion of Ascorbic Acid Decreases Serum Histamine Concentrations in Patients with Allergic and Non-Allergic Diseases." *Naunyn Schmiedebergs Arch Pharmacol* 386(9) (Sep 2013):789–93. Hemilä, H. "Vitamin C and Common Cold-Induced Asthma: A Systematic Review and Statistical Analysis." *Allergy Asthma Clin Immunol* 9(1) (Nov 26, 2013):9–46.

288. Levy, T.E. *Death by Calcium.* Henderson, NV: MedFox Publishing, 2013. Molnar-Kimber, K.L. Rheumatoid-Arthritis-Decisions.com. www.rheumatoid-arthritis-decisions.com (2013) (accessed Jan 2014).

289. McGee, H. *On Food and Cooking: The Science and Lore of the Kitchen.* New York, NY: Scribner, Revised, updated edition, 2004. ISBN-13: 978–0684800011

290. Chai, W., M. Liebman. "Effect of Different Cooking Methods on Vegetable Oxalate Content." *J Agric Food Chem* 53(8) (Apr 20, 2005):3027–30. Paul, V., et al. "Effect of Cooking and Processing Methods on Oxalate Content of Green Leafy Vegetables and Pulses." *As. J. Food Ag-Ind* 5(04) (2012):311–4.

291. Albinhn, P.B.E., G.P. Savage. "The Effect of Cooking on the Location and Concentration of Oxalate in Three Cultivars of New Zealand Grown Ocra (Oxalis tuberose Mol)." *J Sci Food and Agriculture* 81(2001):1027–33. Paul, V., et al. "Effect of Cooking and Processing Methods on Oxalate Content of Green Leafy Vegetables and Pulses." *As. J. Food Ag-Ind* 5(04) (2012):311–4.

292. Gaby, A.R. *Nutritional Medicine.* Concord, NH: Fritz Perlberg Pub, 2011.

293. Ibid.

294. Tareke, E., et al. "Analysis of Acrylamide a Carcinogen Formed in Heated Foodstuffs." *J. Agric. Food Chem* 50(17) (Aug 14, 2002), 4998–5006. Vogt, R., et al. "Cancer and Non-Cancer Health Effects from Food Contaminant Exposures for Children and Adults in California: A Risk Assessment." *Environ Health* 11 (Nov 9, 2012):83.

295. Tareke, E., et al. "Analysis of Acrylamide a Carcinogen Formed in Heated Foodstuffs." *J. Agric. Food Chem* 50(17) (Aug 14, 2002), 4998–5006.

296. Lukac, H., et al. "Influence of Roasting Conditions on the Acrylamide Content and the Color of Roasted Almonds." *J Food Sci* 72(1) (Jan 2007):C033–38.

297. Ibid.

298. Gaby, A.R. *Nutritional Medicine.* Concord, NH: Fritz Perlberg Pub, 2011.

299. Ibid.

300. Dean, C. *The Magnesium Miracle.* New York: Ballantine, 2007. Saul, A. *Doctor Yourself: Natural Healing That Works.* 2nd edition. Laguna Beach, CA: Basic Health Publications, 2012. www.doctoryourself.com.

301. Roberts, H., S. Hickey. *The Vitamin Cure for Heart Disease: How to Prevent and Treat Heart Disease Using Nutrition and Vitamin Supplementation.* Laguna Beach, CA: Basic Health Publications, 2011.

302. Gonzalez, M.J., J.R. Miranda-Massari, A.W. Saul. *I Have Cancer: What Should I Do?: Your Orthomolecular Guide for Cancer Management.* Laguna Beach, CA: Basic Health Publications, 2009.

303. Smith, R.G. *The Vitamin Cure for Eye Disease.* Laguna Beach, CA: Basic Health Publications, 2012.

304. Brighthope, I.E. *The Vitamin Cure for Diabetes: Prevent and Treat Diabetes Using Nutrition and Vitamin Supplementation.* Laguna Beach, CA: Basic Health Publications, 2012. Attia, P. "Is the Obesity Crisis Hiding a Bigger Problem?" TED Talks: TED Partner Series video. 2013 www.ted.com/talks/peter_attia_what_if_we_re_wrong_about_diabetes.html (accessed Jan 2014).

305. Hickey, S, A.W. Saul. *Vitamin C: The Real Story, the Remarkable and Controversial Healing Factor.* Laguna Beach, CA: Basic Health Publications, 2008.

306. Dean, C. *The Magnesium Miracle.* New York: Ballantine, 2007.

307. Roberts, H., S. Hickey. *The Vitamin Cure for Heart Disease: How to Prevent and Treat Heart Disease Using Nutrition and Vitamin Supplementation.* Laguna Beach, CA: Basic Health Publications, 2011.

308. Dean, C. *The Magnesium Miracle.* New York: Ballantine, 2007. Hoffer, A., A.W. Saul. *Orthomolecular Medicine for Everyone: Megavitamin Therapeutics for Families and Physicians.* Laguna Beach, CA: Basic Health Publications, 2008. Gaby, A.R. *Nutritional Medicine.* Concord, NH: Fritz Perlberg Pub, 2011. Roberts, H., S. Hickey. *The Vitamin Cure for Heart Disease: How to Prevent and Treat Heart Disease Using Nutrition and Vitamin Supplementation.* Laguna Beach, CA: Basic Health Publications, 2011. Brighthope, I.E. *The Vitamin Cure for Diabetes: Prevent and Treat Diabetes Using Nutrition and Vitamin Supplementation.* Laguna Beach, CA: Basic Health Publications, 2012. Saul, A. *The Orthomolecular Treatment of Chronic Disease: 65 Experts on Therapeutic and Preventive Nutrition.* Laguna Beach, CA: Basic Health Publications, 2014.

309. Gaby, A.R. *Nutritional Medicine.* Concord, NH: Fritz Perlberg Pub, 2011.

310. Saul, A. *The Orthomolecular Treatment of Chronic Disease: 65 Experts on Therapeutic and Preventive Nutrition.* Laguna Beach, CA: Basic Health Publications, 2014.

311. Attia, P. "Is the Obesity Crisis Hiding a Bigger Problem?" TED Talks: TED Partner Series video. 2013 www.ted.com/talks/peter_attia_what_if_we_re_wrong_about_diabetes.html (accessed Jan 2014).

Appendix. FAVORITE RECIPES

1. Saul, A. *Doctor Yourself: Natural Healing That Works.* 2nd edition. Laguna Beach, CA: Basic Health Publications, 2012. www.doctoryourself.com.

2. Ibid.

INDEX

About the Authors

Robert Smith, Ph.D. received his doctorate from the University of Pennsylvania and is a research scientist studying the function of neural circuits. Dr. Smith's research focuses on how chemical and electrical connections between neurons help to create and shape the sensation of vision. He is an expert in the physiology and biophysical properties of neurons, and in constructing realistic biophysical computational models of neural circuits of the retina. He has also studied nutrition and its importance for preventing age-related disease. Dr. Smith has written many research articles published in scientific journals, has served on review panels for grant applications to the National Institutes for Health, and is a regular attendee at international retina and vision conferences. He recently wrote the book *The Vitamin Cure for Eye Disease* about preventing progressive eye diseases through the use of excellent nutrition.

Todd Penberthy, Ph.D. received his doctorate from the University of Tennessee in biochemistry and is a research scientist studying nutritional biochemistry and developmental genetics. His research is focused on the role of nicotinamide adenine dinucleotide (NAD) and its precursor, niacin, in the metabolic pathways preventing disease. He has collaborated with other basic scientists, clinicians, and leaders in the pharmaceutical industry, specializing in therapy for multiple sclerosis, cancer, cardiovascular disease, and diabetes. Dr. Penberthy has written many research articles, book chapters, reports on medical technologies, and has given presentations at major research hospitals and national and international meetings.